Gray's
Surface Anatomy
and Ultrasound

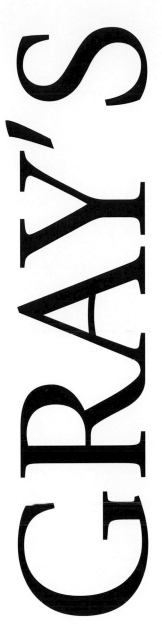

SURFACE ANATOMY AND ULTRASOUND

A Foundation for Clinical Practice

Claire F. Smith
BSc (Hons) PGCE PhD SFHEA FAS FLF
Head of Anatomy
Reader
Brighton and Sussex Medical School
University of Sussex
Brighton, UK

Andrew Dilley
BSc (Hons) PhD
Deputy Head of Anatomy
Senior Lecturer in Anatomy
Brighton and Sussex Medical School
University of Sussex
Brighton, UK

Barry S. Mitchell
BSc (Hons) MSc PhD CBiol FRSB FHEA
Emeritus Professor of Healthcare Sciences
Former Dean Faculty of Health and Life Sciences
De Montfort University
Leicester, UK

Richard L. Drake
PhD FAAA
Director of Anatomy
Professor of Surgery
Cleveland Clinic Lerner College of Medicine
Case Western Reserve University
Cleveland, OH, USA

For additional online content visit StudentConsult.com

ELSEVIER

Edinburgh   London   New York   Oxford   Philadelphia   St Louis   Sydney   Toronto   2018

ELSEVIER

Notices

Knowledge and best practice in this field are constantly changing. As new research and experience broaden our understanding, changes in research methods, professional practices, or medical treatment may become necessary.

Practitioners and researchers must always rely on their own experience and knowledge in evaluating and using any information, methods, compounds or experiments described herein. In using such information or methods they should be mindful of their own safety and the safety of others, including parties for whom they have professional responsibility.

With respect to any drug or pharmaceutical products identified, readers are advised to check the most current information provided (i) on procedures featured or (ii) by the manufacturer of each product to be administered, to verify the recommended dose or formula, the method and duration of administration, and contraindications. It is the responsibility of practitioners, relying on their own experience and knowledge of their patients, to make diagnoses, to determine dosages and the best treatment for each individual patient, and to take all appropriate safety precautions.

To the fullest extent of the law, neither the publisher nor the authors, contributors, or editors, assume any liability for any injury and/or damage to persons or property as a matter of products liability, negligence or otherwise, or from any use or operation of any methods, products, instructions or ideas contained in the material herein.

ISBN: 978-0-7020-7018-1

ELSEVIER your source for books, journals and multimedia in the health sciences
www.elsevierhealth.com

ELSEVIER Book Aid International Working together to grow libraries in developing countries
www.elsevier.com • www.bookaid.org

The publisher's policy is to use **paper manufactured from sustainable forests**

Printed in China

Last digit is the print number: 9 8 7 6 5 4 3 2 1

Content Strategist: *Jeremy Bowes*
Content Development Specialist: *Humayra Rahman Khan/Sharon Nash*
Project Manager: *Joanna Souch*
Design: *Christian Bilbow*
Illustrator: *Richard Tibbitts (Antbits)*
Marketing Manager: *Melissa Darling*

Contents

Contents

Get the most out of your

GRAY'S SURFACE ANATOMY AND ULTRASOUND

Included in your purchase is a variety of **BONUS electronic content**, to supplement and enhance the printed book. The authors have carefully selected additional figures ('eFigs'), videos and expanded tables conveying additional information to enrich your learning experience. Just look out for this icon ▣ throughout the (printed) book – and see the inside front cover for your access instructions.

For a richer learning experience and for no extra charge, find a wealth of enhanced electronic material in the Student Consult eBook that accompanies the print content of this book.

After you redeem your code (see inside front cover) at www.studentconsult. com, you can use the eBook in the browser and/or download it (in the Inkling app) to your mobile device to use anywhere, offline (the videos only play when you're online). The supplementary material is integrated at relevant locations in the enhanced eBook, so you get it right where you need it.

Test your understanding with scored quizzes of single best answer Q&As accompanying each chapter. They're also all collected together in the 'Assessments' chapter, so you can make full use of the self-assessment in one place. Test yourself with some of the figures too, using interactive labels. You can zoom in on high-resolution images, as well as watch videos showing live ultrasound scans as seen in clinical practice. Click through from the 'Learning Resources' chapter to our interactive, animated Surface Anatomy Tool, where you can explore specific parts of areas of the body and make connections with the common clinical procedures related to them.

As with all enhanced eBooks on Student Consult, there's the option to add 'Notes', 'Highlights' and 'Bookmarks'. Select text to easily highlight or make notes, which you can choose to share among other users. By setting your 'Note' to 'Public', you and your friends can share ideas – and reply to them (like on Facebook). Anyone who 'Follows' you can see your public 'Notes'/'Highlights', and if you 'Follow' them, you can see theirs. To 'Follow' someone, click 'Find Friends' near the top of your 'Library' page in Student Consult, and enter the email address that they use for their account. Then you can see their 'Notes' in books that you both have.

Foreword

Until the final years of the 19th century, vizualising anatomical structures deep within the living body non-invasively had seemed an impossible dream: exploring the contents of the body remained the exclusive preserve of the anatomist in the dissecting room and the surgeon in the operating theatre. A few sentences in a London newspaper gave notice of a discovery that would change that perspective and that surely ranks alongside the ability to control pain and infection as a game changer in medicine. *'It is reported from Vienna … Professor Routgen [sic] … has discovered a light which for the purpose of photography will penetrate wood, flesh, cloth, and most other organic substances. The Professor has succeeded in photographing … a man's hand which showed only the bones, the flesh being invisible.'* This news, cabled from the London Standard on 6 January 1896, appears to be the first account in English of Wilhelm Röntgen's momentous discovery of X-rays in November 1895. The clinical potential of his discovery was quickly appreciated: numerous contemporary accounts reveal that clinical practice altered within weeks of the news 'going viral' …*'Never in the history of science has a great discovery received such prompt recognition and has been so quickly utilized in a practical way as the new photography which Professor Roentgen gave to the world only three weeks ago. Already it has been used successfully by European surgeons in locating bullets and other foreign substances in human hands, arms and legs and in diagnosing diseases of the bones in various parts of the body..'* [1]

During the 20th century, developments in physics, electronics and computing continued to exploit X rays and introduced novel ways of displaying internal anatomy in real-time. CT scanning, MRI and ultrasound imaging all revealed levels of anatomical detail acquired non-invasively that had previously been seen only on the pages of atlases of frozen, sectioned cadavers[2].

Ultrasound

In the 1920s and 1930s, ultrasound was used for physical therapy, primarily for members of Europe's soccer teams, for sterilization of vaccines and for cancer therapy in combination with radiation therapy. Karl Theodor Dussik, a neurologist and psychiatrist working in Vienna, is usually credited as the first to apply ultrasound as a potential diagnostic tool and is regarded as the father of ultrasonic diagnosis. In the 1940s, together with his younger brother Friedrich, a physicist, Karl Dussik tried to image the living human brain with ultrasound, calling the process 'hyperphonography'. He interpreted the resulting 2D representations of the intensity attenuation of the waves through the head as 'ventriculograms' that showed the lateral ventricles within the brain. These images were subsequently shown to be artefactual and for a while it seemed as though ultrasound was unlikely to play any further role in diagnostic imaging. The field was re-invigorated in the 1950s when the transmission technique used by Dussik was replaced by the reflection technique. Ultrasound continued to evolve from being a *'.. medical curiosity to a recognized clinical procedure, capable of providing unique diagnostic information'*[3]. Rapid technical developments in electronics, piezoelectric materials and processing power over the last 50 years have produced ultrasound units generating real-time, dynamic grey scale images of anatomy. Karl Dussik's comments in 1953 on the potential use of ultrasound in medicine proved prescient …*However complicated the problems may be the imperative of these possibilities seems so great as to justify any and all efforts to overcome the technical difficulties.'* [4]. Unlike expensive hospital-based CT and MRI scanners, the portability and relatively low cost of modern ultrasound units means that they can brought to the patient at the bedside, in the clinic, on the battlefield and even in orbiting space stations (as part of ADUM, ADvanced Ultrasound in Microgravity, a NASA project[5]). Today, ultrasound is one of the most widely used modalities in medical imaging, regarded by the World Health Organisation as meeting 2/3 of health care imaging needs (WHO 1999). Point of care ultrasound (POCUS) is used as a physical diagnostic tool, to assess, for example, the extent of abdominal trauma following injury (focused abdominal sonography in trauma, FAST) and fetal growth and gestational age during pregnancy, where transabdominal B-mode imaging is regarded as the gold standard protocol. Coloured Doppler ultrasound is used to assess blood flow and vascular pathologies. Non-diagnostic ultrasound imaging to guide interventional procedures such as regional nerve blocks, central venous catheterisation, and cutting-needle and fine needle aspiration biopsies has significantly reduced the risk of iatrogenic injury and is regarded as the gold standard for these applications. POCUS training is now a mandatory

---

[1]Standring S (2016) A brief history of topographical anatomy. J. Anat. (2016) 229, pp32–62

[2]Braune W (1867–1872) Topographisch-Anatomischer Atlas: Nach Durchschnitten an Gefrornen Cadavern. Leipzig: Verlag von Veit & Comp.

[3]Goldberg BB, Gramiak R, Freimanis AK (1993) Early history of diagnostic ultrasound: the role of American radiologists. AJR Am J Roentgenol 160, 189–194.

[4]See: *Classic Papers in Modern Diagnostic Radiology* (Thomas AM, Banerjee AK, Busch U (eds) Springer 2005

[5]https://science.nasa.gov/science-news/science-at-nasa/2005/16feb_ultrasound

component in many postgraduate courses: e.g the Accreditation Council for Graduate Medical Education.

Surface anatomy

It is self-evident that interpreting the images produced by any imaging modality, whether using Xrays, fMRI or ultrasound, is predicated upon relating those images accurately to the relevant topographic anatomy. The bones of Frau Röntgen's hand that appeared in one of her husband's X ray films were identifiable because they corresponded with what was already known about the skeletal anatomy of the hand (no doubt aided by the presence of her wedding ring on her ring finger). Surface anatomy (living anatomy) relates structures under the skin to palpable surface features such as bony protuberances, tendons, muscle bellies or consistent skin creases. The impression that may be gained from most anatomy text books that surface anatomy is an exact science is at variance with everyday clinical experience: relating surface features to the location of underlying deeper structures is significantly influenced by variations in body mass index, height, gender, age and ethnicity and by dynamic factors such as posture and respiration. Recent studies in which surface features have been related to measurements based on modern cross sectional images, rather than measurements based on cadaveric or earlier radiographic studies, have called for a re-appraisal of some markings to take account of these variations. In preparing this book, and in particular in drawing up the instructions in the 'To do' surface anatomy lists, the authors have taken these more recent findings into account. In order to escape the censure of their teachers, students are advised to use these lists to practice on themselves, and their willing friends, before they lay hands on their first patient ... 'Many a student first realizes [the] importance [of surface anatomy] only when brought to the bedside or the operating table of his patient, when the first thing he is faced with is the last and least he has considered'[6].

Diagnostic imaging is an indispensable element of clinical practice. However, learning to interpret the images produced by Xrays, CT, MRI, ultrasound and during endoscopic procedures, takes time, a precious commodity that is in short supply in today's overcrowded medical curricula, particularly in the anatomy lab. This book contains a novel combination of evidence-based surface anatomy and ultrasound anatomy that will help students to reinforce their clinically relevant anatomical knowledge and develop those vital interpretive skills.

Susan Standring MBE PhD DSc FKC Hon FAS Hon FRCS
Emeritus Professor of Anatomy
King's College London
May 2017

[6]Whitnall SE. 1933. *The Study of Anatomy. Written for the Medical Student.* London: Edward Arnold. p 48

Preface

The use of surface anatomy has always been fundamental to clinical practice, for example, for locating a safe injection site or performing an examination of the abdomen. Knowledge of surface anatomy is also essential for using ultrasound. With the introduction of portable ultrasound, there has been a rapid rise in its use in a range of different specialties. As such, there is now a need to ensure that medical and healthcare undergraduate and postgraduate education reflects this service need. In many universities, it is not uncommon to find portable ultrasound units within the anatomy laboratory, where it is being used as an adjunct to more traditional anatomy teaching practices. Its ease of use means that it can be utilized by students. Furthermore, it provides the student with a real-time view of anatomy. For example, the beating of the heart, peristaltic movements within the gastrointestinal tract and muscular contractions during limb movements. Understanding surface anatomy is dependent on understanding the underlying structures, which, unless obscured by bone, can be viewed by ultrasound. Conversely, understanding where to place the ultrasound transducer and how to interpret the image is dependent on knowing the underlying gross anatomy and the overlying surface anatomy. The aim of the book was to develop a resource that blended for the first time surface anatomy and ultrasound.

Expanding the highly esteemed *Gray's* series, this book provides the perfect companion to *Gray's Anatomy for Students, Gray's Basic Anatomy, Gray's Atlas of Anatomy, Gray's Anatomy Review* and the original *Gray's Anatomy*. It is a valuable resource for students studying medicine, physiotherapy, chiropractic, dentistry, nursing and sports therapy, as well as for physician's associates and many other healthcare professionals.

About this book

This book has been designed to offer you the greatest flexibility for your learning. We recommend you start with the introduction chapter, but from there you can move on to whatever region of the body is of interest. In each chapter, we have detailed the surface anatomy first followed by ultrasound. This text is not a full descriptive textbook, and we have only described the anatomy relevant to surface anatomy and what is seen with ultrasound. We therefore recommend other *Gray's* titles for further detail. Within each chapter there are To Do boxes. We recommend that you undertake the activities in these boxes, since they provide a practical approach to learning anatomy that is directly relevant to clinical practice. To Do tasks include the identification of surface features, the drawing of structures and palpation. Use the surface anatomy photographs to assist with locating landmarks. Some palpations can take time to feel, and you may find it helpful to palpate different volunteers to observe normal variation.

All of the surface anatomy illustrations were initially drawn on the models and then computer enhanced during publication. Only tweaks were drawn on afterwards (Fig). This approach was taken because we wanted to demonstrate that all of the illustrations are possible and are based on real surface landmarks that can be felt and located. We used the figures in the text to enable us to write the To Do boxes. By doing so we have demonstrated that all these tasks are possible. Your drawings are not meant to be pieces of artwork. Instead they are creating a road map of important surface features.

Drawing equipment

To undertake the drawings, we used children's face paints, a couple of paintbrushes, a cup of water and some baby wipes.

Ultrasound

Each ultrasound section provides details of the transducer to use and where to position the transducer, as well as a description of the structures that should be visible. It is important to note that in some individuals, these structures will be easier to see than in others. Both body size and fat content make a difference. The descriptions in this book are only a starting point. It is important to spend time scanning over the region of the body that you are examining to build up a picture of the underlying topography. If you cannot find a specific structure, try tilting, rocking or rotating the transducer. Not all anatomical structures that can be seen on ultrasound are detailed in this book. As long as a structure is not obscured by bone, it should be possible to find. An exciting feature of ultrasound is the ability to view anatomy and physiology in action. If you are looking at a muscle or tendon, try moving a limb; if you are looking at blood vessels, use the Doppler function, if available, to visualize the flow of blood.

Consent

It is imperative that in working with colleagues to practice palpation, percussion, drawing and ultrasound that the correct level of consent is in place, that subjects are not made to do anything they do not wish to and that they feel comfortable at all times. Where possible, we have kept the models' clothes in the pictures as they would be during a teaching session to assist with demonstrating how much surface anatomy needs to be exposed for the particular region. Be aware that incidental findings may occur during your sessions and these should always be followed up by routine medical appointment. Working with colleagues offers a fantastic opportunity to practice good communication skills, for example in describing to your colleague what you are going to do: "I am just going to gently press on your shoulder. Please say if it hurts."

Fig. A, Photograph of our drawings during production of the scapula and associated muscles. B, Final illustration of the scapula and associated muscles.

Expert reviewers (in order of contribution)

Jennifer M. McBride PhD
Associate Professor of Surgery
Director of Histology
Cleveland Clinic Lerner College of Medicine of Case
Western Reserve University
Cleveland Clinic
Cleveland, Ohio, USA

Nicki J. G. Delves DCR DMU PgC
Specialist MSK Sonographer & Clinical Tutor
Royal Surrey County Hospital NHS Foundation Trust
Guildford, UK

Kimberly Topp PT PhD FAAA FAS (Hon)
Professor and Chair
Department of Physical Therapy and Rehabilitation
Science
Department of Anatomy
University of California
San Francisco, California, USA

Geoffrey M. Bove DC PhD
Professor
Biomedical Sciences
University of New England College of Osteopathic
Medicine
Biddeford, Maine, USA

Nigel Williams BMedSci BM BS ChM FRCS
Consultant General Surgeon and Colorectal Surgeon
University Hospitals Coventry and Warwickshire
Coventry, UK

Tim Mitchell MA FRCS(ORL-HNS)
Consultant ENT Surgeon
University Hospital Southampton NHS Foundation Trust
Southampton, UK

Andrew N. J. Fish MB BS MD FRCOG
Consultant Gynaecological Oncologist
Honorary Clinical Senior Lecturer
Brighton and Sussex University Hospitals NHS Trust
Brighton, UK

Caroline Alexander MCSP MSc PhD
Adjunct Reader
NIHR Senior Clinical Lecturer
Lead Clinical Academic for Therapies
Imperial College Healthcare NHS Trust
Charing Cross Hospital
London, UK

Richard Ellis PhD BPhty
Senior Lecturer and Associate Head of Research
Department of Physiotherapy
School of Clinical Sciences
Faculty of Health and Environmental Sciences
Auckland University of Technology
Auckland, New Zealand

Mark Goodwin FRCS(Eng) FRCS(Ed) FHEA
Consultant Orthopaedic Surgeon
Royal Bournemouth & Christchurch Hospitals NHS
Foundation Trust
Bournemouth, UK

Malcolm Johnston MRCS FRCR
Consultant and Clinical Lead Interventional Radiologist
Senior Lecturer & Director of Imaging Education
Brighton and Sussex University Hospitals NHS Trust
Brighton, UK

Credits

SURFACE ANATOMY AND ULTRASOUND MODELS (LISTED ALPHABETICALLY)

James Allsopp

Becky Dilley

Lucinda Evans

Catherine Hennessy

Rish Jain

Nicholas Lewis

Vivien Ngo

Ellen Petrovics

Paula Pheby

Jason Pimblett

Gregory Pluck

Jaz Singh

Patrick Tano

Christopher Thornhill

Catherine White

Alex Witek

PHOTOGRAPHERS

Nick White RMIP

Patricia Reid RMIP

Judith Gonzalez-Bernal RMIP

Maytyra Tirén RMIP

Shelley Daber RMIP

Lucy Francis RMIP

Clinical Media Centre
Brighton and Sussex University Hospital NHS Trust
Sussex House
Brighton, UK

Siân Schmidt (Ultrasound Picture page 64)
(fetus 12 weeks)
Advanced Practitioner Sonographer
Worthing Hospital
Western Sussex Hospitals Trust
Worthing, UK

Acknowledgments

We wish to thank a dedicated team of expert reviewers who have helped us bring this first edition to life, as well as all those who agreed to act as ultrasound or surface anatomy models. The authors express their gratitude to Professor Susan Standring for her kind support and words of wisdom. We also thank Cristina Gatti and Anna Fletcher, our student advisers, for their guidance. We would like to thank Nick and his team of photographers for their great work. We would like to kindly acknowledge all figures loaned by *Gray's Anatomy* and *Gray's Anatomy for Students*. Finally, we would like to thank the amazing support of Jeremy, Humayra and Jo at Elsevier, especially in guiding us through this first edition.

Dedications

To my husband, Trevor, my daughters, Hermione and Elodie, my mother, Susan, and in loving memory of my father, Michael, for your unconditional love and support.

Claire F. Smith

To my wife, Becky, for her continued support, and my son, Noah.

Andrew Dilley

To my wife, Jo, and daughter, Lucy, who have both been tremendous supports during the writing of this book.

Barry S. Mitchell

To my wife, Cheryl, who has supported me, and my parents, who have guided me.

Richard L. Drake

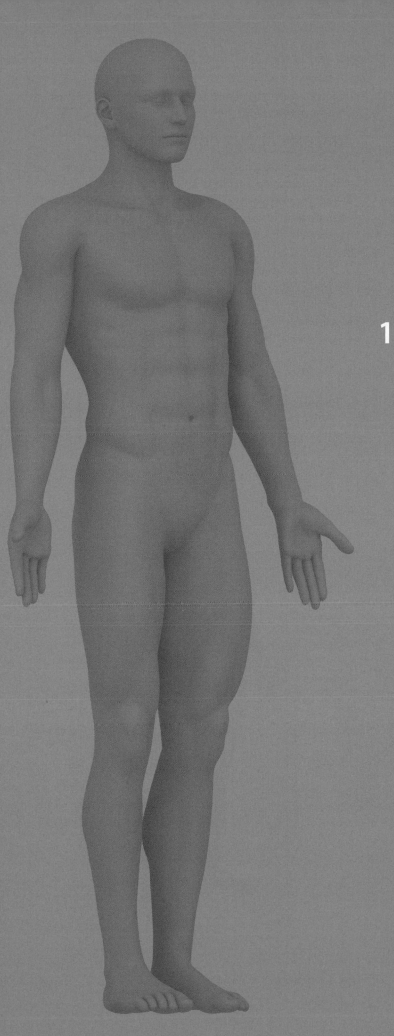

1 Introduction

Conceptual overview

Understanding the human body is essential for safe clinical practice. The human body is a three-dimensional object that can be viewed and examined from the outside and inside. The body is always referred to from the anatomical position, and key anatomical terminology, nomenclature, is used to describe structures. Anatomical language is important for all aspects of medicine and healthcare.

Surface anatomy

Surface anatomy is the study of anatomical structures that can be seen from the outside of the body. It also includes the surface projections and landmarks of deeper structures that are required to perform clinical examinations, investigations and treatments.

ANATOMICAL POSITION AND PLANES

The anatomical position is the reference position from which anatomical relationships are described (Fig. 1.1). In the anatomical position, the individual is standing upright, with the arms at the side and the palms facing forward. The mouth is closed with no facial expression. The eyes are looking forward.

In the anatomical position three planes pass through the body (Fig. 1.2):

- sagittal
- coronal
- transverse (horizontal or axial).

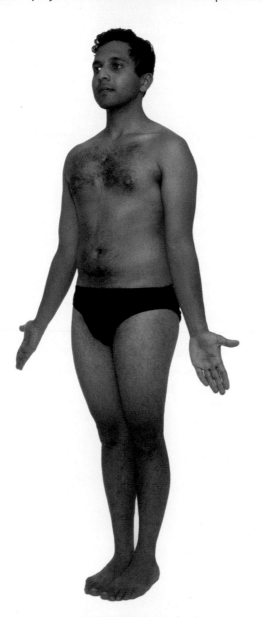

Fig. 1.1 Anatomical position.

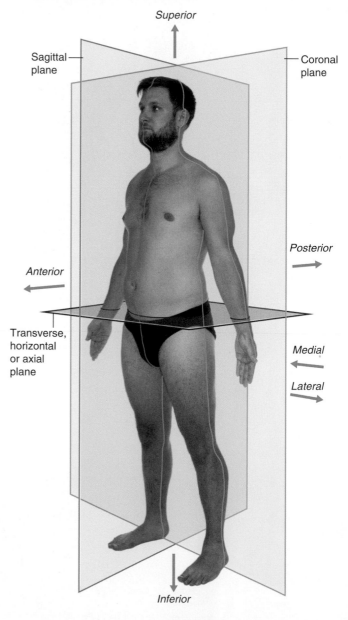

Fig. 1.2 Anatomical planes and terms.

The sagittal plane divides the body from the midline into right and left sides. If it is to the side of the midline, it is referred to as parasagittal. The coronal plane divides the body into anterior and posterior (front and back). The transverse plane divides the body into superior and inferior (upper and lower).

To Do (Figs. 1.1 and 1.2)
- Stand in the anatomical position.
- Using your hand in the air in front of a volunteer make three lines to create the sagittal, coronal and transverse planes.

ANATOMICAL TERMS

Standardized anatomical terms are used to describe structures in relation to each other and are a key part of medical terminology. For example, the hip joint is proximal to the knee joint. Key anatomical terms for describing location are summarized in Table 1.1.

MOVEMENT

Anatomical terms are also used to describe movements of the body. A movement can be aligned to an anatomical plane, or it can occur around a plane. For example, the psoas major muscle is a powerful flexor of the thigh at the hip joint and its movement occurs in the sagittal plane. The terms used for describing movement are considered in opposing pairs; for example, flexion and extension. Key anatomical terms for defining movement are summarized in Table 1.2 (see also Fig. 1.3).

Examination of movement can be performed in three ways: passive, active and against resistance. Passive movement involves asking a patient to relax their limb while it is gently moved by the clinician. Passive movements are used to assess range of motion, which may be limited by deformity. Active movement involves asking a patient to undertake the primary action of the muscle. Active movements are also used to assess the range of motion, as well as joint and muscle function. Movement against resistance is used to produce an isometric contraction, where a muscle contracts without a change in its length or joint angle (Fig. 1.4). In the clinic, it is often performed by asking a patient to push their limb against the clinician's stationary hand, and is part of examination to test for muscle strength. Performing isometric contractions is useful for learning surface anatomy since it assists in the visualization of muscles and tendons.

FASCIA

Fascia is made up of connective tissue and serves to separate and connect anatomical structures. Two types of fascia are found within the body: superficial and deep. Superficial fascia is comprised of loose connective tissue and adipose cells; the amount of adipose tissue together with muscles and

Table 1.1 Anatomical terms

Term	Description
Anterior (ventral)	To the front
Posterior (dorsal)	To the back
Medial	Towards the median sagittal plane
Lateral	Away from the median sagittal plane
Superior	Above
Inferior	Below
Proximal	Closer to origin
Distal	Further from origin
Cranial/cephalic	Towards the head
Caudal	Towards the tail
Superficial	Towards the surface
Deep	Away from the surface

Table 1.2 Movement terms

Term	Description
Flexion	Movement in the sagittal plane decreasing the angle at a joint
Extension	Movement in the sagittal plane increasing the angle at a joint
Adduction	Movement in the coronal plane towards the midline
Abduction	Movement in the coronal plane away from the midline
Medial (internal) rotation	Rotation towards the midline
Lateral (external) rotation	Rotation away from the midline
Pronation	Medial rotation in the forearm so that the palm of the hand faces posteriorly
Supination	Lateral rotation in the forearm so that the palm faces anteriorly
Circumduction	Circular movement
Elevation	Movement superiorly
Depression	Movement inferiorly
Protrusion and protraction	Movement anteriorly
Retrusion and retraction	Movement posteriorly
Eversion	Movement of the sole laterally
Inversion	Movement of the sole medially

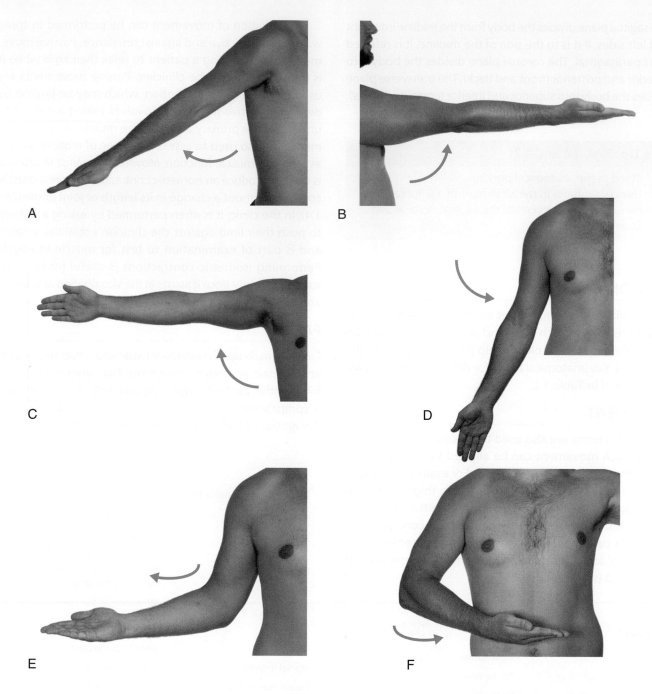

Fig. 1.3 Terms of movement. A, Extension at the shoulder joint. B, Flexion at the shoulder joint. C, Abduction at the shoulder joint. D, Adduction at the shoulder joint. E, Lateral rotation of the shoulder joint. F, Medial rotation at the shoulder joint.

bone make up the surface contours. Deep fascia is comprised of dense connective tissue and does not contain adipose cells. Myofascia forms planes between muscles. In the limbs the myofascia divides groups of muscles into functional compartments. Understanding the arrangement of fascia is important as it often limits the spread of infection and tumors.

SKIN

The skin is the largest organ of the body and is responsible for protection, temperature control and the production of vitamin D. Examination of the skin in clinical practice is an important part of differential diagnosis. The skin is organized into three layers: epidermis, dermis and hypodermis (or

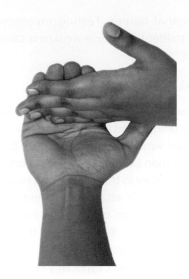

Fig. 1.4 Isometric contraction testing for muscle strength.

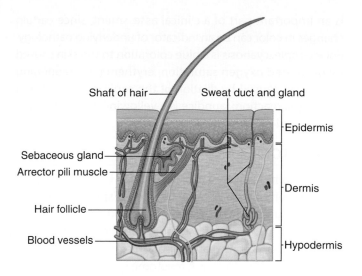

Shaft of hair

Sweat duct and gland

Epidermis

Sebaceous gland

Arrector pili muscle

Dermis

Hair follicle

Blood vessels

Hypodermis

Fig. 1.5 Skin showing the three layers.

subcutaneous tissue) (Fig. 1.5). The epidermis is comprised of keratinous stratified epithelium. It is avascular and varies considerably depending on body region. For example, the epidermis on the sole of the foot is considerably thicker than the epidermis on the eyelid. The dermis contains collagen and elastin fibers and specialized structures, such as the arrector pili muscles, which are responsible for piloerection. The hypodermis is formed of loose connective tissue and adipose (fat) tissue. Within the hypodermis there are many specialized nerve endings that detect pressure, temperature and pain. Superficial blood and lymphatic vessels are also found within this layer. The amount of adipose tissue varies based on the body region. For example, there is little adipose tissue on the back of the hand but more around the abdomen. The amount and distribution of adipose tissue is also dependent on gender. Females tend to deposit more fat around the breasts, hips and thighs, whereas males tend to deposit fat around the abdomen.

The pattern of the collagen and elastin fibers in the dermis creates tension and wrinkle lines (Fig. 1.6). The tension lines are also referred to as natural lines of cleavage (or creases) and run where movement occurs. As skin ages, the amount of collagen and elastin fibers decreases, which deepens the wrinkle lines and causes skin to become thinner. On the palms of the hands and soles of the feet the skin is delineated by small furrows and ridges, known as the papillary ridges. Sweat ducts open at regular intervals along these ridges. The pattern of ridges at the finger tips is unique to each individual.

Hair-bearing skin covers much of the body to varying degrees, except for example the palms of the hand, soles of the feet and parts of the genitals, where glabrous skin is found.

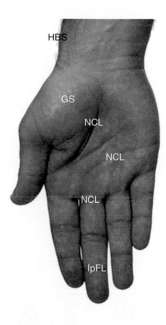

HBS

GS

NCL

NCL

NCL

IpFL

Fig. 1.6 Natural cleavage lines. *GS,* glaborous skin; *HBS,* hair-bearing skin; *IpFL,* interphalangeal flexure line; *NCL,* natural cleavage line.

To Do (Fig. 1.6)

- Examine the natural lines of cleavage as an individual flexes and extends their wrist and digits.
- Examine the hairy skin on the posterior surface of the forearm and the glabrous skin on the anterior surface of the palm.

SKIN COLOR

The color of skin is dependent on both genetic and environmental factors. Melanin is the pigment produced by melanocytes that gives skin its color. Observing skin color is an important part of a clinical assessment, since certain changes in color can be an indicator of underlying pathology. For example, cyanosis is a blue coloration to the skin caused by decreased oxygen saturation; erythema is a reddening of the skin caused by dilation of the capillary beds during an allergic reaction; jaundice is a yellowing of the skin due to the build-up of bilirubin.

DERMATOMES AND MYOTOMES

A dermatome is an area of skin supplied by the anterior or posterior primary rami of an individual spinal nerve (Fig. 1.7). Although dermatome maps can be drawn, there is substantial variation and overlap between individuals. Clinically, dermatomes are important for the diagnosis of nerve or spinal cord injury. A myotome is a group of muscles that are supplied by the anterior or posterior primary rami of an individual spinal nerve. Myotomes are more complex in the limbs, since the large muscle groups are supplied by

multiple spinal nerves. Testing myotomes is clinically important to identify muscle weakness caused by nerve or spinal cord injury.

NATURAL VARIATION

While surface anatomy follows common landmarks, each individual is unique, and therefore it is important to be aware of anatomical variation. In this book we have reported on the most common landmarks. While all bones have a generic shape, they do vary in their detail, and hence in the precise locations of muscle attachments and other associated structures. The pattern of arteries is relatively stable with some known variations, for example in the branching pattern of the coronary arteries. In contrast, the venous network has substantial variation, especially in the superficial veins. Natural variation is also commonly seen between different age groups. In the young, developmental milestones affect anatomical landmarks, for example the bladder in the infant

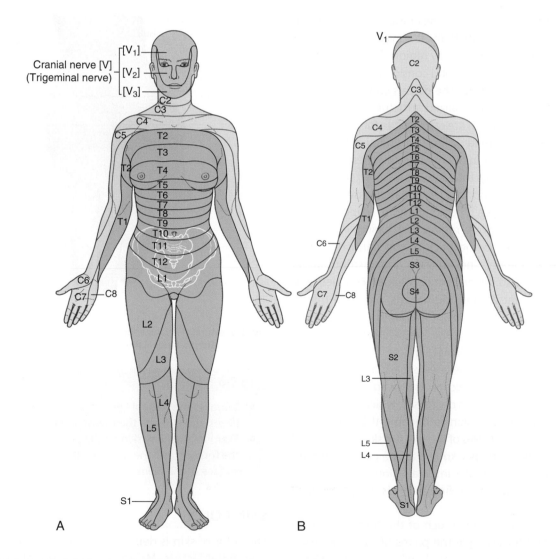

Fig. 1.7 Dermatomes. A, Anterior view. B, Posterior view.
(From Drake, RL, Gray's Anatomy for Students, 3rd ed, 2015, Churchill Livingstone, Elsevier.)

middle finger of the dominant hand is used to tap on the middle phalanx of the middle finger on the other side (Fig. 1.8B). Percussion creates sounds that are resonant or dull. Structures that are hollow produce a more resonant sound, for example the lungs and stomach. Structures that are denser, for example the liver or bone, produce a dull sound.

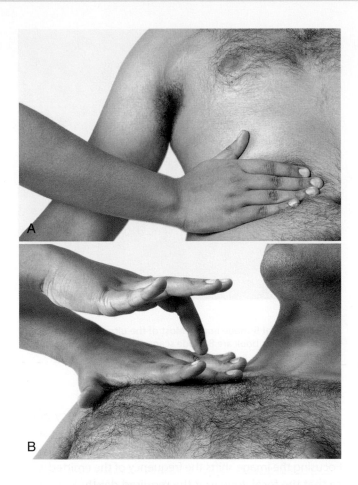

Fig. 1.8 A, Palpation. B, Percussion.

> ### In the Clinic
>
> Scars occur when the skin is damaged through an incision or laceration. During the wound healing process, fibroblasts and keratinocytes invade the area and lay down new extracellular matrix and collagen, which is remodeled to form scar tissue.
>
> Stretch marks (striae cutis distensae) result from damaged collagen fibres in the skin. Puberty, weight gain and pregnancy are frequent causes of stretch marks. At the time of the distension, the affected skin becomes red which later fades to white.
>
> Shingles is caused by reactivation of the varicella zoster virus. Following chickenpox, the virus remains dormant in the cell bodies of the primary sensory neurons that are located within the dorsal root ganglia. After the virus has been reactivated, it is transported to the peripheral terminals of the affected neurons, which leads to a rash within the dermatome supplied by those neurons. Other symptoms include pain.

> ### To Do (Fig. 1.8)
>
> - Practice palpation over the lower ribs and abdomen.
> - Practice percussion over (a) a rib, (b) the abdomen.

is to a greater extent part of the abdominal cavity. During the process of ageing other examples of natural variation can be observed in stature and are especially evident in the skin. During pregnancy the changing body shape brought on by the development of the fetus and by the effect of hormones also affects surface anatomy markings.

PALPATION AND PERCUSSION

Palpation is a technique used to examine underlying structures by gently pressing over the structure. Palpation can be used to assess hardness, size, location and tenderness of structures. It can also be used during dynamic movement to assess joint function (Fig. 1.8A).

Percussion is a technique used to examine structures within the thorax or abdomen by tapping. The indirect method involves placing the middle finger of the non-dominant hand over the area to be percussed, while the

Ultrasound

ULTRASOUND THEORY

In medical diagnostics, ultrasound uses high-frequency soundwaves to produce images of the underlying tissues. The ultrasound transducer is composed of a series of piezoelectric elements that vibrate sequentially in response to an electrical current. The vibrations produce ultrasonic pulses within a range of frequencies between 2 MHz and 20 MHz that travel through the underlying tissues.

Acoustic impedance is a measure of the resistance that ultrasonic waves encounter as they pass through tissue, which is related to the density of tissue and the speed of the sound wave. Whenever there is a change in acoustic impedance, some of the emitted echoes are reflected back to the ultrasound transducer, where they are detected by the piezoelectric elements (Fig. 1.9). Changes in acoustic impedance occur at tissue interfaces. A greater difference in acoustic impedance, such as occurs at soft tissue–bone interfaces, produces stronger echoes. Ultrasonic waves travel at a relatively constant velocity through soft tissue (1540 m/s), therefore the distance traveled by the received echoes can

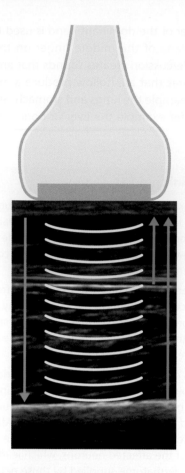

Fig. 1.9 Theory of ultrasound. Ultrasound waves are emitted from the transducer. Whenever there is a change in acoustic impendence, such as at tissue interfaces, echoes are produced that are received by the transducer.

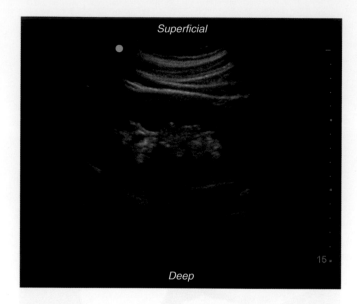

Fig. 1.10 Typical B-mode image. Most of the ultrasound images presented in this book are B-mode scans. (Ultrasound image of the left kidney.)

be accurately measured. The delay in receiving the echo by the piezoelectric elements and the intensity of the echo are used to produce a two-dimensional ultrasound image, called a B (brightness)-mode image (Fig. 1.10). Pixel gray scale values correlate to the strength of the received echoes.

Image resolution is proportional to the frequency of the emitted ultrasonic wave. Higher-frequency transducers produce better lateral and axial resolution. Lateral resolution is the ability to resolve structures at 90 degrees to the ultrasound beam. Axial resolution is the ability to resolve structures in the line of the ultrasound beam. However, higher frequency ultrasonic waves do not penetrate as deep through tissue before the intensity of the wave diminishes. Therefore, there is a fine balance between transducer frequency and required depth. Higher-frequency transducers are better for imaging superficial structures, such as the musculoskeletal system, whereas lower-frequency transducers are better for deep structures, such as the abdomen.

The ultrasound beam is focused within the transducer. The region of optimum lateral resolution is where the beam is at its narrowest. This region is called the focal zone. The

depth of the focal zone is related to the frequency of the emitted wave. Many ultrasound machines allow the user to add focal points at the depth of the structures of interest. Focusing the image shifts the frequency of the emitted wave so that the focal zone is at the required depth.

DOPPLER

Doppler ultrasound is used to examine movement, such as blood flow, within tissue, vessels and the heart. It is based on the Doppler shift principle. When an ultrasound wave is reflected back from an object moving toward or away from the transducer, there is a shift in the frequency of the returning echo. This shift is proportional to the velocity of the moving object. When measuring blood flow, ultrasonic waves are reflected off moving red blood cells at a different frequency to the emitted waves. The displayed velocity of the blood flow is directly related to the perceived Doppler shift. It is important to note that the angle of the ultrasound beam relative to the blood flow is critical. If the blood vessel is perpendicular to the ultrasound beam, there is no Doppler shift. It is best to image a moving object as close to the axial beam as possible, but in practice an angle between 45 degrees and 60 degrees to the axial beam is adequate.

There are several types of Doppler imaging, such as spectral and color Doppler. With spectral Doppler, which includes continuous-wave and pulsed-wave Doppler, the velocities are quantified graphically over time. With color Doppler, the intensity of the Doppler shifts are overlaid on a B-mode image (Fig. 1.11). Pixels are colored relative to the direction (usually red = towards transducer; blue = away

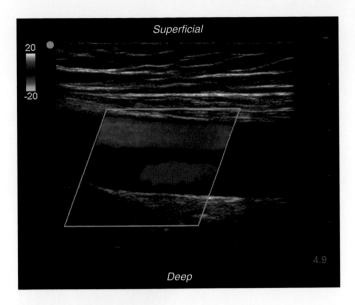

Fig. 1.11 Typical color Doppler image. Doppler data is overlaid on a B-mode image. (Ultrasound image of the femoral artery (red) and vein (blue) in the right thigh.)

from transducer) and strength of flow. It is important to note that color is not necessarily aligned to colors normally used to portray arteries and veins.

TYPES OF TRANSDUCER

The most popular types of ultrasound transducer are the linear, curved (curvilinear or convex) and phased array transducers.

Linear array transducers emit higher frequency ultrasonic waves, typically in the range of 5–18 MHz. They provide better lateral resolution, although the depth of penetration is often limited to less than 5 cm. Linear array transducers are employed in vascular, musculoskeletal, thyroid and breast imaging.

Curved array transducers emit lower frequency ultrasonic waves, typically in the range of 2–9 MHz. They are used to visualize deeper structures. Their curved design results in a wider field of view at deeper depths. Curved array transducers are employed in abdominal, cardiac and obstetric imaging.

Phased array transducers have a smaller footprint than linear and curved array transducers. Their small size means that they can be used between the ribs to examine the heart. They emit lower frequency ultrasound waves and are used to visualize deep structures. Similar to the curved array transducer, they provide a wider field of view at deep depths. They are mainly employed in cardiac imaging.

IMAGING PLANES

Ultrasound planes are the same as the anatomical planes. The main planes are transverse (or axial), sagittal and coronal (Fig. 1.12). The term 'oblique' is used when the transducer is at an angle to the plane (e.g., transverse oblique).

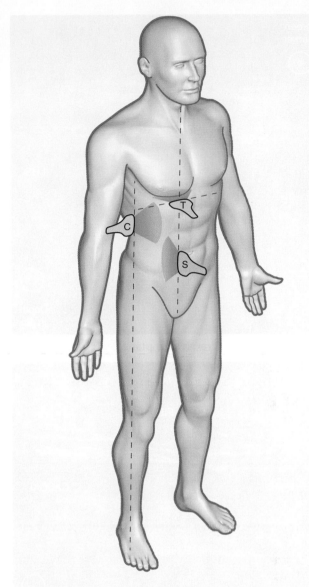

Fig. 1.12 Image planes. *T*, transverse; *S*, sagittal; *C*, coronal.

SCREEN ORIENTATION

For most types of imaging, the screen marker should be on the left-hand side of the image. The exception is in cardiac imaging, where the marker is usually on the right-hand side. Standard orientation of the image should be as the operator is looking at the subject. Generally, the operator is sitting in front of the subject being imaged, with the ultrasound unit behind the subject. During transverse plane imaging, the orientation marker on the transducer should point in the same direction as the screen marker (Figs. 1.13 and 1.14). This means that the screen marker, which is on the left, will correspond to the right side of the subject if they are facing the operator, or the left-hand side of the subject if they have their back to the operator. For sagittal or coronal

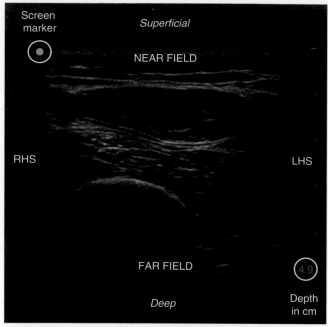

Screen marker

Superficial

NEAR FIELD

RHS

LHS

FAR FIELD

4.9

Deep

Depth in cm

Transverse plane

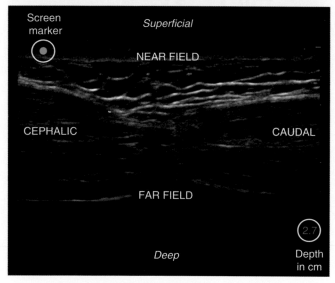

Screen marker

Superficial

NEAR FIELD

CEPHALIC

CAUDAL

FAR FIELD

2.7

Deep

Depth in cm

Sagittal plane

Fig. 1.13 Screen orientation. [Images are of the quadriceps muscles in the right thigh (top) and the rectus abdominis muscle in the anterior abdomen (bottom).]

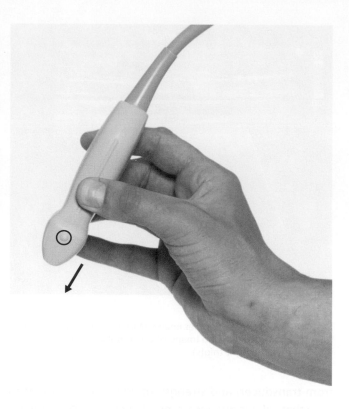

Fig. 1.14 Correct posture for holding the transducer. Note the orientation marker on the side of the transducer (circled).

imaging, the standard practice is that the left side of the image will be cephalic and the right side, caudal.

The direction of the orientation marker on the transducer is shown for each ultrasound figure within this book.

The top of the image is called the near field and is closest to the skin. The bottom of the image is the far field, which is the deepest part of the image (Fig. 1.13). While imaging, adjust the depth setting of the ultrasound so that the region of interest fills the screen. Position the focal points at the same depth as the structure of interest. In some units, this is achieved by altering the depth of the image so that the region of interest is at a midpoint between the top and bottom of the image.

ERGONOMICS

It is important that during imaging both the operator and the subject are comfortable. The operator performing the imaging should sit on a seat adjusted to the correct height. It is also best to use a seat that swivels. The ultrasound unit should be positioned in front of the operator, and the monitor adjusted to a height, or tilted to an angle, that is comfortable for viewing. Make sure the transducer cable is not restricted.

MANIPULATING THE TRANSDUCER

Place sufficient ultrasound gel on the transducer. The gel is required to enable acoustic coupling between the transducer and the skin. Using insufficient gel may lead to artefacts caused by the presence of air, which will scatter the ultrasound echoes away from the probe. Hold the transducer close to the probe face with the first three fingers, similar to holding a pen (Fig. 1.14). Position the transducer on the skin over the region of the body to be examined. Resting the side of the hand on the subject will help to stabilize the transducer.

It is important to apply even pressure with the transducer to the surface of the skin. Care must be taken to use light pressure when imaging superficial structures, since small increases in pressure can suppress superficial veins or disperse tendon synovium or fluid in bursae. The best images are obtained if the transducer is perpendicular (90 degrees) to the structure of interest. It is not always possible to position the transducer directly over the structure of interest. It may be necessary to tilt the transducer so that the beam is directed towards the structure of interest. For example, the liver is partly obscured by the ribs. By positioning the transducer immediately below the costal margin and tilting the transducer superiorly, the liver can be more easily imaged.

Useful transducer movements are:

Sliding: Sliding is when the transducer is moved over the surface of the skin. This is essential for locating structures.

Tilting: Tilting is where the transducer is angled on its short axis (from side to side). This movement is used to extend the field of view.

Rocking: Rocking is where the transducer is angled on its long axis (to and from the orientation marker). This movement is also used to extend the field of view.

Rotating: Rotating is where the transducer is moved from, for example, transverse to sagittal view. Rotating is necessary to move from a short axis to a long axis view of a structure.

Compression: Compression is where more or less pressure is placed on the transducer. It can be used to differentiate veins from arteries. Veins can easily be compressed, whereas arteries cannot.

Transducer movements are shown in Fig. 1.15.

SHORT-AXIS AND LONG-AXIS VIEWS

Structures can be examined in their short axis (transversely) and long axis (longitudinally). In short axis, structures are viewed in cross section, thus a blood vessel would appear as a circle. In long axis, the transducer is positioned along a structure, thus a blood vessel would appear as a tube (Fig. 1.16).

It is generally easier to image a structure in its short axis. To obtain a long-axis view of a structure, start with a short-axis view and, keeping the structure in the middle of the screen, slowly rotate the probe so that it is aligned longitudinally. Blurred edges at the sides of the screen means that the transducer is not aligned longitudinally or the structure of interest is not straight.

IMAGE TERMINOLOGY

Echogenic: A structure that produces echoes. Echogenic structures appear white, e.g., surface of bone.

Anechoic: A structure that does not produce echoes. Anechoic structures will appear black, e.g., lumen of blood vessels, bladder.

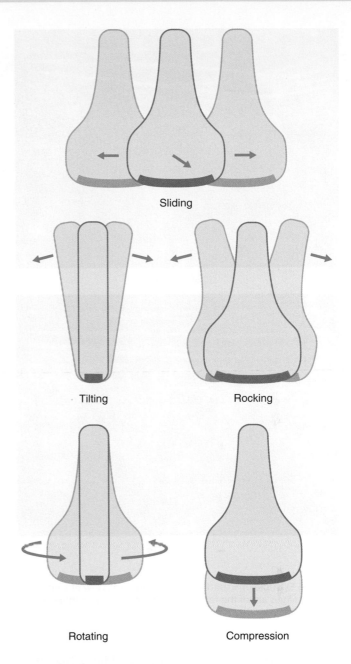

Fig. 1.15 Transducer movements.

Hyperechoic: A structure that produces strong echoes compared to surrounding structures. Hyperechoic structures will appear white.

Hypoechoic: A structure that produces weak echoes compared to surrounding structures. Hypoechoic structures will appear dark gray.

Isoechoic: A structure that produces echoes similar to surrounding structures.

Heterogeneous: An uneven texture pattern of a structure.

Homogeneous: An even (smooth) texture pattern of a structure.

Shadowing: Dark area of image where the ultrasound beam is attenuated by a solid object.

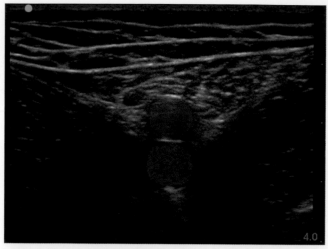

Short-axis

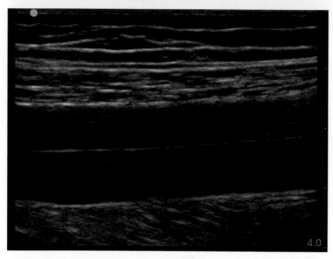

Long-axis

Fig. 1.16 Example of a short-axis and a long-axis view of a blood vessel. [Images are of the femoral artery (red) and vein (blue) in the right thigh.]

Reverberation: Evenly spaced parallel lines caused by ultrasonic waves reflecting back and forth between the transducer and a strong reflecting surface.

Anisotropic artefact: Dark area of image caused when the transducer is not perpendicular to the axis of the structure of interest.

APPEARANCE OF TISSUES

Muscle

Muscle appears hypoechoic (Fig. 1.17A and B). The perimysium, the connective tissue surrounding individual muscle fascicles, appears hyperechoic. A muscle can be identified by moving joints that contract or relax the muscle. During a contraction, the muscle will thicken. Muscles can also be traced to their attachments to help with identification.

Myofascia

Myofascia appears as hyperechoic layers (Fig. 1.17B). The hyperechoic appearance of myofascia makes it easy to delineate muscles.

Subcutaneous fat

Subcutaneous fat appears hypoechoic with characteristic interposed curved hyperechoic lines that are formed by connective tissue septa (Fig. 1.17E). Fat scatters ultrasonic waves, which can diminish the image quality of deeper structures.

Tendon

Tendons appear hyperechoic (light) and in long axis, are striated (Fig. 1.17G).

Hyaline cartilage

Hyaline cartilage appears hypoechoic (Fig. 1.17A).

Fibrocartilage

Fibrocartilage appears hyperechoic and has a homogeneous texture (Fig. 1.17D).

Bone

The surface of bone (the cortex) appears highly echogenic due to the large difference in acoustic impedance between the overlying soft tissue and the bone itself (Fig. 1.17D). Since most ultrasonic waves are reflected back to the surface, underlying bone is devoid of signal.

Nerve

Nerves appear medium gray with a heterogeneous texture. In long axis, they have a striated appearance due to their fascicular structure (Fig. 1.17C). In short axis, nerves have a characteristic honeycomb appearance (Fig. 1.17B).

Blood vessels

The lumen of blood vessels appears anechoic (black), which contrasts with the hyperechoic wall (Fig. 1.17F). Generally, arteries are smaller than veins and have a thicker wall. It is sometimes possible to observe the valves within veins.

Ligaments

Ligaments appear hyperechoic and in long axis, have a laminar appearance (Fig. 1.17D). They are more compact than tendons.

Glands

Glands appear a mid-gray color and have a homogeneous texture (Fig. 1.17F). Fat within glands appears hyperechoic and can suppress transmission deeper into the gland.

Air

Air appears anechoic. Air between the transducer and skin will cause shadowing through the image.

Fluid

Fluid appears anechoic.

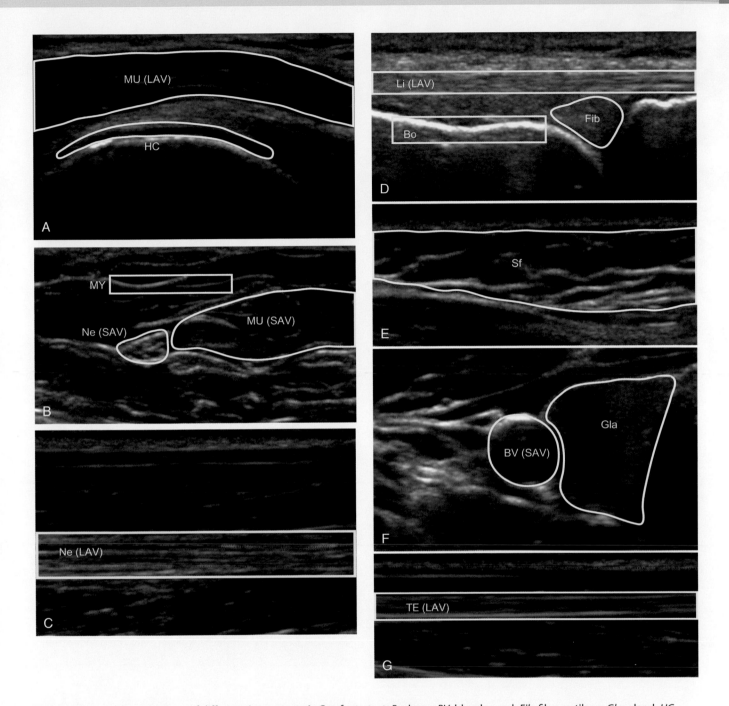

Fig. 1.17 Ultrasound appearance of different tissue types. A–G, refer to text. *Bo*, bone; *BV*, blood vessel; *Fib*, fibrocartilage; *Gla*, gland; *HC*, hyaline cartilage; *LAV*, long-axis view; *Li*, ligament; *MU*, muscle; *MY*, myofascia; *Ne*, nerve; *SAV*, short-axis view; *Sf*, subcutaneous fat; *TE*, tendon.

Summary Checklist

- Anatomical planes and terms
- Skin
- Dermatomes and myotomes
- Ultrasound theory
- Image terminology
- Ultrasound appearance of tissues

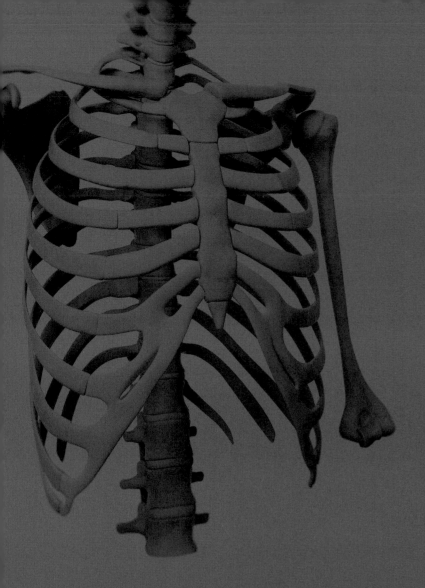

2 Thorax

Conceptual overview

The thorax is a cagelike region that has important roles in protection of the viscera, breathing and movement. It is continuous with the neck superiorly and bounded by the diaphragm inferiorly. The components of the thorax include: bones (sternum, clavicle, ribs and vertebrae), viscera (heart, great vessels, trachea, lungs and esophagus), nerves (vagus and phrenic) and lymphatics. The organs are part of the cardiovascular, respiratory, digestive and lymphatic systems. Clinically, the thorax is a key part of a physical examination for a range of conditions, including valvular diseases of the heart and common infections of the respiratory system.

Surface anatomy

BONES

Anteriorly the bones for examination are the:
- clavicle
- ribs and their costal cartilages
- sternum
- part of the scapula (coracoid process)

On the anterior aspect, the sternum is located in the midline and is divided into the manubrium, body and xiphoid process (Fig. 2.1). The superior border of the manubrium is marked by the jugular notch (suprasternal notch). The division between the manubrium and body of the sternum (manubriosternal joint) can be palpated as a ridge known as the sternal angle, which is where the second costal cartilage articulates. This is a useful landmark for determining which rib you are palpating. If you were to draw an imaginary horizontal line posteriorly from the manubriosternal joint to the vertebral column, the line would usually reach the intervertebral disc between the fourth and fifth thoracic vertebrae (T4 and T5). The manubriosternal joint provides a landmark for locating a number of clinically significant anatomical structures (this may vary due to natural variation):
- the bifurcation of the trachea
- the beginning and ending of the arch of the aorta
- the upper border of the pulmonary trunk
- the point at which the thoracic duct passes from right to left

Moving laterally at the level of the jugular notch, the medial end of the clavicle can be palpated. The clavicle sweeps laterally towards the shoulder region. Adjacent to the sternum, the intercostal spaces can be palpated between the ribs (Fig. 2.2). Palpating intercostal spaces is important for proper placement of a chest drain (see Fig. 2.14).

Posteriorly the bones for examination are the:
- thoracic vertebrae
- ribs
- scapulae

The spinous processes of the vertebrae are located along the midline of the posterior aspect. Flexion of the vertebral column causes the spinous processes to become more prominent. The spinous process of the vertebra prominens, C7, is the first that can be palpated, followed by the prominent spine of the first thoracic vertebra (T1). The scapula sits on the posterior chest wall lateral to the vertebral column. The spine of the scapula lies horizontally and provides a helpful landmark when palpating the supraspinous fossa superiorly and the infraspinous fossa inferiorly. The articulation of the scapula provides the connection between the clavicle and the humerus. The scapula has two main processes, the acromion and the coracoid, which can both be palpated. The medial and lateral borders of the scapula come together inferiorly to form the inferior angle. If a patient is asked to raise their arm above their head, the scapula can be felt rotating laterally, which increases the angle of abduction at the glenohumeral (shoulder) joint (Figs. 2.3 and 2.4).

MUSCLES

The muscles of the thorax are important for movement, to assist respiration and cover the thoracic skeleton. Some abdominal muscles, which are discussed later (Chapter 3), are attached to the inferior portions of the sternum and ribs. During quiet breathing, the muscles of respiration are not easily observed but their location can be palpated.

Anteriorly, the muscles for examination are the:
- pectoralis major
- pectoralis minor
- external intercostal

(Note: Muscles of the back are dealt with in Chapter 5.) The pectoralis major muscle is a sheetlike muscle that can be palpated by tracing the muscle from its origin on the sternum and clavicle, laterally to its insertion on the lateral lip of the intertubercular sulcus of the humerus. The pectoralis major muscle is an important muscle in movement of the upper limb. Although not possible to palpate, the outline of the pectoralis minor muscle can be traced from its origin on the upper margins of the third, fourth and fifth ribs, superiorly and laterally to the coracoid process. The pectoralis minor muscle is an important muscle in stabilizing the pectoral girdle.

The intercostal muscles are important in respiration and run between two adjacent ribs. The intercostal muscles as a group can be palpated by locating any intercostal space in the midaxillary line. At this point, the external, internal

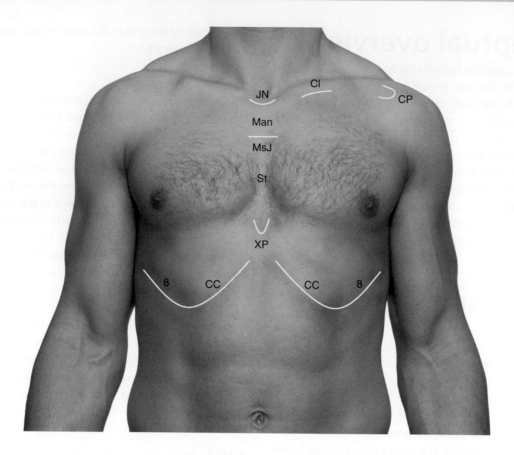

Fig. 2.1 Surface projections of the osteology of the anterior of the thorax. *CC*, costal cartilage; *CI*, clavicle; *CP*, coracoid process; *JN*, jugular notch; *Man*, manubrium; *MsJ*, manubriosternal joint; *St*, sternum; *XP*, xiphoid process; *8*, eighth rib.

To Do (Figs. 2.1, 2.2 and 2.5)

Anterior chest wall:

- Palpate the three component parts of the sternum: the manubrium, the body of the sternum and the xiphoid process.
- Palpate the clavicle from the sternoclavicular joint laterally towards the acromioclavicular joint.
- Palpate the coracoid process below the clavicle, lateral to the midclavicular line.
- Palpate the ribs and the intercostal spaces.
- Palpate the outline of the pectoralis major muscle.
- Palpate an intercostal space in the midaxillary line where the external, internal and innermost muscles are located.
- Undertake a range of movements: flexion, adduction and medial rotation of the humerus, to observe contraction of the pectoralis major muscle.
- Outline the right and left domes of the diaphragm at the fifth intercostal space and sixth rib, respectively.

Posterior chest wall:

- Palpate the spinous processes of the thoracic vertebrae.
- Palpate the spine and borders of the scapula.
- Palpate the acromion above the glenohumeral (shoulder) joint.

and innermost intercostal muscles run from superficial to deep (Table 2.1). Anteriorly, the external intercostal muscle is replaced by a membrane. Posteriorly, the internal intercostal is also replaced by a membrane. The innermost intercostal muscles are especially prominent anteriorly, laterally and posteriorly (Fig. 2.5). They do not extend to the sternum anteriorly or the vertebral column posteriorly.

The diaphragm is a muscular sheet that divides the thoracic and abdominal cavities. The diaphragm has a right and left dome and a central tendon. At rest, the right dome is commonly located at the level of the fifth intercostal space and the left dome at the sixth rib. The left dome is higher than the right due to the presence of the liver. Both domes have been shown to be slightly higher in females. The domes of the diaphragm are affected by respiration

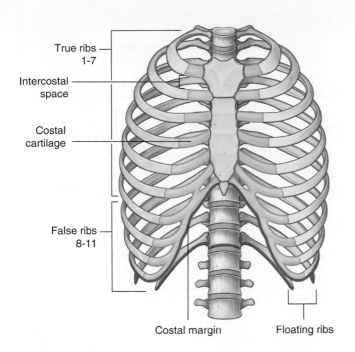

True ribs
1-7

Intercostal
space

Costal
cartilage

False ribs
8-11

Costal margin   Floating ribs

Fig. 2.2 Osteology of the thorax.
(Modified from Drake, RL, Gray's Anatomy for Students, 3rd ed, 2015, Churchill Livingstone, Elsevier.)

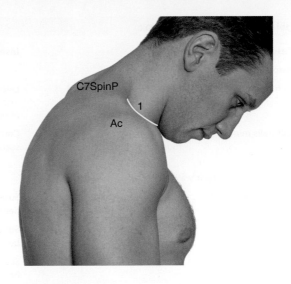

C7SpinP

1

Ac

Fig. 2.4 Lateral view of cervical spine and superior thorax. *Ac,* acromion; *C7SpinP,* C7 spinous process; *1,* first rib.

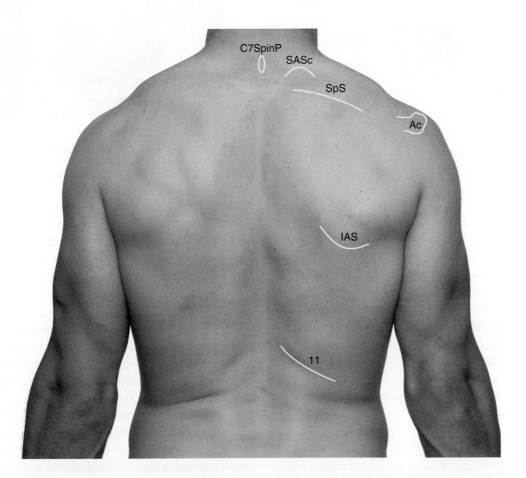

C7SpinP SASc

SpS

Ac

IAS

11

Fig. 2.3 Surface projections of the osteology of the posterior thorax. *Ac,* acromion; *C7SpinP,* C7 spinous process; *IAS,* inferior angle of scapula; *SASc,* superior angle of scapula; *SpS,* spine of scapula; *11,* eleventh rib.

Table 2.1 Muscles of the thorax

Muscle	Origin	Insertion	Innervation	Function
Muscles of the pectoral region				
Pectoralis major	Clavicle and sternum, first seven costal cartilages	Lateral lip of the intertubercular sulcus of humerus	Medial and lateral pectoral nerves C8-T1	Adduction, medial rotation and flexion of the humerus at the shoulder joint
Pectoralis minor	Anterior surfaces of the third, fourth, and fifth ribs	Coracoid process of scapula	Medial pectoral nerves C5-7	Depresses tip of shoulder
Muscles of the thoracic wall				
External intercostal	Inferior margin of rib above	Superior margin of rib below	Intercostal nerves; T1–T11	Most active during inspiration
Internal intercostal	Costal groove of rib above	Superior margin of rib below	Intercostal nerves; T1–T11	Most active during expiration
Innermost intercostal	Costal groove of rib above	Superior margin of rib below	Intercostal nerves; T1–T11	Acts with internal intercostal muscles

Modified from Drake, RL, Gray's Anatomy for Students, 3rd ed, 2015, Churchill Livingstone, Elsevier.

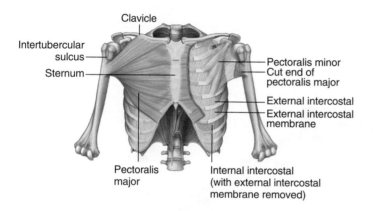

Fig. 2.5 Musculature of the anterior thorax.
(Modified from Drake, RL, Gray's Anatomy for Students, 3rd ed, 2015, Churchill Livingstone, Elsevier.)

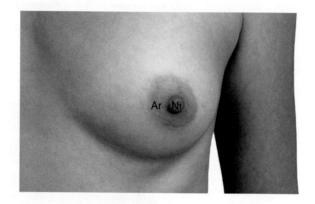

Fig. 2.6 Close-up view of nipple and surrounding areola of the breast. *Ar*, areola; *Ni*, nipple.
(From Drake, RL, Gray's Anatomy for Students, 3rd ed, 2015, Churchill Livingstone, Elsevier.)

and posture, and this should be taken into consideration when examining patients. On the posterior surface, the inferior margin of the diaphragm reaches the twelfth thoracic vertebral level, whereas on the anterior surface, the inferior margin is at the level of subcostal margin. Three main structures traverse through or behind the diaphragm. From superior to inferior, these are the inferior vena cava, the esophagus, and the aorta. Traditionally these structures have been described as passing through at vertebral levels T8, T10 and T12, respectively. However, CT scans have shown for the inferior vena cava there can be variation, with it passing as low as T11.

BREAST

Located superficial to the muscles of the pectoral girdle is breast tissue. The breasts commonly extend from below the clavicle to the sternum and into the axilla. There is natural variation in breast size, which may make surface examination of other thoracic landmarks difficult. The surface anatomy of the breast consists of the central nipple surrounded by the darker pigmented areola (Fig. 2.6).

THORACIC CAVITY

The thoracic cavity is divided into three parts: two lateral pleural cavities, which surround the lungs, and the cavity called the mediastinum. Located in the middle of the thorax, the mediastinum is divided into the superior and inferior mediastinum (Fig. 2.7). The superior mediastinum extends from the manubriosternal plane to the superior thoracic aperture, while the inferior mediastinum extends from the manubriosternal plane to the diaphragm. The inferior mediastinum is further divided into anterior, middle and posterior mediastinum. The anterior mediastinum contains connective tissue, as well as the sternopericardial ligaments

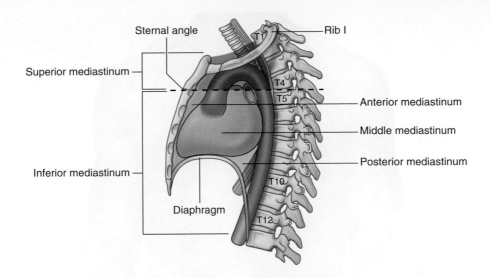

Fig. 2.7 Subdivisions of the mediastinum.
(From Drake, RL, Gray's Anatomy for Students, 3rd ed, 2015, Churchill Livingstone, Elsevier.)

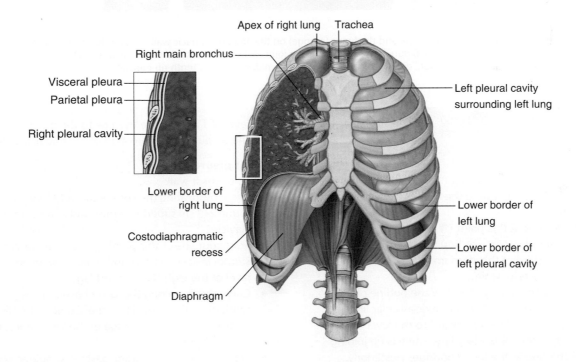

Fig. 2.8 Pleura and borders of the lung.

and remnants of the thymus. The thymus is a lymphoid organ that enlarges during childhood and regresses during adulthood. The middle mediastinum contains the pericardial sac and heart, and the posterior mediastinum contains the four 'tubes', namely the descending aorta, esophagus, azygos vein and thoracic duct.

Pleura

The pleura is a sheetlike structure that comprises two layers: an outer parietal layer, which is adherent to the inner surface of the thoracic wall, and the inner visceral layer (Fig. 2.8). Understanding the extent of the pleura is important clinically and is best understood by tracing it out (Fig. 2.9).

Trachea

As part of the respiratory system, the trachea, with its C-shaped rings of cartilage, passes from the neck into the thorax. The trachea bifurcates approximately 3 cm below the sternal angle, which is located between the fourth and

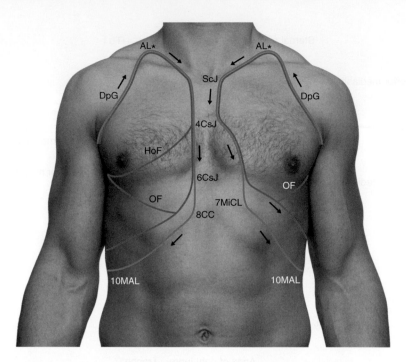

Fig. 2.9 Surface projections of the pleura (blue) and the lungs (orange) on the anterior thoracic wall. *AL*, apex lung; *DpG*, deltopectoral groove; *HoF*, horizontal fissure; *OF*, oblique fissure; *ScJ*, sternoclavicular joint; *4CsJ*, fourth costosternal joint; *6CsJ*, sixth costosternal joint; *7MiCL*, seventh rib in midclavicular line; *8CC*, eighth costal cartilage in the midline; *10MAL*, tenth rib midaxillary line.

To Do (Figs. 2.9 and 2.10)

Left pleura
Anterior chest wall:
- Begin by locating the apex of the left lung, which is found 2–3 cm superior to the middle third of the clavicle.
- Start your line at this point (*) and draw toward the sternoclavicular joint, continuing downward along the lateral third of the sternum to the level of the fourth costosternal joint.
- Make an arch laterally to follow the outline of the heart to the eighth rib in the midclavicular line.
- Now extend the line downward to the level of the tenth rib in the midaxillary line. There is no joining up of this line as the lung continues posteriorly.
- From the axilla, curve a line past the shoulder following the deltopectoral groove to join the starting point.

Posterior chest wall:
- Make a dot at a point 2 cm lateral to the spinous process of the second thoracic vertebra. Note that this is at the articulation of the costotransverse joint.
- Make a line from this point inferiorly to the level of the twelfth thoracic vertebra.
- Make an arch superiorly toward the lateral part of the ribs, ending at the midaxillary line.
- At your starting point, draw a curved line forming the apex of the lung. Ensure the apex reaches the

level of T1. Continue this line to the inferior angle of the scapula in the direction of the midaxillary line.

Right pleura
Anterior chest wall:
- Begin by locating the apex of the right lung, which is found 2–3 cm superior to the middle third of the clavicle.
- Start your line at this point (*) and draw toward the sternoclavicular joint, continuing downward to the level of the eighth costal cartilage.
- Curve the line along the lower costal cartilages to the tenth rib in the midaxillary line. Do not join this line up because the lateral edge of the lung curves to continue posteriorly.
- From the axilla, curve a line past the shoulder following the deltopectoral groove to join the starting point.

Posterior chest wall:
- Make a dot at a point 2 cm lateral to the spinous process of the second thoracic vertebra. Note that this is at the articulation of the costotransverse joint.
- Make a line from this point inferiorly to the level of the twelfth thoracic vertebra.
- Make an arch superiorly toward the lateral part of the ribs, ending at the midaxillary line.
- At your starting point, draw a curved line forming the apex of the lung. Ensure the apex reaches the level of T1. Do not join this line up because the lateral edge of the lung curves to continue anteriorly.

Left lung
Anterior chest wall:
- Start at the apex of the left lung, 2–3 cm above the middle third of the clavicle, draw a line toward the sternoclavicular joint. Continue the line along the lateral border of the sternum to the level of the fourth costosternal joint.
- Make an arch laterally to follow the outline of the heart to the sixth rib in the midclavicular line.
- Extend the line to the eighth rib in the midaxillary line and the tenth rib in the paravertebral line.
- From the axilla, curve a line past the shoulder, following the deltopectoral groove, to join the starting point. The marking of the lungs should be within the markings made to represent the pleura.

Posterior chest wall:
- Starting at the apex of the pleura, create a line just inside the parietal pleura. In the midline, extend this line inferiorly to the level of T10. At this level, draw a line laterally representing the base of the lung.
- To represent the oblique fissure, locate the spinous process of T2 and draw a line inferiorly and laterally to join the border of the lung at the level of the inferior angle of the scapula.

Right lung
Anterior chest wall:
- Starting at the apex of the right lung, 2–3 cm above the middle third of the clavicle, draw a line toward the sternoclavicular joint. Continue the line along the lateral border of the sternum to the level of the sixth costosternal joint.
- To mark out the oblique fissure, take a line from the eighth costal cartilage 2–3 cm medial to the midclavicular line, and draw obliquely upward and backward toward the axilla.
- To mark out the horizontal fissure, draw a horizontal line from the fourth costosternal joint to meet the oblique fissure in the axilla.
- Extend the line to the eighth rib in the midaxillary line and the tenth rib in the paravertebral line.
- From the axilla, curve a line past the shoulder, following the deltopectoral groove, to join the starting point. The marking of the lungs should be within the markings made to represent the pleura.

Posterior chest wall:
- Starting at the apex of the pleura, create a line just inside and following the parietal pleura. Stop at the level of T10 and draw a line laterally to represent the base of the lung.
- To represent the oblique fissure, locate the spinous process of T2 and draw a line inferiorly and laterally to join the border of the lung at the level of the inferior angle of the scapula. Note that the horizontal fissure does not project to the posterior surface.

Trachea
Anterior chest wall:
- Draw a line medially through the jugular notch.
- Divide this line into two branches at the level of the manubriosternal joint, each directed downward and laterally, to represent the bifurcation.

fifth thoracic vertebrae. The trachea bifurcates into the primary bronchi (the bifurcation has been shown to be slightly higher in females). The right bronchus is wider and shorter and more vertical than the left. The left bronchus is narrower and less vertical.

Lungs

The lungs are the principal organs of respiration. They are located within the pleural cavities and vary in form. The right lung has three lobes: the superior, middle and inferior, which are divided by oblique and horizontal fissures. The left lung has only two lobes: the superior and inferior, which are separated by an oblique fissure. Both lungs have a superior border, known as the apex, that sits just above the clavicle in the midclavicular line. The borders of the lungs follow those of the pleura with the exception that the inferior border of the lungs are more superior, thereby creating the costodiaphragmatic recesses. The lower borders of the lungs differ. The right lower border in the midclavicular line is at the fifth rib or sixth intercostal space whereas the left lower border is at the sixth rib or seventh intercostal space (Figs. 2.8–2.10).

Heart

The heart is a muscular four-chamber pump. It is enclosed within its own cavity, the pericardial cavity, which is surrounded by a small amount of serous fluid that enables the heart to beat in a friction-free environment. The pericardial cavity is surrounded by the fibrous pericardium and the serous layer of parietal pericardium, which is adhered inferiorly to the diaphragm and anteriorly to the sternum via the sternopericardial ligaments. The heart has two receiving chambers, namely the right and left atria, which empty into the right and left ventricles through the tricuspid and bicuspid valves respectively. The orientation of the heart is such that the right border is formed by the right atrium. The inferior border is formed predominantly by the right ventricle and a portion of the left ventricle towards the apex. The left border is formed by the left ventricle inferiorly and the left atrium superiorly. The superior border is formed by

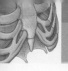
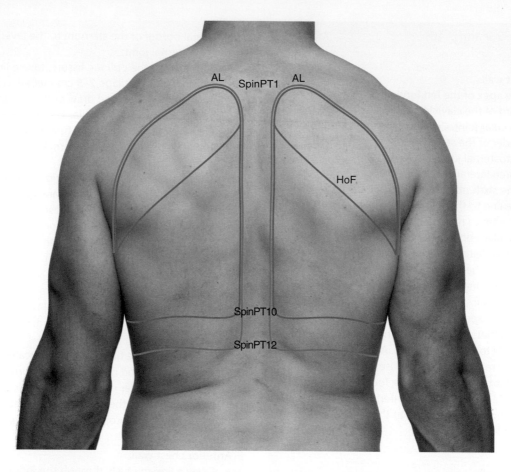

Fig. 2.10 Surface projections of the pleura (blue) and lungs (orange) on the posterior thorax. *AL*, apex lung; *HoF*, horizontal fissure; *SpinPT1*, spinous process of T1; *SpinPT10*, spinous process of T10; *SpinPT12*, spinous process of T12.

the upper parts of the atria and the great vessels. Hearts vary in size between individuals, and their position ranges from the second or third costal cartilage to the fifth or sixth costal cartilage, with the apex typically located in the midclavicular line at the fifth or sixth intercostal space. Pathological enlargement of the heart (cardiomegaly) is common and can result from a range of conditions, such as hypertension and mitral valve disease. Understanding the normal position is important in recognizing cardiomegaly (Fig. 2.11).

The surface projections of the heart valves lie in an oblique line behind the sternum. This alignment is very helpful for auscultation of heart sounds. The tricuspid valve lies just above the level of the plane of the fifth costal cartilage to the right lateral edge of the sternum, whereas the mitral valve lies just left of the midline adjacent to the left inferior fourth costal cartilage and fourth intercostal space. The aortic valve lies adjacent to the third intercostal space roughly in the midline of the sternum, and the pulmonary valve lies in the plane of the third costal cartilage to the left lateral edge of the sternum. To listen to the heart valves there sure key places to place a stethoscope, which are not simply overlying the valves (Fig. 2.12).

Great vessels

The great vessels project superiorly and pass out of, or into, the thorax to and from the neck, upper limb and abdomen. The brachiocephalic veins are the most anterior of the great vessels and are located just behind the manubrium of the sternum. The brachiocephalic veins are formed from the fusion of the subclavian and internal jugular veins. The fusion lies just behind the sternoclavicular joints. The superior vena cava is formed from the union of the right and left brachiocephalic veins just behind the right second costal cartilage or the first intercostal space. The formation of the superior vena cava has been found to be higher in females and in young adults. The internal jugular veins run inferiorly, lateral to the trachea. The arch of the aorta is also located behind the sternum. The aorta curves superiorly, laterally and posteriorly, passing behind the pulmonary arteries and bronchi on the left. The concavity of the arch of the aorta is either at the sternal angle or just below it. The brachiocephalic trunk is usually the first arterial branch off the arch of the aorta. The trunk divides into the right common carotid artery and the right subclavian artery (Fig. 2.13).

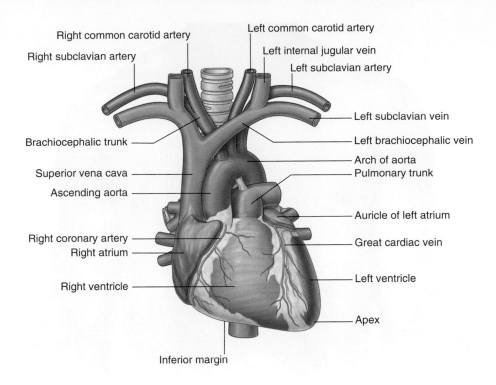

Fig. 2.11 Anterior view of the heart.
(Modified from Drake, RL, Gray's Anatomy for Students, 3rd ed, 2015, Churchill Livingstone, Elsevier.)

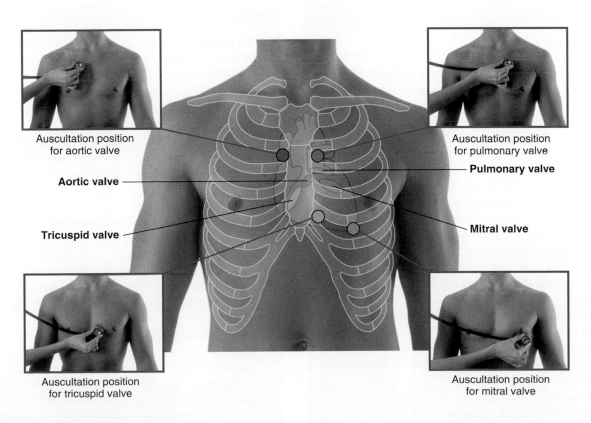

Fig. 2.12 Surface projections of heart valves.
(From Drake, RL, Gray's Anatomy for Students, 3rd ed, 2015, Churchill Livingstone, Elsevier.)

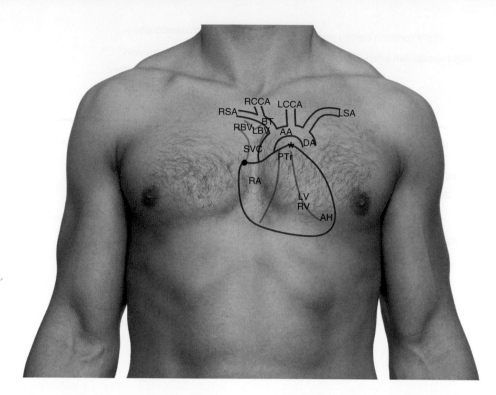

Fig. 2.13 Surface projections of the heart and the great vessels on the anterior chest wall. *AA*, arch aorta; *AH*, apex heart; *BT*, brachiocephalic trunk; *DA*, descending aorta; *LBV*, left brachiocephalic vein; *LCCA*, left common carotid artery; *LSA*, left subclavian artery; *LV*, left ventricle; *PTr*, pulmonary trunk; *RA*, right atrium; *RBV*, right brachiocephalic vein; *RCCA*, right common carotid artery; *RSA*, right subclavian artery; *RV*, right ventricle; *SVC*, superior vena cava.

To Do (Fig. 2.13)

Heart borders
Anterior chest wall:
- Mark a point 2 cm lateral from the sternum at the level of the second costal cartilage on the subject's left side *.
- Mark a second point 1 cm lateral from the sternum at the level of the third costal cartilage on the right hand side of the subject •. Join these points together.
- On the right, draw a line inferiorly, bulging slightly laterally, down to the sixth right costal cartilage to form the lateral border of the right atrium.
- To represent the base of the heart, draw a line laterally to the left, ending at the fifth left intercostal space in the midclavicular region (to the edge of the nipple in a male, in a female take this line as far as is comfortable at the level of the fifth intercostal space).
- To complete the heart, draw a line curving from the fifth intercostal space in the midclavicular region superiorly and medially to join your starting point 2 cm lateral to the sternum at the second left costal cartilage.

Heart valves
- Draw a small ellipse to demarcate the approximate location of each of the valves (Fig. 2.12).

To Do (Fig. 2.13)

Great vessels
Anterior chest wall:

Aortic arch
- Draw two curved lines about 2.5 cm apart starting at the subject's right half of the sternal angle.
- The apex of the aortic arch curves 3–4 cm lateral to the sternum at the lower border of the first rib. The arch should curve sharply due to the aortic arch running posteriorly.

Superior vena cava
- Continue the line from the subject's third right costal cartilage superiorly for 4 cm to mark the right border of the superior vena cava.
- Draw on the right and left brachiocephalic veins as they drain into the superior vena cava. Note the left brachiocephalic vein continues anterior to the arch of the aorta.

Brachiocephalic trunk
- Draw two curved lines about 1.5 cm apart starting just right of the highest point of the aortic arch and continuing toward the right sternoclavicular joint. At this point, the trunk divides into the right common carotid artery and the right subclavian artery.

Right common carotid artery
- Draw two lines about 1 cm apart, starting at the brachiocephalic bifurcation, to the right sternoclavicular joint, and continue superiorly to the upper border of the thyroid cartilage (level of C3/C4). Here, the artery divides into the internal and external carotid arteries.

Left common carotid artery
- Draw two lines about 1 cm apart, beginning at the highest part of the aortic arch, lateral to the brachiocephalic trunk and continue the line to the left sternoclavicular joint. From this point take the lines superiorly to the upper border of the thyroid cartilage at the left lateral edge. At this point, the artery divides into the internal and external carotid arteries.

Left subclavian artery
- Draw two lines 1 cm apart lateral to the left common carotid artery to represent the left subclavian artery.

Percussion of the chest
Tapping the chest wall produces a hollow, drumlike sound over air filled spaces, such as the lung, but a dull sound over solid organs, such as the heart, or over fluid.
- Spread the fingers of one hand flat against the subject's chest and tap the middle phalanx of the middle finger with the middle finger of the other hand.
- Explore the chest surface in this way and decide whether the resonant areas defined by percussion coincide with the lung outlines you have already marked.

Listening to the chest
- There are key locations to use when listening to the chest with a stethoscope. Use Fig. 2.12 to try listening at these points.

In the Clinic

Pneumothorax
In emergency medicine, a chest drain may be required to drain fluid or air from the pleural cavities. The most common position for the insertion of a chest drain is anterior to the midaxillary line, in the 'safe triangle'. The triangle is delineated by the anterior border of the latissimus dorsi muscle, the lateral border of the pectoralis major muscle, a line superior to the horizontal level of the nipple and an apex below the axilla (Fig. 2.14).

Pneumonia
Pneumonia is inflammation of the lung, often resulting from infection. Common symptoms include difficulty breathing, a cough with mucus and a fever. The surface markings of the lungs are important in listening to the chest and establishing which lobes are affected. Commonly, pneumonia presents in one or two bronchopulmonary segments (defined subdivisions within each lung lobe), but may extend to one whole lobe. When listening to a patient's chest with pneumonia, rattles that are crackling or bubbling can be heard as the fluid within the lungs moves.

Pleural effusion
Pleural effusion occurs when fluid becomes trapped between the parietal and visceral pleural layers. A drain may be placed, guided by ultrasound, at the point where the greatest amount of fluid is seen, commonly at the lowest level.

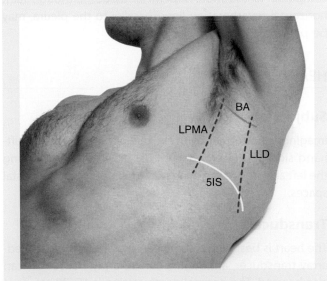

Fig. 2.14 Schematic diagram showing safe triangle for insertions of chest drain. *BA*, base of axilla; *LLD*, lateral edge of latissimus dorsi; *LPMA*, lateral edge of pectoralis major; *5IS*, fifth intercostal space.

Ultrasound

ANTERIOR MUSCLES OF THE THORAX AND LUNGS

Subject position

Imaging can be performed either lying supine or sitting.

Transducer

Use a linear array transducer. Set the depth setting to 3–5 cm.

Transducer position

Position the transducer in the transverse plane on the anterior thoracic wall (left or right side) along the midclavicular line in the second or third intercostal space. In a female it may be necessary to go below the breast tissue (Fig. 2.15).

Image features

Three layers of muscle should be in view. These muscles are the pectoralis major, pectoralis minor and the intercostal muscles. Surrounding these muscles, hyperechoic myofascia will be visible. Superficial to the pectoralis major muscle there will be a layer of subcutaneous fat. The bright relatively thick hyperechoic line below the intercostal muscles is the pleura, which, during live imaging, will move synchronously with respiration. The lung appears hypoechoic compared to the more superficial tissues, although faint horizontal reverberation lines, parallel to the pleura, may be present (Fig. 2.15).

HEART

Subject position

Imaging is performed with the subject lying on their left-hand side (left lateral decubitus) or supine. Positioning the left arm above the head may help open the intercostal spaces.

Transducer

The heart is best viewed between the ribs using a phased-array transducer, although a curved-array transducer can also be used. The optimal depth setting is 15–20 cm.

Apical view

Transducer position

Position the transducer on the left side of the thorax in the fifth or sixth intercostal space along the midclavicular line. This location is the point of maximal impulse, which can be

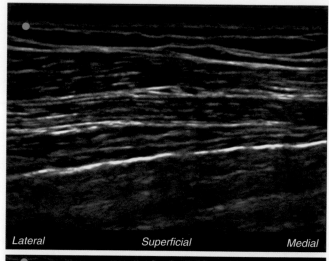

Lateral　　　*Superficial*　　　*Medial*

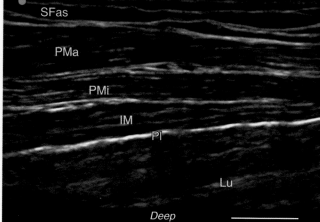

SFas

PMa

PMi

IM

Pl

Lu

Deep

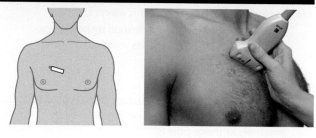

Fig. 2.15 Ultrasound image of the anterior muscles of the thorax and lungs. *IM*, intercostal muscle; *Lu*, lung; *Pl*, pleura; *PMa*, pectoralis major; *PMi*, pectoralis minor; *SFas*, superficial fascia. Scale bar = 1 cm.

located by palpating the thorax. With the screen orientation marker on the right-hand side of the image (which is the convention for echocardiography), rotate the transducer until the orientation marker is pointing to the left side of the subject (3 o'clock position; Fig. 2.16). The transducer should be tilted slightly upward, so that the beam is passing through the long axis of the heart from the apex to the base. If the screen orientation marker is on the left-hand side of the screen, the probe orientation marker should point towards the right side of the subject (9 o'clock position).

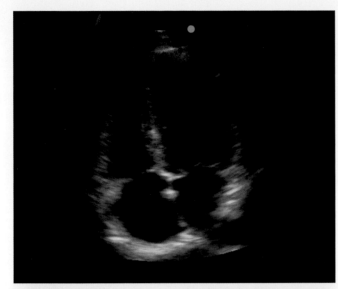

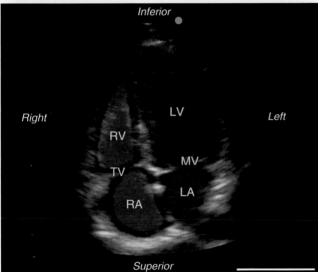

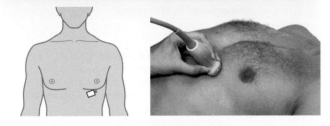

Fig. 2.16 Ultrasound image of the heart – apical view. *LA*, left atrium; *LV*, left ventricle; *MV*, mitral valve; *RA*, right atrium; *RV*, right ventricle; *TV*, tricuspid valve. Scale bar = 5 cm.

Image features

The four chambers of the heart should be visible. The pericardium and cardiac muscle will appear hyperechoic compared to the fluid-filled chambers of the heart. The heart is viewed upside down, with the apex at the top of the image (closest to the transducer) and the base/atria towards the bottom of the image. At the top of the image, the left and right ventricles will be in view. The left ventricle appears approximately twice the size of the right ventricle. Between the atria and the ventricles, movements of the tricuspid and mitral valves can be visualized during live imaging (Fig. 2.16 and Video 2.1).

Long axis parasternal view

Transducer position

Position the transducer on the left side of the thorax in the third or fourth intercostal space close to the sternum. With the screen orientation marker on the right-hand side of the image, rotate the transducer until the orientation marker points to the right shoulder (10 o'clock position) (Fig. 2.17). If the screen orientation marker is on the left-hand side of the screen, the probe orientation marker should point towards the left anterior superior iliac spine (4 o'clock position).

Image features

In this view, the heart is visualized along its long axis, from inferior (left-hand side of the image) to superior (right-hand side of image). The left side of the heart can be seen towards the bottom of the image. The right side of the heart is at the top of the image. The long axis parasternal view provides a detailed window into the left side of the heart. The hypoechoic left atrium and ventricle can be observed. Superior (right on image) to the left ventricle, above the left atrium, the aorta and aortic valve should also be in view. The pericardium is easily visualized as a bright hyperechoic curved feature toward the bottom of the image. Adjacent to the pericardium, it may be possible to observe a short axis view of the descending aorta (Fig. 2.17).

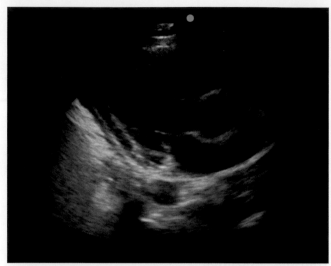

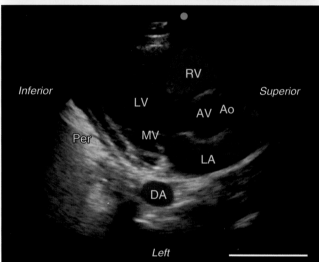

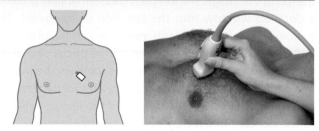

Fig. 2.17 Ultrasound image of the heart – long axis parasternal view. *Ao*, aorta; *AV*, atrioventricular valve; *DA*, descending aorta; *LA*, left atrium; *LV*, left ventricle; *MV*, mitral valve; *Per*, pericardium; *RV*, right ventricle. Scale bar = 5 cm.

Summary Checklist

- Surface projections of the bones related to the thorax
- Surface projections of the pleura and markings of the lungs
- Surface projections of the heart and its valves
- Ultrasound imaging of the muscles of the chest wall
- Ultrasound imaging of the pleura
- Ultrasound imaging of the heart

In the Clinic

Ultrasound imaging of the heart is known as echocardiography. Conventional B- and M-mode imaging and Doppler are used to assess the integrity of the organ (Video 2.1). Doppler techniques, for example pulse wave and continuous Doppler, have the advantage of providing a measure of blood flow and valve movements. As well as imaging through the skin (transthoracic approach), the heart can be imaged using a specialized transducer that is inserted into the esophagus (transesophageal approach).

Ultrasound can be used to assess pathologies affecting both the pleura and the lungs, such as pleural effusions, mesothelioma and hematothorax. Although a healthy air-filled lung appears hypoechoic due to the lack of acoustic echo beyond the pleura, consolidation of the lung caused by infection (e.g., in pleural disease) can be seen. To allow a more extensive view of the lung parenchyma, lower frequency phased-array or curved transducers are frequently used in the clinic. Real-time imaging during respiration can aid assessment of pleural effusion and diaphragm paralysis. Ultrasound is also frequently used in the clinic for breast imaging.

Other clinical applications in the thorax include monitoring the placement of central venous catheters and needle guidance during aspiration of fluid from the pleural space (thoracentesis) or pericardium (pericardiocentesis), as well as during biopsies of the pleura, mediastinal lymph nodes or breast. Table 2.2 provides an overview of the some of the thoracic conditions that can be diagnosed or monitored by ultrasound.

Table 2.2	Thoracic pathologies that are can be diagnosed or monitored by ultrasound
Viscera	**Pathology**
Heart	Valvular disease (e.g., valvular insufficiency or stenosis), cardiomyopathy (e.g., dilated or hypertrophic cardiomyopathy), congenital disease (e.g., atrial or ventricular septal defects), ischemic heart disease, pulmonary hypertension, pericarditis
Lungs	Pleural effusion, pneumothorax, pneumonia, neoplasms
Diaphragm	Diaphragm paralysis
Ribs	Rib fractures

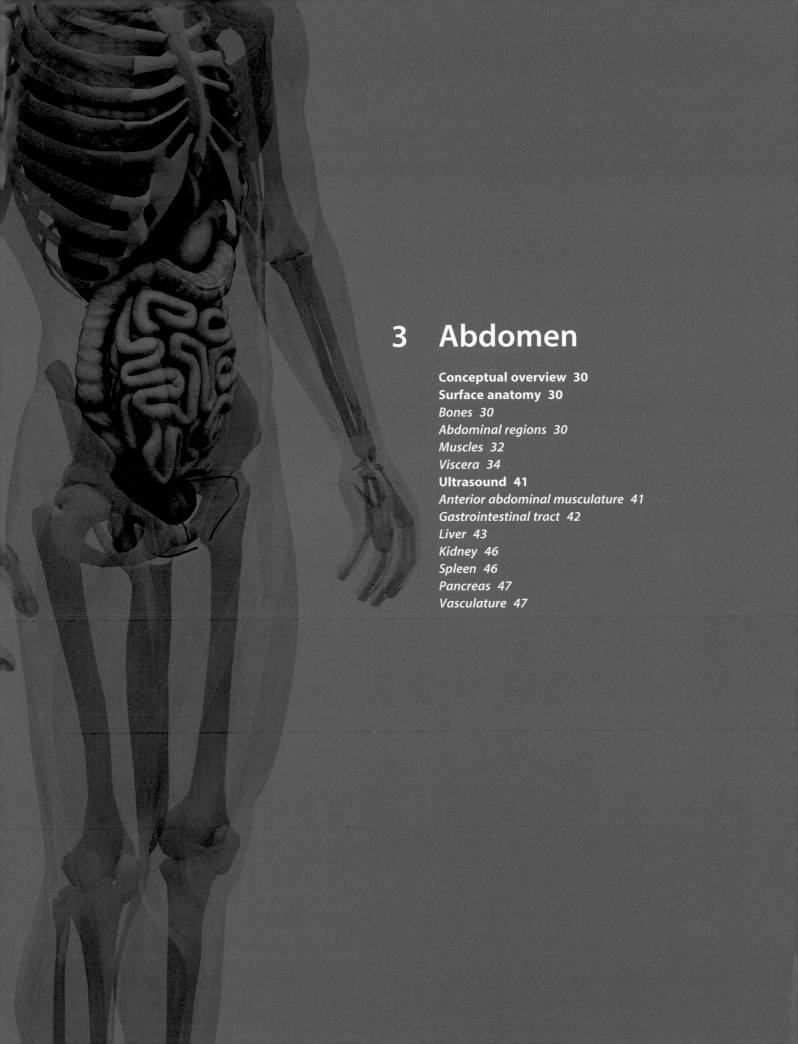

3 Abdomen

Conceptual overview

The abdomen is a rectangular-shaped cavity that is continuous inferiorly with the pelvic cavity and superiorly with the thorax. The abdominal cavity is bounded superiorly by the diaphragm and surrounded on its anterior, lateral and posterior sides by fascia and musculature. The components of the abdomen include bones (vertebrae, lower ribs and their associated costal cartilages) and viscera (stomach, small and large intestines, liver, gallbladder, pancreas, spleen, suprarenal glands and kidneys). The viscera are part of the gastrointestinal, hepatobiliary, endocrine and urinary systems. The abdomen can be examined to see if it is distended or flat, symmetrical or asymmetrical and if any abdominal scars are present. These are helpful observations for visual assessment during palpation for enlarged organs or fluid accumulations. Clinically, the abdomen is an important region in a physical examination for a range of conditions, including appendicitis, autoimmune conditions, such as ulcerative colitis, and diseases of the liver, for example cirrhosis. Abdominal examination is key to the detection of abdominal organomegaly (whether physiological or pathological).

Surface anatomy

BONES

The osteology of the abdomen consists of bones associated with the thoracic cavity, pelvic girdle and the vertebrae. On the anterior aspect, the superior part of the abdominal cavity is protected by the sixth to tenth ribs and associated costal cartilages, and by the xiphoid process of the sternum in the midline. Inferiorly, the iliac crests of the pelvic girdle form a bony boundary both posteriorly and laterally. The iliac crests end anteriorly as the anterior superior iliac spines (ASIS). The pubic tubercle of the pubic bone lies on either side of the midline anteriorly. Posteriorly, the thoracic (T10–T12) and lumbar vertebrae (L1–L5) provide support for the viscera and attachment points for muscles (Fig. 3.1).

ABDOMINAL REGIONS

When viewing the abdomen from the front, there are two organizational patterns, the four quadrant and the nine region, that are used to divide the abdomen in order to

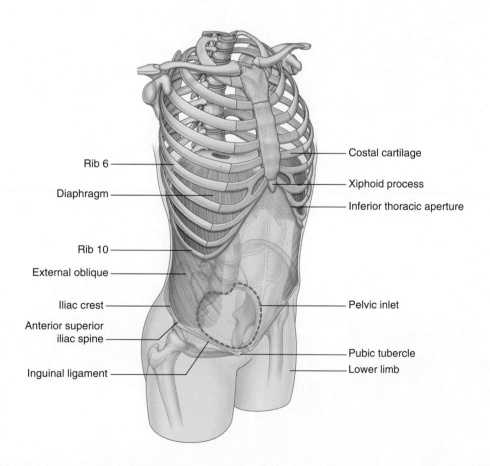

Rib 6		Costal cartilage
Diaphragm		Xiphoid process
		Inferior thoracic aperture
Rib 10		
External oblique		
Iliac crest		Pelvic inlet
Anterior superior iliac spine		
		Pubic tubercle
Inguinal ligament		Lower limb

Fig. 3.1 Osteology associated with the abdominal cavity.
(Modified from Drake, RL, Gray's Anatomy for Students, 3rd ed, 2015, Churchill Livingstone, Elsevier.)

assist with clinical descriptions. The four quadrant pattern is formed by a median plane passing through the midline from the xiphoid process to the pubic symphysis. A second plane passes horizontally through the umbilicus (transumbilical plane). These two planes create four quadrants known as the right upper quadrant, the left upper quadrant, the right lower quadrant and the left lower quadrant (Fig. 3.2). The umbilicus is commonly at the level of the L4, but can vary from the L2 to S1 level. The nine region pattern is formed by right and left midclavicular planes that pass from the middle of each clavicle, to a point midway between the anterior superior iliac spine and the pubic tubercle on each side. Two horizontal planes cross the abdomen. The subcostal plane is at the lower border of the costal cartilage of the tenth rib, posteriorly at the level of the third lumbar vertebra. The second horizontal plane, the intertubercular plane, extends between the right and left iliac crests, posteriorly at the level of the L5. The nine regions created are the right

hypochondrium, epigastric, left hypochondrium, flank (lateral or lumbar region), umbilical, and groin (inguinal or iliac region) (Fig. 3.3). An additional plane used clinically is the transpyloric (transduodenal) plane, which is at the level of the first lumbar vertebra and passes through the first part of the duodenum.

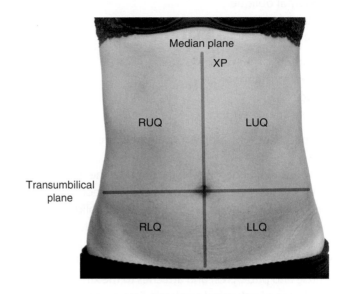

Fig. 3.2 Surface projections of the four quadrant organizational pattern. *LLQ*, left lower quadrant; *LUQ*, left upper quadrant; *RLQ*, right lower quadrant; *RUQ*, right upper quadrant; *XP*, xiphoid process.

To Do (Figs. 3.2 and 3.3)

Anterior abdominal wall:
- Palpate the xiphoid process.
- Palpate the sixth to tenth ribs and their associated costal cartilages.

Surface organization of the four quadrants.
- Starting from the xiphoid process, trace the median plane inferiorly towards the pubic symphysis.
- Locate the transumbilical plane.
- Examine the four quadrants (right upper quadrant, left upper quadrant, right lower quadrant and left lower quadrant).

Surface organization of the nine regions.
- Start from the lowest point of the costal cartilage of the tenth rib and draw the horizontal subcostal plane.
- From the top of the iliac crests, draw the horizontal intertubercular plane.
- Draw two lines that run inferiorly from the middle of both clavicles towards the pelvis.
- Examine the nine regions created (right hypochondrium, epigastric, left hypochondrium, right flank (lateral), umbilical, left flank (lateral), right groin (inguinal), pubic and left groin (inguinal).
- Half-way between the xiphisternal joint and the umbilicus add the transpyloric (transduodenal) plane, which will be 2–3 cm above the subcostal plane. In the majority of individuals this passes through the lower borders of the ninth costal cartilages.

Posterior abdominal wall:
- Palpate the spinous processes of the lower thoracic and lumbar vertebrae.
- Palpate the iliac crest and follow it laterally and anteriorly to the anterior superior iliac spine.

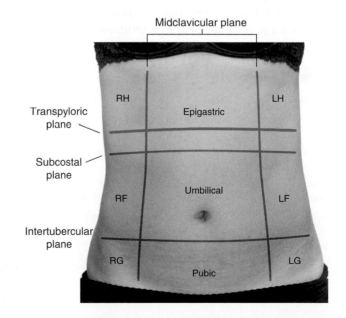

Fig. 3.3 Surface projections of the nine region organizational pattern (plus transpyloric). *LF*, left flank; *LG*, left groin; *LH*, left hypochondrium; *RF*, right flank; *RG*, right groin; *RH*, right hypochondrium.

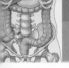

MUSCLES

The muscles of the abdominal wall (Table 3.1) are important for movement and protecting the viscera, and can act to increase the intraabdominal pressure during micturition, defecation or parturition (Fig. 3.4).

Anterior abdominal muscles:

- rectus abdominis
- external oblique
- internal oblique
- transversus abdominis

Posterior abdominal muscles:

- quadratus lumborum
- iliacus
- psoas major

(Note that muscles of the back are described in Chapter 5.)

The anterior abdominal wall comprises the rectus sheath as well as the muscles listed above. The rectus sheath is formed by the aponeuroses of the external oblique, internal oblique and the transversus abdominis muscle. The rectus abdominis muscle is contained within the sheath. The rectus abdominis muscles arise from the pubic symphysis, pubic tubercle and pubic crest and attaches to the xiphoid process and fifth to seventh costal cartilages. Each muscle is separated in the midline by the linea alba. The linea alba is a fibrous band comprised of fibers from the rectus sheath that run from the xiphoid process to the pubic symphysis. The linea alba can sometimes be seen on the surface as an indentation and feels more fibrous to palpate than the neighboring rectus abdominis muscle. The rectus abdominis muscle contains three or four horizontal tendinous intersections that blend with the rectus sheath. The lateral edge of the rectus abdominis is marked by the linea semilunaris (Fig. 3.5). The linea semilunaris runs from the ninth rib to the pubic tubercle. At the level of the umbilicus the linea semilunaris is found approximately 7 cm laterally. The umbilicus is the scar tissue left after the detachment of the umbilical cord. The umbilicus is circular or oval in shape, although the precise shape of the umbilicus varies according to age and size and may protrude or be depressed. The external oblique muscle is a flat muscle that sweeps anteriorly and inferiorly. It has a large aponeurosis, which contributes to the linea alba and forms the inguinal ligament. The external oblique muscle can be palpated on the anterolateral aspect of the abdominal wall. The internal oblique muscle sweeps superiorly and anteriorly and also has an aponeurosis that contributes to the rectus sheath. The transversus abdominis muscle is the innermost layer, which runs transversely and has an aponeurosis that contributes to the rectus sheath. On the posterior abdominal wall the quadratus lumborum muscle lies between the twelfth rib and the iliac crest. The iliacus and psoas major muscles act on the hip joint and will be considered in Chapter 7 (Fig. 3.5).

Inguinal canal

The inguinal canal is formed on its anterior border by the aponeurosis of the external oblique muscle and internal oblique muscle. The arching roof is formed by the transversalis fascia and the internal oblique and transversus muscles. The posterior border is formed by the transversalis fascia. The floor is formed by the inguinal and lacunar ligaments.

Table 3.1 Abdominal wall muscles

Muscle	Origin	Insertion	Innervation	Function
External oblique	Lower eight ribs (ribs 5–12)	Iliac crest	Thoracic spinal	Compress abdominal contents; flex trunk
Internal oblique	Thoracolumbar fascia; iliac crest	Lower three or four ribs	Thoracic spinal nerves (T7–T12) and L1	Compress abdominal contents
Transversus abdominis	Thoracolumbar fascia; costal cartilages lower six ribs (ribs 7–12)	Aponeurosis	Thoracic spinal nerves (T7–T12) and L1	Compress abdominal contents
Rectus abdominis	Pubic crest, pubic tubercle, and pubic symphysis	Costal cartilages of ribs 5–7; xiphoid process	Thoracic spinal nerves (T7–T12)	Compress abdominal contents
Posterior abdominal wall muscles				
Psoas major	T12 and L1–L5 vertebrae, and disc	Lesser trochanter of the femur	L1–L3	Flexion of thigh at hip joint
Quadratus lumborum	Iliac crest	Transverse processes of L1–L4	T12 and L1–L4	Stabilize rib 12 and lateral bending
Iliacus	Iliac fossa, upper lateral surface of sacrum	Lesser trochanter of femur	Femoral nerve (L2–L4)	Flexion of thigh at hip joint

Modified from Drake, RL, Gray's Anatomy for Students, 3rd ed, 2015, Churchill Livingstone, Elsevier.

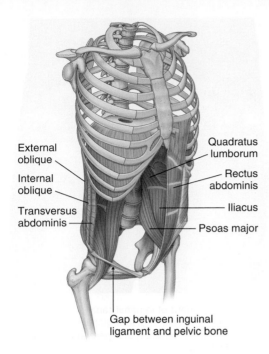

External oblique

Internal oblique

Transversus abdominis

Quadratus lumborum

Rectus abdominis

Iliacus

Psoas major

Gap between inguinal ligament and pelvic bone

Fig. 3.4 Musculature of the anterior abdominal wall. *ASIS,* anterior superior iliac spine; *EO,* external oblique; *IL,* inguinal ligament; *LiA,* linea alba; *LS,* linea semilunaris; *ReA,* rectus abdominus. *(From Drake, RL, Gray's Anatomy for Students, 3rd ed, 2015, Churchill Livingstone, Elsevier.)*

Anterior abdominal wall:
- Lying supine, palpate the linea alba in the midline. Moving laterally, outline the rectus abdominis muscle in the resting subject and feel the muscle contract as the subject tries to sit up, especially against resistance.
- On the anterolateral aspect of the abdominal wall palpate the external oblique muscle.osterior abdominal wall:
- Locate the iliac crests. From the midline, move laterally 5 cm. Moving superiorly, palpate the quadratus lumborum muscle up to the twelfth rib.

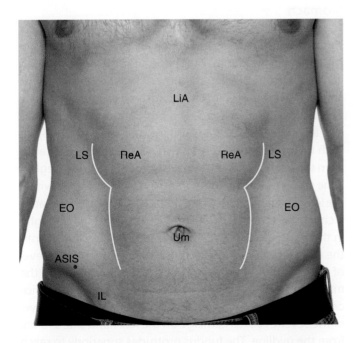

LiA

LS ReA ReA LS

EO EO

Um

ASIS

IL

Fig. 3.5 Surface projections of the anterior abdominal wall. *ASIS,* anterior superior iliac spine; *EO,* external oblique; *IL,* inguinal ligament; *LiA,* linea alba; *LS,* linea semilunaris; *ReA,* rectus abdominus; *Um,* umbilicus.

The inguinal canal is an important structure during embryonic development as it allows for the passage of the testes and their associated neurovascular bundles into the scrotum. In females, it contains the round ligament of the uterus. Early in development, the gonads (testes and ovaries) start developing on the posterior abdominal wall at the level of L1. The final position of the ovaries is variable; the most consistent feature is the relationship of the ovaries to the uterus. If the uterus is large, the ovaries are located at a higher landmark. The testes descend further, led by the gubernaculum, through the inguinal canal and into the scrotum. To exit the peritoneal cavity the testes traverse the anterior abdominal wall musculature. Their point of exit is the deep inguinal ring, which is located midway between, and just above, the pubic symphysis and the anterior superior iliac spine (Figs. 3.6 and 3.7). The canal continues medially to the superficial inguinal ring, lateral to the pubic tubercle.

The inguinal canal can be palpated to determine the presence of an inguinal hernia. With the subject standing, place the index finger on the scrotum and follow the spermatic cord superiorly to the superficial inguinal ring. It will be felt as a slitlike opening just lateral to the pubic tubercle. Ask the subject to cough, which will increase their intraabdominal pressure and feel for any bulges.

Peritoneum

The peritoneum is a thin, sheetlike serous membrane that lines the abdominal cavity and at certain points is reflected onto the abdominal viscera. Peritoneum lining the walls of the abdominal cavity is known as parietal peritoneum, and peritoneum covering the viscera is known as visceral peritoneum. In between the visceral and parietal peritoneum there is usually a small amount of peritoneal fluid. The reflections of peritoneum result in viscera being either

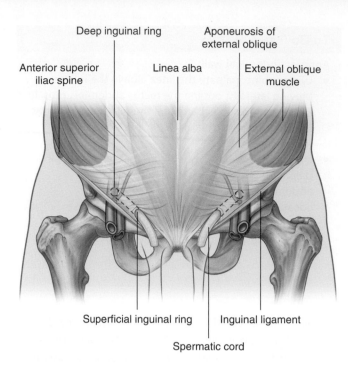

Fig. 3.6 Inguinal canal.
(From Drake, RL, Gray's Anatomy for Students, 3rd ed, 2015, Churchill Livingstone, Elsevier.)

To Do (Figs. 3.6 and 3.7)

Anterior abdominal wall:
- Locate the deep inguinal ring by placing a measuring tape between the pubic symphysis and the anterior superior iliac spine. The deep inguinal ring is located at the midpoint between these landmarks. The pulse of the femoral artery may be felt here.
- Locate the superficial inguinal ring just lateral to the pubic tubercle, it may be felt as a slitlike defect.

---

completely covered (intraperitoneal), partially covered or not covered at all (retroperitoneal). Two peritoneal recesses are created on the right and left lateral sides of the ascending and descending colons. These recesses are known as the paracolic gutters and are clinically important as they can potentially spread infection and cancer cells and are sites of ascitic fluid accumulation.

VISCERA

The viscera within the abdomen include the:
- gastrointestinal tract (stomach, duodenum, jejunum, ileum, cecum and colon)
- liver and gallbladder
- appendix

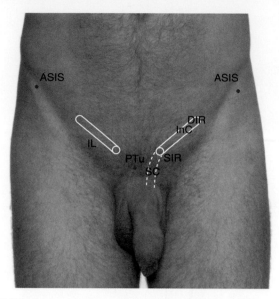

Fig. 3.7 Surface projections of inguinal canal. *ASIS*, anterior superior iliac spine; *DIR*, deep inguinal ring; *IL*, inguinal ligament; *InC*, inguinal canal; *PTu*, pubic tubercle; *SC*, spermatic cord; *SIR*, superficial inguinal ring.

- kidneys
- spleen
- pancreas
- suprarenal glands

Gastrointestinal tract

Stomach

The stomach is a dilated portion of the gastrointestinal tract situated under the left lower ribs and costal cartilages in the left hypochondrium. The shape and size of the stomach varies considerably depending on general body habitus and on the contents within the stomach; it can accommodate two to three liters of food. The position of the stomach is also affected by respiration and the position of the subject. With the subject in the erect position, the stomach extends from the left hypochondrium down to the umbilical region. If the subject is supine the stomach is more contained within the left hypochondrium. The pylorus is located approximately 3 cm above the level of the umbilicus, slightly to the right, in the transpyloric plane. The stomach can be divided into the cardiac region where the esophagus enters (at the level of the twelfth thoracic vertebra), the fundus, the body (the main part of the stomach) and the pylorus. The cardiac orifice can be identified on the anterior abdominal wall at the level of the seventh costal cartilage on the left-hand side 2–3 cm from the midline. The fundus protrudes superiorly to reach as high as the fifth intercostal space. The body of the stomach has greater and lesser curvatures. The greater curvature turns medially and, depending on the individual, may dip into the left flank region. The pylorus is orientated horizontally, at the level of the transpyloric plane (Figs. 3.8 and 3.9).

Small intestine

The small intestine consists of the duodenum, jejunum and ileum and is approximately six meters in length. The small intestine passes through the umbilical region as the duodenum, the left flank as the jejunum and the umbilical, right flank and right groin regions as the ileum. The duodenum is the most proximal component and is approximately 30 cm in length arranged in a C-shape around the pancreas. The duodenum is predominately located in the superior part of the umbilical region and consists of four parts, with only the first part being intraperitoneal. The first part begins immediately distal to the pyloric sphincter and continues in a transverse direction along the transpyloric plane towards the right midclavicular line. The second part starts at the level of the L2, where the duodenum takes a 90 degree turn inferiorly to the level of L3. At this point, it becomes the third part as it turns another 90 degree to the left to become the fourth part, which runs superiorly to the level of L2. The fourth part is continuous with the jejunum. The duodeno-jejunal flexure is found 2.5 cm to the left of midline (Fig. 3.9). The jejunum is predominantly located in the left flank and left groin regions. The jejunum has a larger diameter than the ileum. There is no external landmark that identifies the transition from jejunum to ileum. The ileum is mainly located in the right flank and the umbilical region, as well as the right iliac fossa. At the end of the ileum is the ileocecal junction which is located in the right groin region.

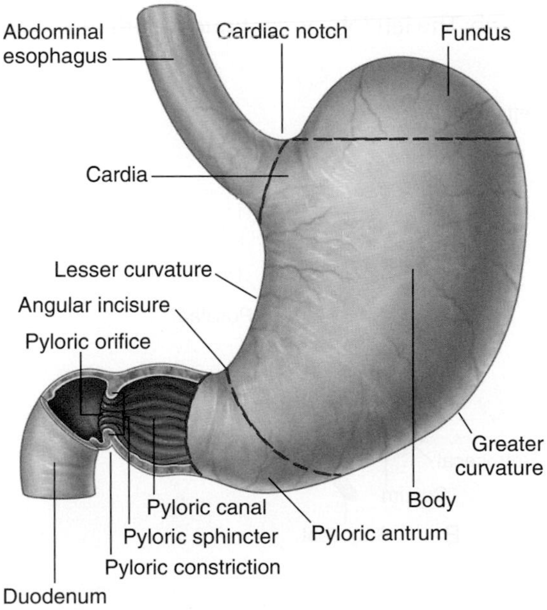

Large intestine

The large intestine consists of the cecum, and the ascending, transverse, descending and sigmoid sections of the colon (Fig. 3.10A). The large intestine is approximately 1.5 meters long. The appendix is an oval- or tail-shaped appendage primarily comprised of lymphoid tissue with a central lumen.

To Do (Fig. 3.9)

Stomach
Anterior abdominal wall:
- Within the left hypochondrium, start by drawing the fundus of the stomach as a dome at the fifth intercostal space at the level of the midclavicular line.
- Follow the lateral edge of the stomach as it forms the greater curvature, which sweeps medially immediately below the transpyloric plane just past the midline.
- Create a line from this point(*) horizontally at the level of the transpyloric plane to outline the pylorus.
- Make a small coin-shaped ending here to represent the pyloric orifice.
- At the top of this shape, continue the horizontal line back to the left of the subject, and then take the line superiorly curving upwards to represent the lesser curvature of the stomach.
- Terminate this line at the level of the seventh costal cartilage and draw the esophagus, which joins the stomach here at the cardiac orifice.

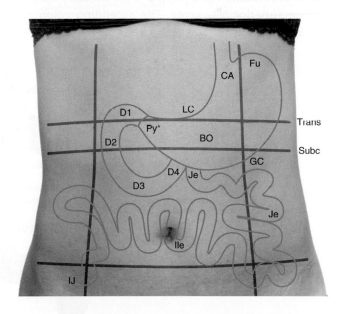

Fig. 3.8 Stomach.
(From Drake, RL, Gray's Anatomy for Students, 3rd ed, 2015, Churchill Livingstone, Elsevier.)

Fig. 3.9 Surface projections of stomach and duodenum. Regions of the stomach. *BO*, body; *CA*, cardia; *D1–D4*, four parts of the duodenum; *Fu*, fundus; *GC*, greater curvature; *IJ*, ileocecal junction; *Ile*, illeum; *Je*, jejunum; *LC*, lesser curvature; *Py*, pylorus; *Subc*, subcostal plane; *Trans*, transpyloric plane.

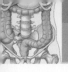

The appendix may be located in the right inguinal (right iliac fossa), though its position can vary (Fig. 3.10B). The appendix is usually located a third of the way along a line from the right anterior superior iliac spine to the umbilicus. Maximum tenderness can be felt at this point during inflammation of the appendix. The ascending colon begins at the ileocecal junction in the right inguinal region (right iliac fossa). The cecum is situated in the right inguinal region (right iliac fossa) and may be palpated depending on the degree of distention at a point 2–3 cm medially from the anterior superior iliac spine. The ascending colon rises superiorly through the right flank to the right hypochondrium

where it makes a 90 degree turn (hepatic flexure) to the left to continue as the transverse colon. The hepatic flexure is marked by the intersection of the midclavicular line and the subcostal plane. The transverse colon crosses the midline of the body below the transpyloric plane and reaches the left hypochondrium. There is great variation in the degree of curvature of the transverse colon; in some individuals the transverse colon hangs down into the pubic region, but for most it is confined to the lower part of the epigastric and umbilical regions. In the lateral aspect of the left hypochondrium the transverse colon is located immediately inferior to the spleen, where it turns to run inferiorly through the left flank as the descending colon. This turn is referred to as the left colic or splenic flexure. The descending colon passes through the left flank region and into the left groin region (left iliac fossa). The course of the descending colon is lateral to the midclavicular line. The descending colon is continuous with the sigmoid colon, which lies mainly in the left groin region (left iliac fossa), before passing medially into the pubic region to continue as the rectum and anal canal (Fig 3.11). Details of the rectum and anal canal are described in Chapter 4.

Liver and gallbladder
The liver lies in the right hypochondrium, epigastrium and left hypochondrium. The liver is anatomically divided into right and left lobes by the presence of the falciform ligament (Figs. 3.12 and 3.13). The right lobe lies superiorly against the diaphragm at the level of the fourth intercostal space. It continues towards the midline, at the level of the xiphisternal junction, and as far inferiorly as the level of the seventh rib. The left lobe is continuous with the right lobe,

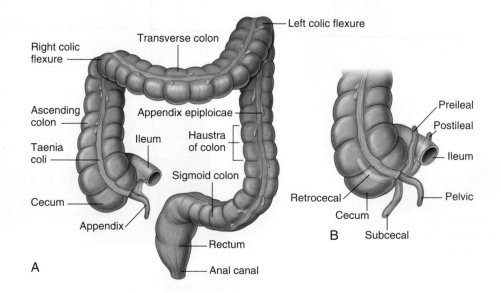

Fig. 3.10 A, Large intestine. B, Orientations of the appendix.
(From Drake, RL, Gray's Anatomy for Students, 3rd ed, 2015, Churchill Livingstone, Elsevier.)

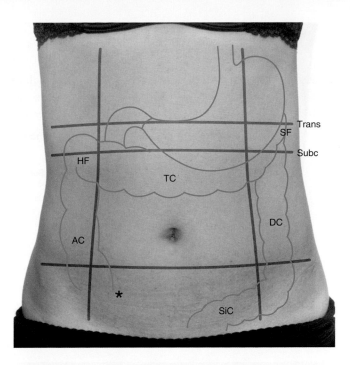

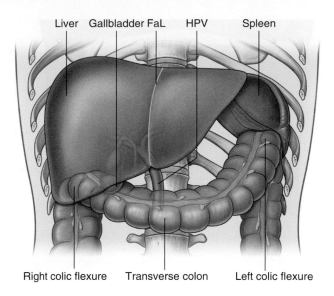

Fig. 3.12 The liver and its major relations. *FaL*, falciform ligament; *HPV*, hepatic portal vein.
(Modified from Drake, RL, Gray's Anatomy for Students, 3rd ed, 2015, Churchill Livingstone, Elsevier.)

Fig. 3.11 Surface projections large intestine. *, appendix; *AC*, ascending colon; *DC*, descending colon; *HF*, hepatic flexure (right colic flexure); *SiC*, sigmoid colon; *SF*, splenic flexure (left colic flexure); *Subc*, subcostal plane; *TC*, transverse colon; *Trans*, transpyloric plane.

To Do (Fig. 3.11)

Large intestine
Anterior abdominal wall:
- To draw the ascending colon, locate the right anterior superior iliac spine. 2–3 cm medially from this point draw a line superiorly through the right flank region up to the hepatic flexure at the intersection of the midclavicular line and the subcostal plane.
- From the hepatic flexure, draw a line that curves slightly inferiorly across the body through the superior part of the epigastrium and into the left hypochondrium; this represents the transverse colon. Note that the extent to which the transverse colon passes inferiorly varies significantly between individuals.
- Continue the line as it turns 90 degrees inferiorly and passes through the left flank region and into the left iliac fossa; this represents the descending colon.
- Create a superior curve towards the midline to represent the sigmoid colon. Continue this line down to the pubic tubercle.
- Trace a line from the right anterior superior iliac spine to the umbilicus and locate McBurney's point. The appendix usually lies deep to this.

extending approximately 5 cm across the midline into the left hypochondrium. In a thin individual, the liver edge may be palpated. The liver makes a dull sound on percussion. Draining into the liver is the hepatic portal vein. The hepatic portal vein is formed at the level of L1 by the confluence of the splenic and superior mesenteric veins. The gallbladder is located just inferior to the liver and is adherent to the undersurface of the right lobe of the liver. The fundus of the gallbladder lies at the midclavicular line on the transpyloric plane at the level of the ninth costal cartilage (Murphy's point), close to the lateral margin of the right rectus abdominis muscle. The bile duct forms when the cystic and the common hepatic ducts join and drains for 5–10 cm towards the medial aspect of the second part of the duodenum.

Spleen

The spleen is located in the left hypochondrium, inferior to the diaphragm on the posterior abdominal wall, between the ninth and eleventh ribs. Its most superior point is at the level of the spinous process of the ninth thoracic vertebra (Fig. 3.14). The most inferior point is at the level of the first lumbar vertebra. The spleen is not palpable unless it is enlarged by up to three times its normal size. An enlarged spleen may be caused by infection, liver disease or hematological disorders.

Pancreas

The pancreas is a retroperitoneal organ consisting of a head, neck, body, uncinate process and tail. It lies at the level of the second lumbar vertebra, posterior to the stomach. The head of the pancreas sits within the C-shape of the

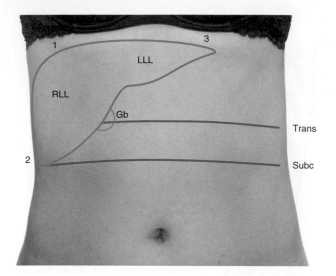

Fig. 3.13 Surface projections of the liver. *Gb*, gallbladder; *LLL*, left lobe of the liver; *RLL*, right lobe of the liver; *Subc*, subcostal plane; *Trans*, transpyloric plane. Numbers refer to To Do list below.

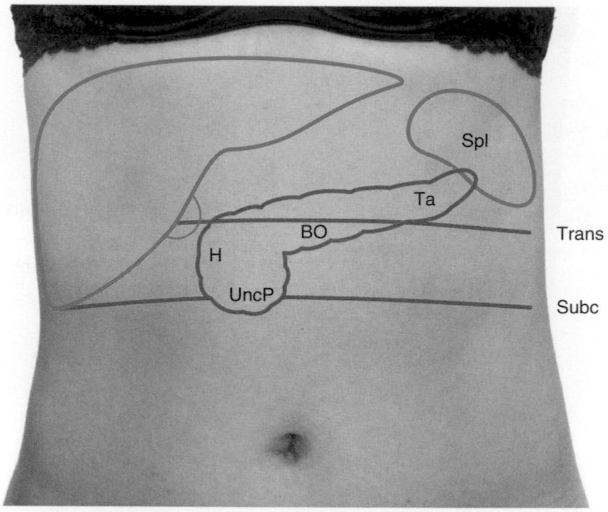

Fig. 3.14 Surface projections of the spleen and pancreas. *BO*, body; *H*, head; *Spl*, spleen; *Subc*, subcostal plane; *Ta*, tail; *Trans*, transpyloric plane; *UncP*, uncinate process.

To Do (Fig. 3.13)

Liver
Anterior abdominal wall:
- To draw out the liver mark out three points: Point 1. 2 cm below the right nipple. Point 2. 2–3 cm below the level of the subcostal plane in the midaxillary line. Point 3. 2–3 cm below the left nipple. Join points 1 and 3 with a line curving superiorly to mark the superior border. Join points 1 and 2 to form the lateral border. Join points 2 and 3.
- Add in the position of the gallbladder at the midclavicular line on the transpyloric plane on the right side.

To Do (Fig. 3.14)

Spleen
Anterior abdominal wall:
- On the anterior aspect in the left hypochondrium, start 1–2 cm from the left tip of the liver and draw a slightly curved line laterally; this forms the superior aspect of the spleen. Continue the line to just above the transpyloric plane and then curve the line back to the starting point.

Pancreas
Anterior abdominal wall:
- Having drawn the liver and spleen, draw a line at a slight inclination superior to the transpyloric plane from the gallbladder to the spleen.
- Continue this line back towards the midline. In the midline take this line inferiorly and then round towards the right of the subject to represent the uncinate process.

duodenum. The body and tail of the pancreas continue along the transpyloric line. The head, uncinate process and body lie within the epigastric region with the tail extending into the left hypochondrium (Fig. 3.14). The pancreas is not palpable.

Kidney

The kidneys are paired retroperitoneal organs located on the posterior abdominal wall. They are approximately 10 cm in length. The renal hilum is most commonly located at L2. The left kidney is located between T12 and L3. The right kidney is slightly lower and located between L1 and L4 because of the position of the liver. The ureter leaves each kidney at its hilum and passes just infero-laterally parallel to the tips of the lumbar transverse processes (Fig. 3.15).

Suprarenal glands

The suprarenal glands are paired endocrine glands located at the superior pole of the kidneys. They extend superiorly

for 2–3 cm. The suprarenal glands consist of an inner medulla and an outer cortex.

Vasculature

Within the abdominal cavity, the main arterial supply is from the aorta. The aorta is situated on the posterior abdominal wall in the midline. It passes posterior to the diaphragm, between its crura, at the level of T12, beneath the median arcuate ligament. The aorta has three main anterior branches—the celiac trunk and the superior and inferior mesenteric arteries (T12, L1 and L3, respectively)—before bifurcating into the common iliac arteries at the level of L4.

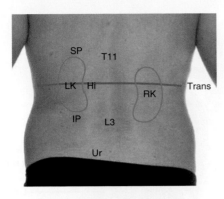

Fig. 3.15 Surface projections of the kidneys projected onto the skin of the back. *Hi,* hilum; *IP,* inferior pole; *LK,* left kidney; *RK,* right kidney; *SP,* superior pole; *Trans,* transpyloric plane; *Ur,* ureter. *(Modified from Drake, RL, Gray's Anatomy for Students, 3rd ed, 2015, Churchill Livingstone, Elsevier.)*

To Do (Fig. 3.15)

Kidney

Anterior abdominal wall:

- Locate the position of the kidneys. The hilum of the right kidney is located below the transplyoric plane, roughly 5 cm lateral form the midline. The hilum of the left kidney is located above the transpyloric plane, roughly 5 cm laterally from the midline.

Posterior abdominal wall:

- Locate T11 by counting down from C7. To check you are at the correct level, locate the twelfth rib and follow this back to T12. Move your finger superiorly one level to T11.
- On the left side trace a horizontal line from the eleventh vertebra laterally 5–6 cm. This location will be the superior pole of the kidney. Add a mark here.
- Count down from T11 to locate L3.
- On the left side, trace a horizontal line 5–6 cm. This location will be the inferior pole of the kidney. Add a mark here.
- Draw two arcs from the superior to lateral poles in order to form the lateral and medial margins. The lateral arc marking the lateral border should be 9–10 cm from the midline.
- Repeat on the right side but note that the right kidney will be slightly lower by 2–3 cm.
- You will find that the markings will be affected by the person's posture.

The aorta gives off two lateral branches, the renal arteries, between the vertebral level of L1–2 (Figs. 3.16A and 3.17). In addition the aorta gives off two gonadal arteries and four paired segmental lumbar arteries.

The inferior vena cava drains venous blood from the lower limbs and is formed by the confluence of the common iliac veins at the level of the fifth lumbar vertebra. It runs superiorly, and passes through the caval opening in the diaphragm at the level of T8. The venous blood from the gastrointestinal tract within the abdomen passes via the portal vein to the liver (Fig. 3.16B).

In the Clinic

Hernia

The abdomen may be palpated to determine whether it is flat, distended or has any outpouchings. A hernia is an outpouching of the abdominal viscera or omentum that has pushed itself through a weakness in the muscular abdominal wall. Hernias are classified by their different locations as umbilical, diaphragmatic or inguinal. An inguinal hernia may be further classified as being direct or indirect.

Biliary colic and cholecystitis

In some individuals, gallstones can form within the gallbladder. A gallstone can temporarily block the cystic duct and cause the gallbladder to contract. This results in pain, which is referred to as biliary colic. The pain is typically referred to the right hypochondrium and may also be referred to the right shoulder or parasternal area. Symptoms can be triggered by meals with an especially high fat content, although this is not absolute. The pain may last from minutes to several hours. Cholecystitis is inflammation of the gallbladder, which is caused by infection following blockage of the cystic duct by a gallstone. Symptoms include pain in the right upper quadrant, nausea, vomiting and fever. In both conditions the diagnosis is made by medical history, examination and by using ultrasound to establish the presence of gallstones. The shoulder pain is a referred pain and is attributed to innervation of the diaphragm by the phrenic nerve, which originates from spinal cord levels C3, C4, and C5. The same spinal cord levels also innervate the skin over the neck and shoulder. Inflammation of the diaphragm in these patients can therefore lead to pain that is referred to the tip of the shoulder.

Appendicitis

An appendicitis is caused by inflammation of the appendix, which is nearly always from infection within the lumen. The early clinical presentation includes pain in the umbilical region that may be transient. This is followed by more severe pain in the right groin region. The pain is increased on palpation. Other symptoms include nausea and vomiting. Ultrasound imaging may be used as part of the diagnosis, especially in children.

Kidney stones

Kidney stones, or renal calculi, are formed from the minerals in urine. Small stones may go unnoticed and pass out of the body during urination. Larger stones may become lodged, which can cause back pain, nausea and hematuria (blood in the urine). Ultrasound imaging may reveal a dilated renal pelvis or point of obstruction.

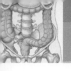

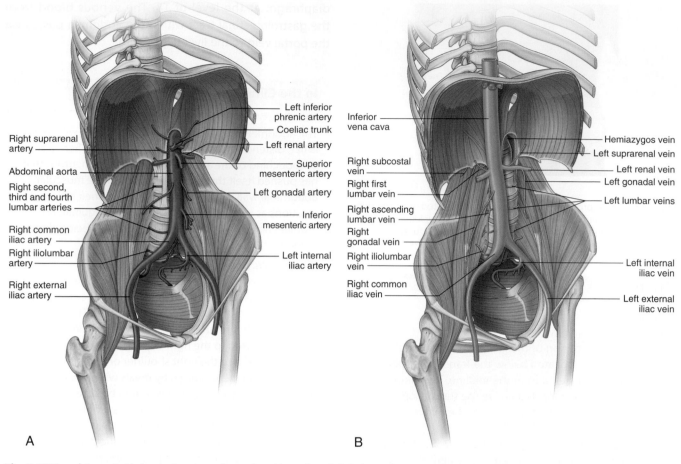

A

B

Fig. 3.16 Vasculature. A, Abdominal aorta and associated branches. B, Inferior vena cava and associated tributaries. *(From Standring, S, ed. Gray's Anatomy, 41e, 2015, Elsevier.)*

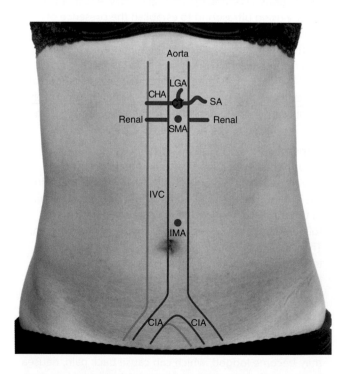

Fig. 3.17 Surface projections of the abdominal vasculature. *CHA*, common hepatic artery; *CIA*, common iliac artery; *CT*, celiac trunk; *IMA*, inferior mesenteric artery; *IVC*, inferior vena cava; *LGA*, left gastric artery; *SA*, splenic artery; *SMA*, superior mesenteric artery.

To Do (Fig. 3.17)

Vasculature

Anterior abdominal wall:

- Draw a midline tube extending from the xiphoid process to 3–4 cm above the pubic tubercle. This is the outline of the abdominal aorta.
- To represent the celiac trunk, draw a circle at vertebral level T12. To locate this level, move superiorly from the subcostal margin 3–4 cm.
- Add to the celiac trunk three points to mark out the left gastric, splenic and common hepatic arteries.
- Move 1 cm inferiorly and add a circle to represent the superior mesenteric artery.
- At the same point add two arteries laterally to represent the renal arteries.
- Add the inferior mesenteric artery by finding a point 3–4 cm above the bifurcation landmark.
- Inferior to the bifurcation of the aorta, and 2–3 cm to the right, add two tubes to represent the formation of the inferior vena cava by the common iliac veins at vertebral level L5.
- Continue the tube representing the inferior vena cava superiorly to the level of T8 where the inferior vena cava pierces the diaphragm.

To Do (Fig. 3.17)

Palpation

Palpation of the abdomen should be performed in a systematic way following the nine segments. If there is pain in the abdomen, guarding (protecting) of the anterior abdominal wall may occur, making palpation difficult.

- Place your hand flat over each region, and with flexion at the metacarpophalangeal joints, feel the structures below the skin.
- On the right side, locate the subcostal margin. Palpate the liver edge. Ask the subject to take a deep breath because the liver descends on inspiration making palpation easier.
- Palpation of the small intestine should be undertaken along with observation of the subject's face. Look for changes in facial expression due to pain during palpation. Begin with light palpation using the fingers. Deep palpation may be performed by using the palm of the hand, at all times being aware of guarding and any painful responses.
- Locate the left anterior superior iliac spine. Just a few centimeters medially, the sigmoid colon may be palpated when filled with feces by using index and middle fingers on the dominant hand, moving over the colon.

To Do (Fig. 3.17)

Percussion

Percussion of the stomach produces tympany due to gas within the stomach. Percussion of the small intestine is very useful in determining any distention due to gas, fluid or tumor.

- To percuss the small intestine, begin over the umbilical region. Resonance suggests gas, whereas dull areas suggest fluid.

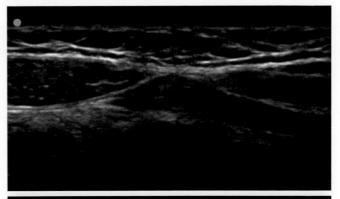

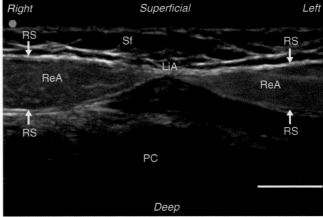

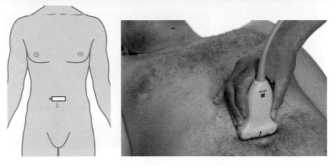

Fig. 3.18 Ultrasound of the anterior abdominal musculature. *LiA*, linea alba; *PC*, peritoneal cavity; *ReA*, rectus abdominus; *RS*, rectus sheath; *Sf*, subcutaneous fat. Scale bar = 1 cm.

Ultrasound

ANTERIOR ABDOMINAL MUSCULATURE

Subject position

Imaging is performed with the subject lying supine.

Transducer

Use a linear array transducer. Set the depth setting to 3–5 cm.

Transducer position

To image the rectus abdominis muscle, position the transducer in the transverse plane for short-axis views over the midline of the anterior abdomen immediately inferior to the xiphoid process of the sternum scan inferiorly towards the pubic symphysis. In Fig. 3.18, the transducer was positioned 5 cm below the xiphoid process.

To image the external oblique, internal oblique and transversus abdominus muscles, position the transducer in transverse plane for short-axis views over the anterolateral aspect of the abdomen. In Fig. 3.20, the transducer was positioned on the left side at the level of the umbilicus, along a vertical line extending from the anterior superior iliac spine.

Image features

Anterior abdominal wall

In the transverse plane, the paired rectus abdominis muscles can be seen surrounded by the bright hyperechoic rectus

41

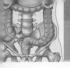

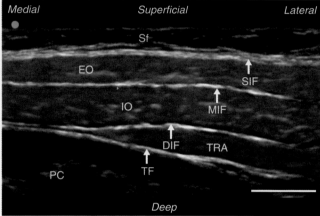

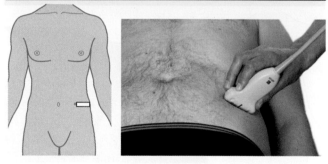

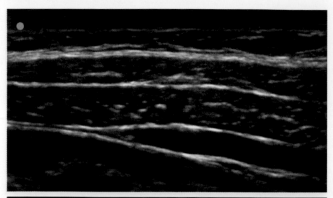

Fig. 3.19 Ultrasound of the anterolateral abdominal musculature. *DIF*, deep investing fascia; *EO*, external oblique; *IO*, internal oblique; *MIF*, middle investing fascia; *PC*, peritoneal cavity; *Sf*, subcutaneous fat; *SIF*, superficial investing fascia; *TF*, transversalis fascia; *TRA*, transversus abdominis. Scale bar = 1 cm.

sheath (Fig. 3.18). The linea alba will be in view in the midline marking the right and left muscle belly on each side. It may be possible to differentiate the individual layers of the fascia forming the rectus sheath. The hypoechoic region deep to the rectus abdominis muscle is the peritoneal cavity.

Anterolateral abdominal wall

In the transverse plane, the three muscle layers formed by the external oblique, internal oblique and transversus abdominis muscles will be in view (Fig. 3.19). Above the external oblique muscle there is a layer of subcutaneous fat. Surrounding the three muscles, the superficial,

intermediate and deep layers of investing fascia can be seen as bright hyperechoic lines. Deep to the transversus abdominis muscle, the hyperechoic transversalis fascia extends medially with the deep layer of investing fascia. Deep to this fascia, the peritoneal cavity will be in view, which appears hypoechoic.

GASTROINTESTINAL TRACT

Subject position

Imaging is performed with the subject lying supine.

Transducer

Use a curved array transducer. Set the depth setting to 5–12 cm. The stomach is best viewed during deep inspiration.

Transducer position

Most major parts of the gastrointestinal tract can be visualized using ultrasound. The stomach, jejunum, ileum, cecum and colon can be easily imaged from the anterior abdomen (Figs. 3.20 and 3.21). The stomach can be viewed immediately inferior to the subcostal margin on the left side, the jejunum within the upper left quadrant, the ileum below the umbilicus and the cecum in the lower right quadrant. The complete length of the colon can be tracked as it passes superiorly along the right flank (ascending colon), in the subcostal plane (transverse colon) and as it descends the left flank (descending colon). The transducer can be positioned so that the structures can be visualized either in their long-axis or short-axis. The duodenum is difficult to observe using ultrasound, although it can be imaged in transverse view immediately to the right of the pancreas.

Image features

Stomach

The anterior curved wall of the stomach will appear as a bright hyperechoic convex line (Fig. 3.20). It should be possible to locate the fundus as well as the greater and lesser curvatures. The interior of the stomach appears hypoechoic.

Jejunum

With the transducer aligned longitudinally, the jejunum appears as a long tube, approximately 2–4 cm in diameter, with many flexures (Fig. 3.21A). The walls are hyperechoic and the interior appears gray interspersed with white transverse hyperechoic streaks, which are produced by the prominent mucosal folds that circle the lumen (plicae circulares). During real-time imaging, there will be observable peristaltic movements (Video 3.1).

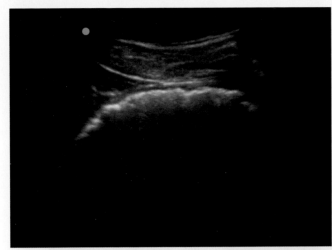

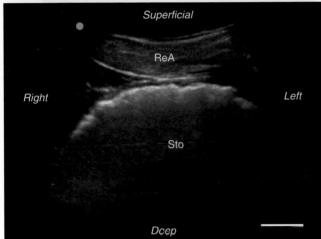

Superficial

ReA

Right   *Left*

Sto

Deep

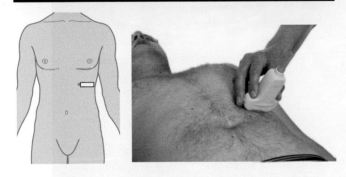

Fig. 3.20 Ultrasound of the stomach. *ReA*, rectus abdominus; *Sto*, stomach. Scale bar = 2 cm.

Ileum

With the transducer aligned longitudinally, the ileum appears as a long tube with many flexures (Fig. 3.21B). It is narrower than the jejunum, approximately 2–3 cm in diameter. The walls are hyperechoic and the interior is mainly isoechoic due to fewer mucosal folds compared to the jejunum. As with the jejunum, during real-time imaging, there will be observable peristaltic movements.

Cecum and colon

With the transducer aligned longitudinally, the walls of both the cecum and colon are characterized by prominent hyperechoic sacculations, known as the haustra (Fig. 3.21C). The interior of these structures appears hypoechoic.

LIVER

Subject position

Imaging is performed with the subject lying supine. Deep inspiration will help visualize of the liver.

Transducer

Use a curved array transducer. Set the depth setting to 12–15 cm.

Transducer position

The liver is imaged on the right side of the abdomen, immediately below the subcostal margin in the right hypochondrium and epigastric regions (Fig. 3.22). Starting with the transducer in the transverse plane towards the midline, scan laterally to observe the main features. For examination of the right lobe of the liver, it may be necessary to align the transducer over the sixth or seventh intercostal spaces. Angle the probe slightly cephalically and apply moderate pressure.

Image features

In Fig. 3.22, the liver is viewed in transverse plane. With the probe in the midline (Fig. 3.22A), towards the bottom of the image, the bodies of the lumbar vertebrae will be in view. The anterior surface of each bone will appear as a convex hyperechoic arc. Immediately anterior to the bodies of the vertebrae, the aorta and inferior vena cava can be seen in their short axis as two hypoechoic circles. Filling the image, above these vessels, the liver will appear isoechoic. A noticeable feature surrounding the posterior contours of the liver is the diaphragm, which appears hyperechoic. The left lobe of the liver can be seen within the midline. Posterior to the left lobe and anterior to the aorta and inferior vena cava, the ligamentum venosum appears as a bright hyperechoic streak. The portal vein is visible within the approximate center of the liver, lateral to the ligamentum venosum. It is clearly defined by its bright hyperechoic lining and can be seen in its short axis as it enters the liver and, angling the probe cephalic, its long axis, as it divides into the left and right branches. Scanning laterally (Fig. 3.22B), the hepatic veins will come into view. In contrast to the portal vein, these do not have an obvious hyperechoic lining. The left, medial and right hepatic veins will appear as three hypoechoic longitudinal projections feeding into the inferior

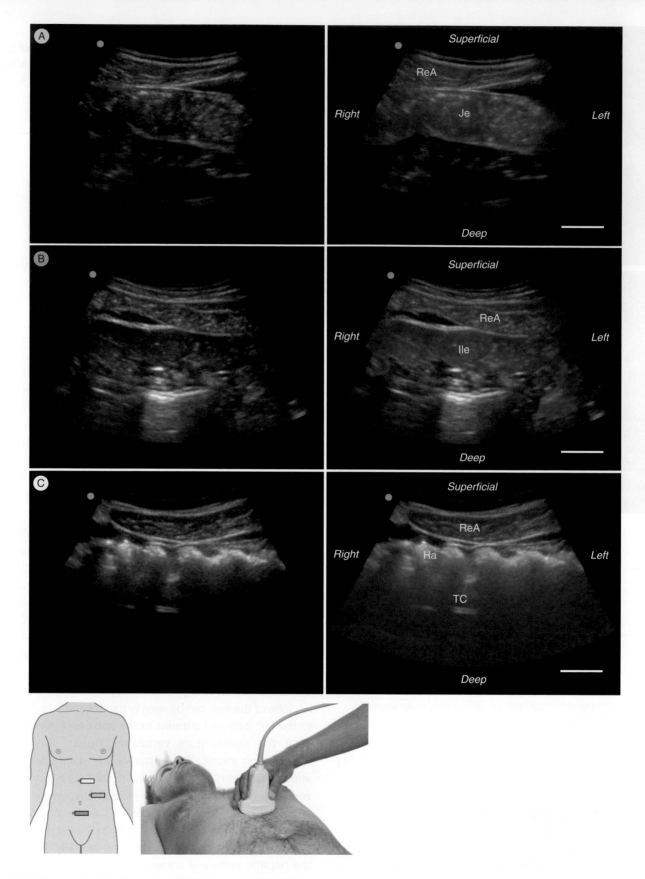

Fig. 3.21 Ultrasound of (A) the jejunum, (B) the ileum and (C) the transverse colon. *Ha*, haustra; *Ile*, ilieum; *Je*, jejunum; *ReA*, rectus abdominus; *TC*, transverse colon. Scale bar = 2 cm.

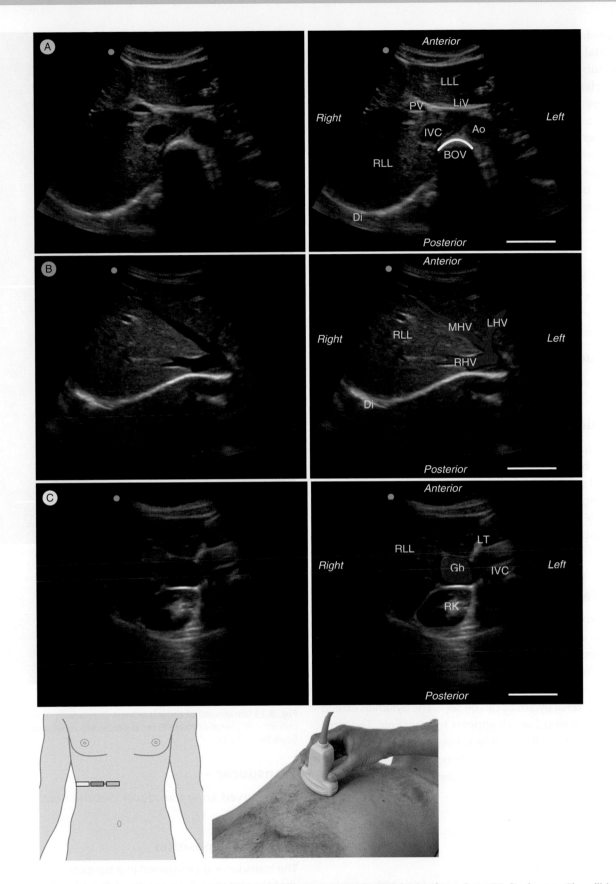

Fig. 3.22 Ultrasound of the liver. A, Left lobe. B, Right lobe. C, Gallbladder. *Ao*, aorta; *BOV*, body of vertebrae; *Di*, diaphragm; *Gb*, gallbladder; *IVC*, inferior vena cava; *LHV*, left hepatic vein; *LiV*, ligamentum venosum; *LLL*, left lobe of the liver; *LT*, ligamentum teres; *MHV*, middle hepatic vein; *PV*, portal vein; *RHV*, right hepatic vein; *RK*, right kidney; *RLL*, right lobe of the liver. Scale bar = 4 cm.

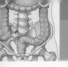
vena cava. The hepatic veins are best observed from the intercostal space. Moving the transducer towards the right of the subject (Fig. 3.22C), the fundus and body of the gallbladder will come into view. The gallbladder appears as a large clearly defined hypoechoic structure on the posterior aspect of the liver. Sitting posterior to the gallbladder, the right kidney is seen. The outer cortex appears similar in texture to the liver, whereas the pyramids will appear hypoechoic, and the renal sinus will be hyperechoic. During scanning of the liver, it will be possible to observe several of the ligaments. These will appear hyperechoic.

KIDNEY

Subject position

Imaging is performed with the subject lying supine or in the right or left lateral decubitus positions. Deep inspiration will help visualize the kidney.

Transducer

Use a curved array transducer. Set the depth setting to 10–15 cm.

Transducer position

The transducer should be positioned slightly posterior (7 cm) to the left or right midaxillary line, either in the most inferior intercostal space, or immediately below the subcostal margin, depending upon whether the subject has taken a deep breath in (Fig. 3.23). The kidney is best viewed in the coronal plane. Angling the transducer will help avoid shadows produced by the ribs. Firm pressure will also help avoid shadows.

Image features

In the coronal plane, the internal structure of the kidney should be easily identifiable (Fig. 3.23). Each kidney will be surrounded by a bright hyperechoic fibrous capsule. Below the capsule, the renal cortex and its extensions, the columns, appear isoechoic. Sitting between the renal columns, the hypoechoic renal pyramids can be seen. The pyramids extend into the renal sinus, which appears hyperechoic. The renal pelvis and ureter will be visible as they exit the kidney. Both structures appear hypoechoic, although the ureter will have a bright hyperechoic lining. The ureter extends inferiorly (towards the right of the screen).

SPLEEN

Subject position

Imaging is performed with the subject lying either supine or in the right lateral decubitus position. Deep inspiration will help visualize the spleen.

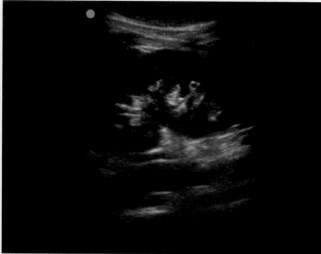

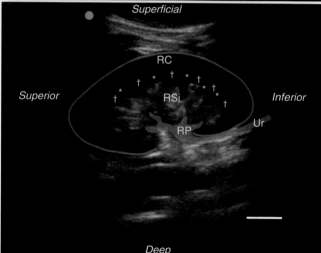

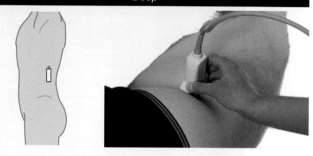

Fig. 3.23 Ultrasound of the left kidney. *, pyramids; †, renal columns; *RC*, renal cortex; *RP*, renal pelvis; *RSi*, renal sinus; *Ur*, ureter. Scale bar = 2 cm.

Transducer

Use a curved array transducer. Set the depth setting to 12–15 cm.

Transducer position

The transducer is positioned in a transverse oblique plane, slightly posterior (5 cm) to the left midaxillary line in the most inferior, or adjacent, intercostal space (Fig. 3.24). The spleen sits lateral, and immediately anterior, to the left kidney.

Image features

In the transverse plane, the spleen appears as a large isoechoic wedge-shaped structure (Fig. 3.24). On the medial surface, branches of the splenic vessels can be seen entering the organ at the splenic hilum. The walls of the vessels appear hyperechoic. On the posterior wall of the spleen, the left kidney may be in view.

PANCREAS

Subject position

Imaging is performed with the subject lying supine. Deep inspiration will help visualize the pancreas.

Transducer

Use a curved array transducer. Set the depth setting to 8–15 cm.

Transducer position

Position the transducer in the transverse plane over the midline immediately inferior to the xiphoid process of the sternum (Fig. 3.25). Scan inferiorly 2–4 cm from the sternum to locate the pancreas. It is located in the transpyloric plane.

Image features

The pancreas appears as a mottled structure sitting deep to the left lobe of the liver and above the aorta. In the transverse plane, the curve of the uncinate process can be observed, with the body and tail extending to the left of the subject (Fig. 3.25). The hypoechoic splenic vein can be seen immediately below the pancreas, following the inferior surface of the body.

VASCULATURE

Subject position

Imaging is performed with the subject lying supine.

Transducer

Use a curved array transducer. Set the depth setting to 10–15 cm.

Transducer position

Position the ultrasound transducer in the transverse plane for short axis views of the aorta and vena cava in the midline of the anterior abdomen below the xiphoid process of the sternum (Fig. 3.26). Scanning inferiorly, the abdominal aorta can be tracked through the abdomen.

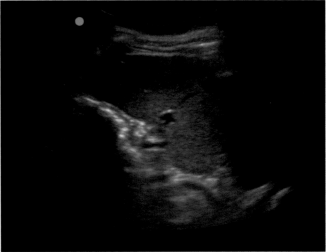

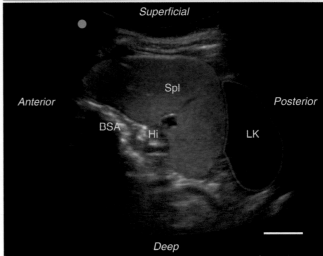

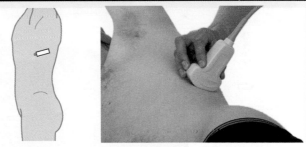

Fig. 3.24 Ultrasound of the spleen. *BSA*, branches of splenic artery; *Hi*, hilum; *LK*, left kidney; *Spl*, spleen. Scale bar = 2 cm.

Image features

In the transverse plane, the abdominal aorta and inferior vena cava are visible as two small hypoechoic circles, with the abdominal aorta sitting on the anterior surface of the bodies of the vertebrae (Fig. 3.26).The aorta lies to the left side of the inferior vena cava (right on image). The walls of both vessels appear hyperechoic. Scanning caudally along the length of the vessels, several branches can be

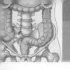

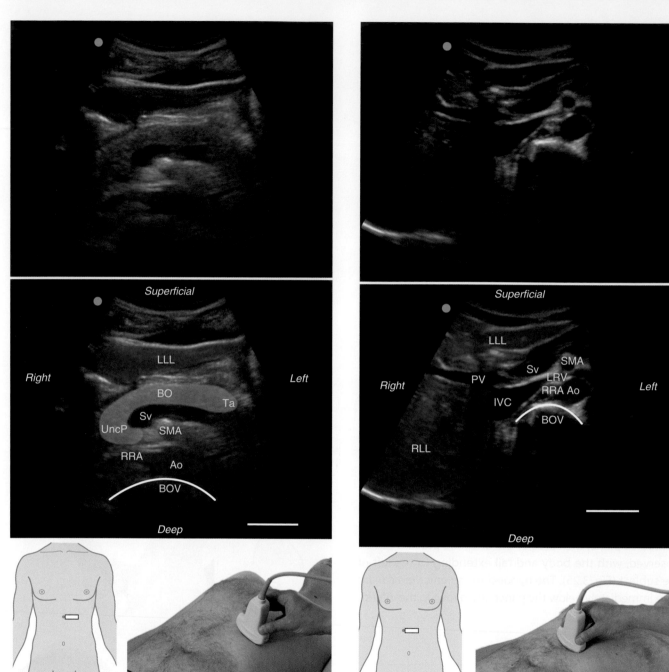

Fig. 3.25 Ultrasound of the pancreas. *Ao*, aorta; *BO*, body of the pancreas; *BOV*, body of vertebra; *LLL*, left lobe of the liver; *RRA*, right renal artery; *SMA*, superior mesenteric artery; *Sv*, splenic vein; *Ta*, tail of the pancreas; *UncP*, uncinate process. Scale bar = 3 cm.

Fig. 3.26 Ultrasound of the abdominal aorta and associated structures at the level of the left renal vein. *Ao*, aorta; *BOV*, body of vertebra; *IVC*, inferior vena cava; *LLL*, left lobe of the liver; *LRV*, left renal vein; *PV*, portal vein; *RLL*, right lobe of the liver; *RRA*, right renal artery; *SMA*, superior mesenteric artery; *Sv*, splenic vein. Scale bar = 3 cm.

identified. Immediately inferior to the transpyloric plane, the left renal vein can be seen extending anterior to the abdominal aorta from the left kidney towards the inferior vena cava (Fig. 3.26). Below the left renal vein, part of the right renal artery will be in view passing from the aorta towards the right kidney. Anterior to the left renal vein,

the superior mesenteric artery, which has a clearly defined hyperechoic wall, can be seen in a short-axis view. At this location, the portal and splenic veins should also be visible. The liver can be observed as a large isointense structure to the right side of the inferior vena cava.

In the Clinic

Ultrasound can be used to diagnose and monitor a diverse range of conditions that affect the abdomen. B-mode imaging is frequently used to identify cysts, carcinomas, hemangiomas, metastases and abscesses. It can also be used to identify sites of infection and fatty deposits, as well as to assess organ size in conditions such as hepatomegaly (enlargement of the liver). B-mode imaging is routinely used for needle guidance during biopsies and to evaluate the extent of abdominal trauma following injury. Doppler ultrasound provides an important tool for the assessment of vascular pathologies, for example, abdominal aortic aneurysms (a bulge in a weakened area of the wall of the abdominal aorta, usually where it branches) and stenosis (narrowing of blood vessels) as well as thrombosis (blood clots within vessels). Table 3.2 provides an overview of some of the abdominal conditions that can be diagnosed or monitored by ultrasound.

Table 3.2 Abdominal pathologies that are routinely diagnosed by ultrasound

Viscera	Pathology
Liver	Cirrhosis, portal hypertension, portal or hepatic vein thrombosis, fatty liver
Gallbladder	Gallstones, cholecystitis
Pancreas	Pancreatitis
Kidney	Polycystic kidney disease, hydronephrosis, ureteric stones
Gastrointestinal tract	Appendicitis, diverticulitis

Summary Checklist

- Four quadrants and nine regions of the abdomen
- Surface projections of the gastrointestinal tract
- Surface projections of abdominal viscera: liver, kidneys, pancreas, spleen
- Surface projections of the aorta and inferior vena cava
- Ultrasound imaging of the abdominal musculature
- Ultrasound imaging of the stomach, small and large intestines
- Ultrasound imaging of the liver, gallbladder, spleen and kidneys
- Ultrasound imaging of the abdominal vasculature

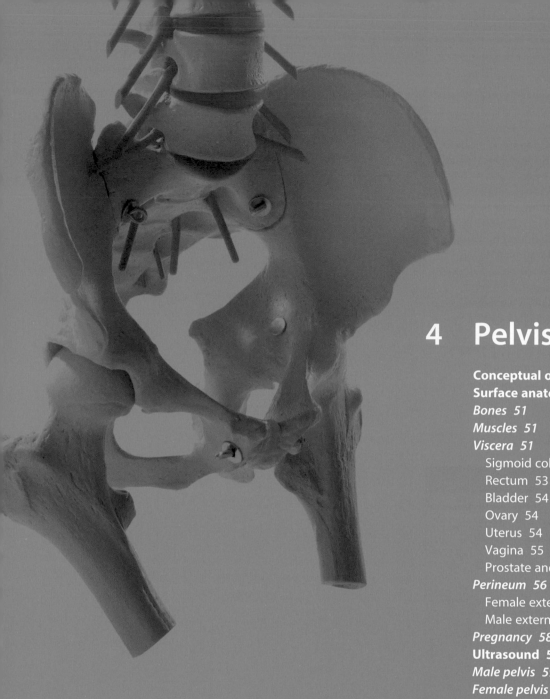

4 Pelvis and perineum

Conceptual overview

The pelvis is a bowl-shaped bony frame that is continuous superiorly with the abdominal cavity and inferiorly with the lower limbs and gluteal region. The pelvic cavity is bounded inferiorly by the pelvic diaphragm and surrounded on its lateral and posterior walls by the bones that form the pelvic girdle, and anteriorly by musculature. The components of the pelvic cavity include bones (sacrum, ilium, ischium and pubis) and viscera (sigmoid colon, rectum, uterus, ovaries, vagina, distal ureters, bladder, seminal vesicles and prostate). These organs are parts of the gastrointestinal, urinary and reproductive systems. Clinically, the pelvis is a key region in physical examination during pregnancy, and for a range of conditions that include fibroids of the uterus and hyperplasia of the prostate. The pelvic cavity is easily accessible to palpate from the anterior. Examination of pelvic contents may also be performed through the rectum (PR – per rectum) and vagina (PV – per vaginam).

Surface anatomy

BONES

The osteology of the pelvis consists of the bones that form the pelvic girdle and sacrum. The bones of the pelvic girdle are the ilium, ischium and pubis. The pubis bones are anterior and articulate at the pubic symphysis within the midline. Immediately lateral to the pubic symphysis are the pubic tubercles, which can be palpated. The superior border of the pubis is marked by the pecten pubis (pectineal line). Lying laterally and superiorly is the ilium. On the anterior aspect of the ilium is a very noticeable prominence, the anterior superior iliac spine. The ilium has an iliac crest which continues medially to the sacroiliac joint (Fig. 4.1). On the superior medial surface of the ilium is the arcuate line. Lying laterally and posteriorly is the ischium. The ischium has two projections on its posterior surface: a large ischial tuberosity and a smaller ischial spine. Between these two projections are two notches: the greater and lesser sciatic notches. These are converted into foramina by the presence of ligaments. The foramina contain important neurovascular bundles that supply the perineum, gluteal regions and lower limb. The ischium has a protruding ischial spine which points medially. This is a key palpable landmark for midwifery purposes to determine the descent of the fetal head and progress of labor, as well as for administering local anesthesia, such as a pudendal nerve block. The ilium, pubis and ischium all articulate in the acetabulum. Located posteriorly in the

midline, the sacrum consists of five fused vertebrae. Each sacral vertebra has a spinous process that can be palpated in the intergluteal cleft. On the anterior aspect, the sacrum projects forward as the sacral promontory. The sacrum articulates with the coccyx at the sacrococcygeal joint. Typically, there are three, four or five coccygeal vertebrae. The coccyx is difficult to palpate, since it lies towards the end of the intergluteal cleft, posterior to the anal orifice.

The sacral promontory, arcuate line and pectineal line (pecten pubis) are used to demarcate a true (lesser) and false (greater) pelvic cavity (Fig. 4.2). The false or greater pelvic cavity is part of the abdominal cavity. The true pelvic cavity is, as its name implies, part of the pelvic cavity and lies below the level of the pelvic brim. The pelvic brim is also known as the pelvic inlet and is marked by a line passing posteriorly from the upper margin of the pubic tubercle to the sacral promontory. In the anatomical position, the anterior superior iliac spine and the upper margin of the pubic symphysis are in the same vertical plane. The pelvic inlet is inclined obliquely at an angle of about 50 to 60 degrees to the horizontal. The plane of the pelvic outlet is much less oblique, at an angle of about 10 to 15 degrees to the horizontal. Anteriorly, the pubic arch marks the most anterior part of the perineum, and the tip of the coccyx marks the most posterior point. The perineum is a diamond-shaped area between the inferior border of the pubic symphysis anteriorly, the coccyx posteriorly, and the ischial tuberosities on each side.

MUSCLES

The muscles of the pelvis are important for movement of the lower limbs and for protection of the abdomino-pelvic viscera, and can act to increase intraabdominal pressure. Two muscles are associated with the pelvic wall: the obturator internus muscle and the piriformis muscle. The muscles associated with the pelvic floor are collectively referred to as the pelvic diaphragm, and consist of levator ani muscles and the coccygeus muscle. These muscles are not palpable (Table 4.1). The muscles of the anterior abdominal wall have already been described in Chapter 3. Muscles that act on the hip joint are covered in Chapter 6.

VISCERA

The viscera within the pelvis are components of the gastrointestinal, urinary and reproductive systems. The pelvic cavity can be examined to determine whether it is distended or flat, and whether it is symmetrical or has any abdominal scars from previous surgical procedures.

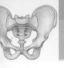
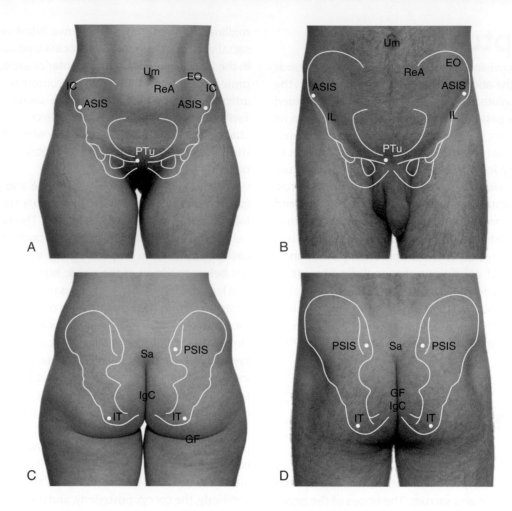

Fig. 4.1 Surface projections of the osteology of the pelvis. A, Anterior female. B, Anterior male. C, Posterior female. D, Posterior male. *ASIS*, anterior superior iliac spine; *EO*, external oblique; *GF*, gluteal fold; *IC*, iliac crest; *IgC*, intergluteal cleft; *IL*, inguinal ligament; *IT*, ischial tuberosity; *PSIS*, posterior superior iliac spine; *PTu*, pubic tubercle; *ReA*, rectus abdominus; *Sa*, sacrum; *Um*, umbilicus.

To Do (Fig. 4.1)

Anterior pelvic wall:
- In the midline, follow the linea alba inferiorly. Locate and gently palpate the pubic tubercles.
- Moving laterally, palpate the bony prominence of the ilium at the anterior superior iliac spine.
- Compare the orientation of the pelvis in standing and sitting by placing finger tips on the anterior superior iliac spine with one hand and the pubic tubercle with the other.

Posterior pelvic wall:
- In the midline, palpate the spinous processes of the lumbar vertebrae.
- Palpate the iliac crests and follow them laterally.
- Palpate the quadratus lumborum muscle approximately 5 cm lateral to the spinous processes, between the iliac crest and the twelfth rib.

- Sit on a chair and place your hands on the seat with the palms facing up. Move so that you are sitting on your own hands and palpate the ischial tuberosities.

The viscera include the:
- sigmoid colon
- rectum and anal canal
- urinary bladder
- ovaries
- uterus
- vagina
- prostate and seminal vesicles

Sigmoid colon

The sigmoid colon takes an S-shaped course of variable length and is located in the superior aspect of the left groin.

It descends in contact with the left pelvic wall and then crosses the pelvic cavity where it is continuous with the rectum (Fig. 4.3). It is frequently seen when imaging this region. The sigmoid colon is more easily palpable on the anterior surface when it contains feces.

Rectum

The rectum begins at the level of S3 (Fig. 4.3) and is continuous with the anal canal at the anorectal junction. It is loosely attached by fascia to the anterior surface of the sacrum.

However, the main support for the rectum (and its fecal contents) is provided by the pelvic diaphragm. There are several bends in the rectum, and at the anorectal junction there is a sharp bend, the perineal flexure, which is formed by the tonic contraction of the slinglike arrangement of the puborectalis muscle. This arrangement is important in maintaining fecal continence. Many of the contents of the pelvis can be palpated by a rectal examination. With a subject lying on their left side, the right index finger of a gloved hand can be inserted into the rectum. At the point of entry,

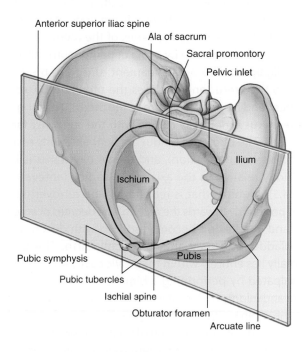

Fig. 4.2 Osteology of the pelvis.
(With permission from Drake, RL, Gray's Anatomy for Students, 3rd ed, 2015, Churchill Livingstone, Elsevier.)

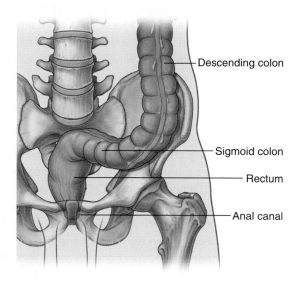

Fig. 4.3 Sigmoid colon and rectum.
(With permission from Drake, RL, Gray's Anatomy for Students, 3rd ed, 2015, Churchill Livingstone, Elsevier.)

Table 4.1 Muscles of the pelvic walls and diaphragm

Muscle	Origin	Insertion	Innervation	Function
Obturator internus	Anterolateral wall of true pelvis	Greater trochanter of femur	Nerve to obturator internus L5, S1	Lateral rotation of the extended hip joint; abduction of flexed hip
Piriformis	Anterior surface of sacrum	Greater trochanter of femur	Branches from S1 and S2	Lateral rotation of the extended hip joint; abduction of flexed hip
Levator ani	In a line around the pelvic wall as a condensation of obturator internus fascia	Perineal membrane, perineal body	Branches from S4 and from inferior rectal (pudendal nerve S2–4)	Forms pelvic floor which supports plevic viscera and reinforces pelvic sphincters
Coccygeus	Ischial spine, sacrospinous ligament	Coccyx, sacrum	Branches from the anterior rami of S3 and S4	Contributes to the formation of the pelvic floor

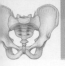

the tone of the anal sphincter muscles can be assessed. In the male, the prostate can be palpated anteriorly, and in the female, the uterus and if enlarged, the ovaries. Abnormalities of the rectum, such as polyps or tumors, may also be palpated.

Bladder

The bladder is a muscular sac and is the most anterior of the pelvic organs. The bladder is retroperitoneal. When the bladder is empty it is located within the pelvic cavity; as it fills it rises, and when full it extends into the abdominal cavity. As the bladder fills, the peritoneum covering the bladder also rises creating an area on the anterior aspect of the bladder that is void of peritoneum; this is clinically relevant as a suprapubic catheter may be inserted into the bladder at this point without piercing the peritoneum. The most superior aspect of a full bladder lies at a point between the pubic symphysis and the umbilicus. If a urethral catheter is not possible, a full bladder may have a suprapubic catheter inserted 2.5 cm superior to the pubic symphysis.

Ovary

The ovaries are ovoid in shape and are approximately 3–4 cm in length. Each ovary contains follicles with developing oocytes. The ovaries are attached to the posterosuperior surface of the broad ligament by a stalk of peritoneum called the mesovarium. Laterally, each ovary is closely related to the parietal peritoneum which covers the side wall of the pelvic cavity and lies between the internal and external iliac arteries. The posterior lateral aspect of each ovary is in close proximity to the fimbriae of the uterine tube. Enlarged ovaries, preovulation or with pathological cysts, can descend

into the recto-uterine pouch (pouch of Douglas). At ovulation, an oocyte is released from the surface of an ovary into the peritoneal cavity and, normally, it immediately enters the open end of a uterine tube.

Uterus

The uterus is a thick-walled muscular organ. The nulliparous (not having borne a child) uterus is about 7.5 cm long, 1–2 cm thick and about 5 cm at its widest and lies entirely within the pelvic cavity. During pregnancy, the uterus becomes enlarged and extends into the abdomen. The uterine tubes open into the lateral sides of the uterus. The part of the uterus superior to the openings of the uterine tubes is termed the fundus. Inferior to the fundus is the body of the uterus, which caudally becomes the cervix of the uterus (Fig. 4.4).

The uterus is covered by a fold of peritoneum called the broad ligament. The broad ligament runs from the pelvic walls to the uterus and encloses the uterine tube, round ligament and neurovasculature of the uterus. The long axis of the uterus is normally curved with the concavity facing anteriorly. The body and fundus are bent anteriorly relative to the cervix (anteflexion), and the whole uterus is bent anteriorly relative to the axis of the vagina (anteversion) (Fig. 4.5). A uterus that is retroflexed and retroverted will point posteriorly towards the rectum. The degrees of anteversion and anteflexion become reduced with distension of the bladder and may alter after childbirth. The uterus normally lies entirely within the pelvic cavity and may only be palpated by performing a bimanual examination. The index and middle fingers of a gloved right hand are inserted into the vagina with the thumb pointing towards the pubis. Using the right hand, the internal fingers allow for palpation of the uterus to determine whether it is anteverted or

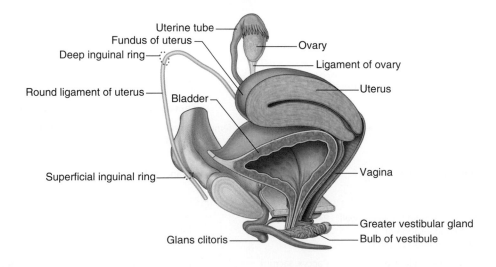

Fig. 4.4 Female reproductive system.
(Modified with permission from Drake, RL, Gray's Anatomy for Students, 3rd ed, 2015, Churchill Livingstone, Elsevier.)

retroverted. The internal fingers can gently elevate the uterus to aid the palpation from the surface. The left hand is placed over the abdomen at the midpoint between the pubis and the umbilicus and gentle pressure is applied. There are no specific surface landmarks for the uterus as its position varies according to the degree of distension of the bladder.

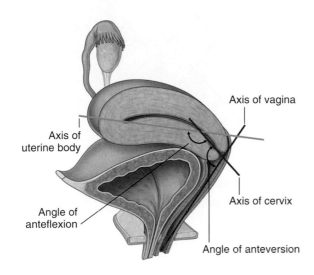

Fig. 4.5 Uterus angles of anteflexion and anteversion.
(With permission from Drake, RL, Gray's Anatomy for Students, 3rd ed, 2015, Churchill Livingstone, Elsevier.)

Vagina

The vagina is a thin-walled fibromuscular tube that extends inferiorly and anteriorly from the cervix and opens inferiorly into the vestibule. The cervix projects into the vagina and the surrounding 'spaces' of the vagina are known as fornices. A vaginal examination can be performed by inserting the index and middle fingers of a gloved hand into the vagina with the thumb pointing towards the pubis and the ring and little finger flexed. This allows the vagina to be expanded for examination for any nodules. Anteriorly, the bladder may be palpated. The cervix can be palpated and may be moved slightly to enable the fornices to be felt. The shape and size of the cervix should be noted. An ultrasound transducer may also be used to image the reproductive organs (see In the Clinic box, p. 64).

Prostate and seminal vesicles

The prostate lies immediately inferior to the bladder and surrounds the prostatic part of the urethra. It is composed of a glandular part (accounting for approximately two-thirds) and a fibromuscular part. The prostate is divided into right and left lobes that are separated anteriorly by the isthmus. Paired seminal vesicles are sacs that lie lateral to the ductus deferens. Each seminal vesicle consists of a coiled tube (Fig. 4.6). The posterior surface of the prostate may be palpated via a rectal examination.

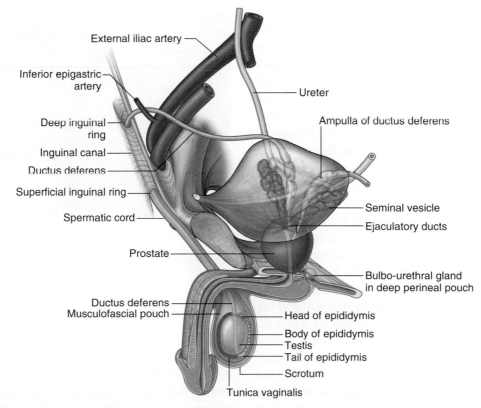

Fig. 4.6 Prostate and seminal vesicles.
(Modified from Drake, RL, Gray's Anatomy for Students, 3rd ed, 2015, Churchill Livingstone, Elsevier.)

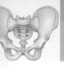

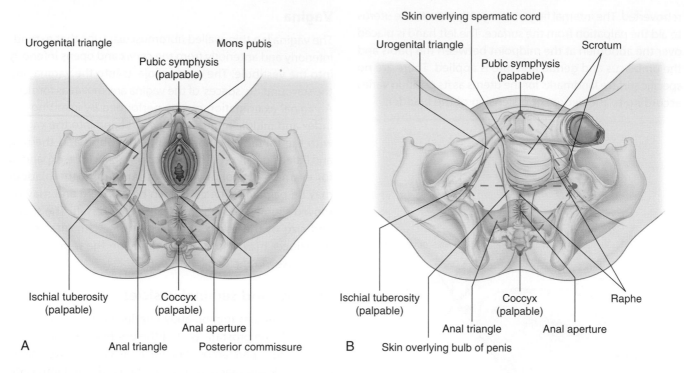

Fig. 4.7 A, Perineum in females. B, Perineum in males.
(Modified from Drake, RL, Gray's Anatomy for Students, 3rd ed, 2015, Churchill Livingstone, Elsevier.)

PERINEUM

The perineum is the region between the most superior aspect of the thighs that overlies the outlet of the bony pelvis. It is a diamond-shaped area that extends anteriorly from the inferior border of the pubic symphysis, posteriorly to the coccyx and laterally to the ischial tuberosities. It is divided into an anal triangle posteriorly and a urogenital triangle anteriorly, separated by an imaginary line that joins the two ischial tuberosities. The perineum includes the anal orifice and the external genitalia (Fig. 4.7). The urogenital triangle is closed by the perineal membrane. The membrane is perforated by the vagina and urethra in the female and the urethra in the male. The membrane and ischiopubic rami provide key attachment points for the erectile bodies and muscles of the external genitalia in both males and females. The fibers of the muscles of the the external genitalia, perineum and anal sphincter converge at a midline point of dense connective tissue known as the perineal body, which can be palpated between the posterior margin of the scrotum and the anal orifice in the male (Fig. 4.8) and the ischial tuberosities and the vagina in the female (Fig. 4.9).

The anal triangle can be further divided into two ischio-anal fossae or ischiorectal fossae with the fibrofatty anococcygeal body in the midline between the anal orifice and the tip of the coccyx. The fossae contain adipose tissue and neurovascular bundles that supply the perineum and external genitalia.

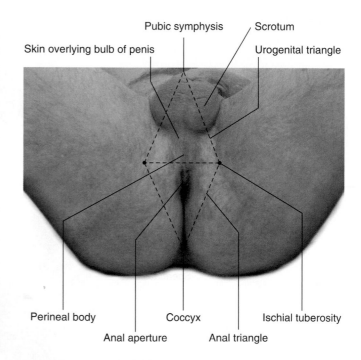

Fig. 4.8 Surface projections of the male perineum.

The pelvic diaphragm forms the muscular floor of the pelvic cavity. Its main function is to support the pelvic viscera, and it is important in resisting the rise in intrapelvic pressure that occurs when the abdominal wall muscles contract during expulsive efforts, such as in coughing, defecation and

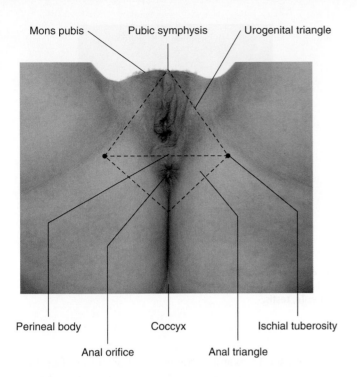

Mons pubis | Pubic symphysis | Urogenital triangle

Perineal body | Coccyx | Ischial tuberosity
Anal orifice | Anal triangle

Fig. 4.9 Surface projections of the female perineum.

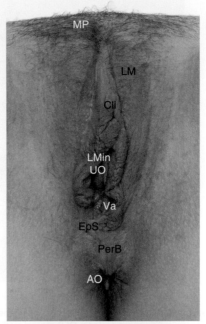

A

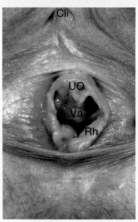

B

Fig. 4.10 A, Surface anatomy of the female external genitalia. B, Inferior view. *AO*, anal orifice; *Cli*, clitoris; *EpS*, episiotomy scar; *LM*, labia majora; *LMin*, labia minora; *MP*, mons pubis; *PerB*, perineal body; *Rh*, remnants of hymen; *UO*, urethral orifice; *Va*, vagina. *(B, from Drake, RL, Gray's Anatomy for Students, 3rd ed, 2015, Churchill Livingstone, Elsevier.)*

parturition. Superficial to the pelvic diagram in the perineum are structures associated with the external genitalia.

Female external genitalia

The mons pubis is the raised eminence anterior to the pubic symphysis. The mons pubis contains adipose tissue. The amount of adipose tissue varies and typically decreases after the menopause. The mons pubis in the postpubescent individual is covered with pubic hair. The vulva is the name given to the structures of the female external genitalia. The labia majora are folds of hair-bearing skin which join anteriorly in the mons pubis and posteriorly between the vaginal and anal orifices. The pudendal cleft lies between the medial margins of the labia majora. The labia minora are two thin folds of hairless skin within the labia majora. The labia minora contain erectile tissue at their base and are characterized by typically pink, moist thin skin. The vestibule lies between the inner surfaces of the labia minora and contains the urethral and vaginal orifices and vestibular glands. The skin of the vestibule is moist and hairless. The most anterior orifice is the opening of the urethra, the external urethral orifice. The clitoris is a body of erectile tissue lying anterior and superior to the urethral orifice. The clitoris consists of two crura, body and glans. The glans clitoris is partly covered by the anterior margins of the labia minora that form the prepuce (foreskin) of the clitoris (Fig. 4.10). The vaginal orifice varies in appearance depending on age and after vaginal delivery. The hymen is a mucous membrane that may partially or completely occlude the vaginal orifice. After rupture, hymenal caruncles may be visible. The contents of the pelvis may be palpated via vaginal examination where a right index and middle fingers are inserted into the vagina as described above.

Male external genitalia

Penis

The penis consists of a shaft, or body, a root and glans. In the anatomical position, the penis is considered to be erect. The body of the penis consists of three cylindrical masses of erectile tissue. These are the two adjacent corpora cavernosa and the corpus spongiosum, which lies ventrally and surrounds the spongy part of the urethra. Each corpus is surrounded by a fascial sheath. The distal end of the corpus

57

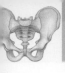

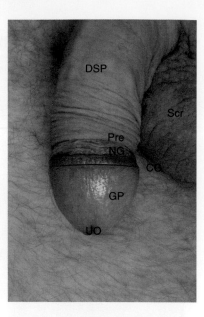

Fig. 4.11 Surface anatomy of the dorsal aspect of the penis. Non circumcised penis. *CG*, corona glans; *DSP*, dorsal surface penis; *GP*, glans penis; *NG*, neck glans; *Pre*, prepuce; *Scr*, scrotum; *UO*, urethral orifice.

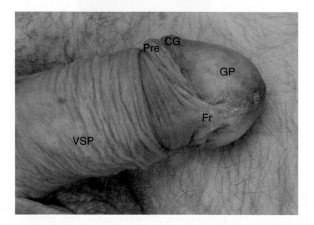

Fig. 4.12 Surface anatomy of the ventral aspect of the penis. *CG*, corona glans; *Fr*, frenulum; *GP*, glans penis; *Pre*, prepuce; *VSP*, ventral surface penis.

spongiosum is enlarged as the caplike glans penis, which has a margin known as the corona glandis (Fig. 4.11). The skin covering the shaft of the penis is mobile, particularly where it extends over the glans penis as a double fold, the prepuce or foreskin. The prepuce is attached on the ventral surface at the junction between the glans and body, forming the frenulum (Fig. 4.12). The skin of the glans and corona glandis is firmly attached to the underlying fibrous sheath. The skin over the penis is thin and may have darker pigmentation to adjacent skin. Examination of the penis includes inspection of the skin, prepuce and the glans to check for any sign of infection, unusual discharge, inflammation, scars

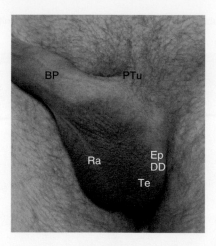

Fig. 4.13 Surface projections of the scrotum and testis. *BP*, body penis; *DD*, ductus deferens; *Ep*, epididymis; *PTu*, pubic tubercle; *Ra*, raphe; *Te*, testis.

or neoplasia. To examine the external urethra orifice, hold the glans between the index finger and thumb and apply gentle pressure.

Scrotum

The scrotum is a muscular sac containing the testes that is located posterior to the penis. The skin over the scrotum is rough and appears corrugated. The scrotum is divided into two compartments by a connective tissue scrotal septum or raphe (Fig. 4.13). Each compartment contains a testis and its associated structures. The thin-walled scrotum helps ensure the testes are kept just below body temperature. Visual examination of the scrotum may reveal small local movements as a result of dartos muscle contractions. These contractions are different from the cremaster reflex, which pulls the testis towards the body to increase temperature or for protection. The superficial fascia of the scrotum contains smooth muscle fibers of the dartos muscle.

Testis

Each testis is ovoid in shape and contains many coiled, continuous seminiferous tubules where spermatozoa are produced. Spermatozoa then pass into the epididymis, which is continuous with the ductus deferens. Visual examination and palpation of the scrotum can assess for any swellings or lumps that may indicate a hydrocele (accumulation of fluid around the testis) or testicular tumor. To palpate the testis, take the testis between the index finger, middle finger and thumb. The epididymis feels like a cordlike structure on the posterior superior surface.

PREGNANCY

During pregnancy many changes occur in the woman's body, some of which affect the normal surface anatomy. In

from around 18 weeks and by a healthcare professional from around 24 weeks. Palpating the location of the fetal head and back can help establish a good location for auscultation of the fetal heart rate. Towards the later stages of pregnancy, the degree of lumbar lordosis increases in response to the changing line of gravity.

Increased vascularity in pregnancy means that the vagina may appear 'blue' especially in the later months when the pressure caused by the developing fetus on the venous system can cause pelvic congestion. The superficial veins, previously unnoticeable, may become more pronounced.

Pregnant individuals should not be asked to lie supine for a long time as it puts pressure on the aorta and inferior vena cava that can reduce arterial and venous flow.

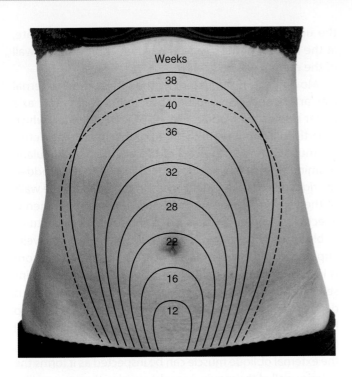

Fig. 4.14 Surface projections of the height of the fundus of the uterus during pregnancy.

particular, the breasts enlarge and there can be increased pigmentation of the areolae. The breasts may be more sensitive during examination. In late pregnancy, colostrum may be expressed. Stretch marks (striae distensae) may be seen on the skin of the breasts, hips and abdomen. Stretch marks that are a result of pregnancy are referred to as striae gravidarum. The skin in the region of the linea alba may develop pigmentation known as linea nigra.

The most notable changes are in the abdomen. During pregnancy, the fundus of the uterus can be palpated on the anterior abdominal wall above the pubic symphysis by 12 weeks and at the level of the umbilicus at 24 weeks. By 36 weeks, the fundus of the uterus extends to the xiphisternum (Fig. 4.14). As it expands, the uterus pushes the abdominal contents laterally. The round ligaments of the uterus become stretched and in some subjects this may be felt as pain extending down to the labia majora.

The uterus is predominantly angled anteriorly, with the body of the uterus anterior to the line of gravity. As it enlarges during pregnancy, the line of gravity of the female moves anteriorly with a resultant change in posture. As pregnancy progresses, the muscles of the anterior abdominal wall, especially the rectus abdominis muscle, passively spread laterally, and the width of the linea alba increases temporarily. The remaining gap provides a space for palpation of the fetus. Fetal movements can usually be felt by the mother

In the Clinic

Benign prostatic hyperplasia
Benign prostatic hyperplasia is an enlargement of the prostate that is commonly associated with aging. The gland may feel enlarged when palpated and may protrude into the rectum. A tumor of the prostate is often felt as a hard, irregular-shaped nodule.

Episiotomies/perineal tears
An episiotomy may be used to increase the diameter of the vaginal outlet during childbirth, providing greater control over blood loss and repair to the perineum. An incision is made from the vaginal orifice to the right lateral side. Perineal tears frequently occur in the midline. Both episiotomies and tears are surgically repaired with local anesthetic and sutures.

Ultrasound

MALE PELVIS

Subject position

Imaging is performed with the subject lying supine. The bladder should be full, since this improves visualization by providing an acoustic window. It is recommended that the subject drinks approximately 500 ml of water 1 hour before imaging.

Transducer

Use a curved array transducer. Set the depth setting to 12–15 cm, or 4–10 cm to observe the external iliac vessels

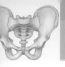

and spermatic cord. A linear array transducer can also be used to inspect these more superficial structures.

Transducer position

The transducer should be positioned immediately above the pubis in the midline. The male pelvis can be imaged in either the sagittal or transverse plane. Tilt the probe to optimize the image and to scan through the pelvis. To image the prostate, angle the transducer inferiorly. To image the iliac vessels, move the transducer to the left or right of the midline. Firm pressure should be applied.

Image features

Sagittal plane view

The rectus abdominis muscle can be seen at the top of the image (Fig. 4.15A). Deep to the muscle, the balloon-shaped bladder will be in view filling most of the image (when full). The detrusor muscle that forms the bladder wall appears relatively hyperechoic compared to the anechoic cavity. Directly inferior to the bladder (on the right-hand side of the image) the prostate can be seen protruding into the bladder. It has an isoechoic mid-gray appearance with a hyperechoic wall. Passing inferiorly from the bladder through the posterior third of the prostate, the urethra appears as a bright horizontal streak. The seminal vesicles sit posterior to the bladder and may be visible. The seminal vesicles are variable in size and are characterized by their curved tapered appearance as they follow the contours of the posterior wall of the bladder. The seminal vesicles have a dark gray appearance and are surrounded by a hyperechoic wall. Since these structures do not sit directly along the midline, it may be necessary to tilt the probe slightly to the left or right. Towards the base of the seminal vesicle, the ejaculatory duct can be seen as a light streak passing towards the urethra. With the probe on the midline, the ductus deferens may be in view. The ductus deferens appear as small hypoechoic tubelike structures. Posterior to the seminal vesicles, at the bottom of the image, the ampulla of the rectum can be inspected. The anterior wall appears hyperechoic, whereas the cavity is hypoechoic due to the presence of gas.

Transverse plane view

Posterior to the rectus abdominis muscle, the full bladder appears as a large rectangular-shaped structure (Fig. 4.15B). On the posterolateral wall of the bladder, the two seminal vesicles can be observed in their short axis, which are circular in appearance. Medial to the seminal vesicles, the ductus deferens will be in view. With the transducer tilted inferiorly, the prostate appears to sit behind the bladder (although this is related to the orientation of the probe). It is a relatively hypoechoic structure, and in the center,

the urethra can be observed. Posterior to the prostate, at the bottom of the image, the hyperechoic anterior wall of the rectum will be in view.

Moving the probe laterally, the left or right external iliac artery and vein can be observed in their short axis either side of the bladder (Fig. 4.15C). The bladder, which is partly full, is in view to the right of the image. The detrusor muscle forming the wall of the bladder is particularly prominent since it is not stretched. Lateral to the bladder, the right external iliac artery and vein can be seen. The walls of the vessels appear hyperechoic, whereas the lumen is anechoic. Doppler can be used to confirm these structures as blood vessels and to distinguish the artery from the vein. Superficial to the external iliac vessels, the spermatic cord is in view. It has a medium gray appearance and contains several smaller hypoechoic structures, namely the ductus deferens and testicular vessels. The spermatic cord can also be seen in its long view passing through the inguinal canal (left on image). Lying over the top of the spermatic cord, the external oblique muscle can be inspected as it forms the anterior wall of the inguinal canal. Lateral to the external iliac vessels, the iliacus muscle is seen in short axis. A bright white streak may be observed deep to the external iliac vessels and iliacus muscle. This streak is echo from the surface of the iliac crests.

FEMALE PELVIS

Subject position

Imaging is performed with the subject lying supine. The bladder should be full, since as well as improving image quality, a full bladder pushes the bowel away from the uterus. It is recommended that the subject drinks approximately 500 ml of water 1 hour before imaging.

Transducer

Use a curved array transducer. Set the depth setting to 12–15 cm.

Transducer position

The transducer should be positioned approximately halfway between the umbilicus and the pubis along the midline. The female pelvis can be imaged in either the sagittal or transverse plane. Tilt the probe to optimize the image and to scan through the pelvis. To inspect the left and right ovaries, tilt, rock or slide the transducer (in transverse orientation) to the left or right, respectively. Angling the transducer so that its most lateral edge is slightly cephalic can improve visualization of the ovaries. Note that the ovaries can be difficult to locate and there is variability in their anatomical position. Moving the transducer to the left or right of the

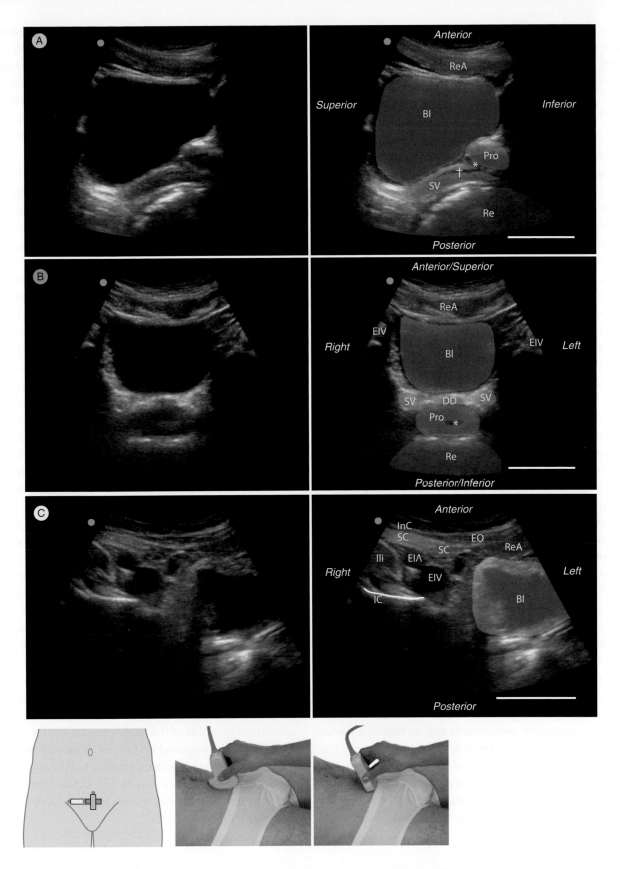

Fig. 4.15 Ultrasound of the male pelvis. A, Midsagittal. B, Transverse with the transducer tilted inferiorly. C, Transverse to the right of the midline. †, *ejaculatory duct*; *, *urethra*; *Bl*, bladder; *DD*, ductus deferens; *EIA*, external iliac artery; *EIV*, external iliac vein; *EO*, external oblique; *IC*, iliac crest; *Ili*, iliacus; *InC*, inguinal canal; *Pro*, prostate; *Re*, rectum; *ReA*, rectus abdominus; *SC*, spermatic cord; *SV*, seminal vesicle. Scale bar = 3 cm.

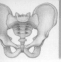
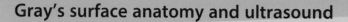
midline will also enable visualization of the external iliac vessels. By moving the transducer towards the pubis, and angling inferiorly, it is possible (in some subjects) to view the pelvic floor. Firm pressure should be applied.

Image features

Sagittal plane view

The rectus abdominis muscle can be seen at the very top of the image (Fig. 4.16A). When full, the balloon-shaped bladder fills much of the image. The pear-shaped uterus, approximately 6–10 cm in length, sits behind the bladder. The normal anteverted and anteflexed uterus will curve superiorly over the bladder, whereas a retroverted and retroflexed uterus will curve posteriorly away from the bladder (eFig. 4.17). Both the myometrium (muscular wall) and endometrium (inner lining) can be distinguished on ultrasound. The myometrium has a fairly dark gray isoechoic appearance, whereas the appearance of the endometrium changes throughout the menstrual cycle (eFig. 4.18). During the menstrual and early follicular stage (days 1–8), it appears as a very thin hyperechoic line. In the later follicular stage (days 9–14), it has a laminar appearance, where the middle hyperechoic central canal is surrounded by a hypoechoic functional zone and an outer hyperechoic basal layer. During the luteal phase (days 15–28), it is at its thickest and appears hyperechoic compared to the myometrium. In a postmenopausal individual who is not on hormone replacement therapy, the endometrium should be thin. The cervix forms the most inferior part of the uterus. The dome-shaped curve of the cervix should be visible at the most inferior aspect of the uterus, but may appear to merge with the vagina. Continuous with the cervix, the vagina can be seen extending down the posterior length of the bladder (approximately horizontally across image). The muscular wall of the vagina appears relatively darker compared to the bright streak of the central vaginal canal. The enlarged vaginal vault can be seen at the most superior end of the vagina. Superior and posterior to the uterus, the ileum of the small intestine will be present and will be in close proximity to the uterus. It should be easily distinguished from the uterus due to the presence of peristaltic movements and its heterogeneous texture. Posterior to the uterus and vagina, towards the bottom of the image, the sigmoid colon or rectum can be seen. The position of the sigmoid colon and coils of small intestine may sometimes make visualization of the uterus and ovaries difficult, especially visualization of small

postmenopausal ovaries. Below the bright hyperechoic anterior wall of these structures, the image may appear anechoic due to the presence of gas. Although not obvious in the figure, the anechoic recto-uterine pouch can sometimes be seen sitting between the uterus and large intestine. It is extremely difficult to observe the ureters on ultrasound. However, Doppler can be used to view urine entering the bladder from the ureteral orifice (Video 4.1).

Transverse plane view

The uterus can be seen in its short axis either lying posteriorly or superiorly in relation to the bladder. It will appear oval in shape and characterized by its dark gray myometrium (Fig. 4.16B). The right or left ovaries will come in to view as the probe is rocked or moved towards the right or left, respectively. The almond-shaped ovaries are approximately 3 cm in length and 1–2 cm wide. They have a relatively dark appearance, and depending upon the time point during the menstrual cycle, dark hypoechoic follicles may be present. It should be possible to see the uterine tube extending from the anterolateral aspect of the uterus towards the ovary. The lumen of the uterine tube has a hypoechoic appearance. The broad ligament can be easily identified surrounding the uterus, uterine tubes and ovaries. It appears as a hyperechoic lining, which helps identify these anatomical structures. In close proximity to the uterus and ovaries, peristaltic movements of the ileum can be observed. Posterior to the uterus, a hyperechoic streak will be visible, which is formed by the anterior wall of the sigmoid colon or rectum.

Moving the transducer closer to the pubis and angling it inferiorly, the pelvic floor structures come into view (Fig. 4.16C). At the top of the image, the rectus abdominis muscle is observed. Sitting posterior to this muscle, the bladder appears almost rectangular in shape. Immediately posterior to the bladder, the vagina is seen in short axis. The vaginal canal appears as a bright streak compared to the surrounding hypoechoic muscular wall of the vagina. Behind the vagina, the anal sphincter can be viewed. It is relatively circular and has a hyperechoic central region, the anal mucosa, which is surrounded by a dark hypoechoic ring, the internal anal sphincter, and a narrow gray colored ring, the external anal sphincter. Either side of the anal canal, the levator ani muscle (specifically, the puborectalis portion) is seen as an isoechoic band converging immediately posterior of the anal sphincter. Lateral to the levator ani muscle, the ischiorectal fossae can be inspected. These fossae appear heterogeneous in texture due to the presence of fat.

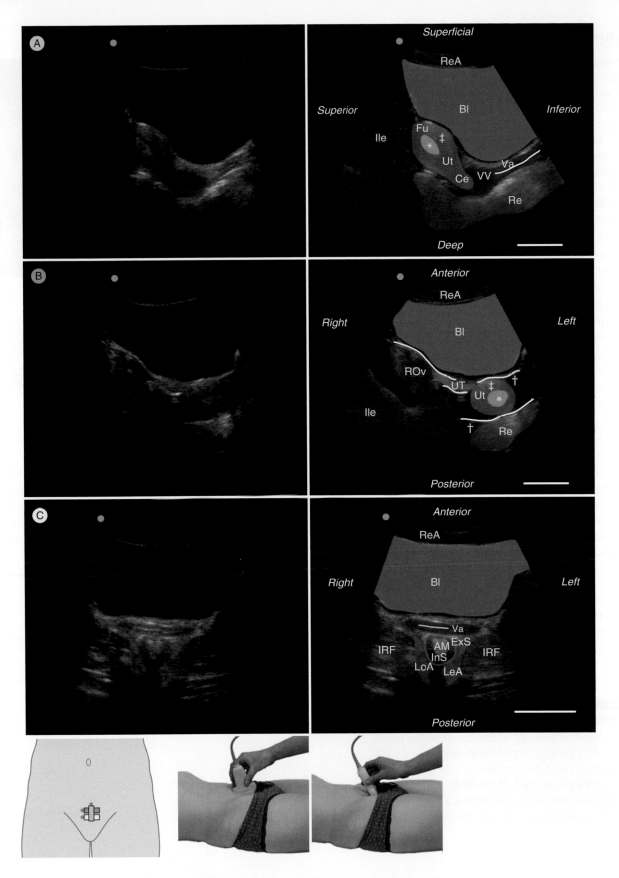

Fig. 4.16 Ultrasound of the female pelvis. A, Midsagittal. B, Transverse to the right of the midline. C, Transverse with the transducer tilted inferiorly. †, *broad ligament*; *, *endometrium*; ‡, *myometrium*; *AM*, anal mucosa; *Bl*, bladder; *Ce*, cervix; *ExS*, external sphincter; *Fu*, fundus; *Ile*, ileum; *InS*, internal sphincter; *IRF*, ischiorectal fossa; *LeA*, levator ani; *Re*, rectum; *ReA*, rectus abdominus; *ROv*, right ovary; *UT*, uterine tubes; *Ut*, uterus; *Va*, vagina; *VV*, vaginal vault. Scale bar = 3 cm.

In the Clinic

Ultrasound provides an important tool for clinical assessment of the pelvis in both males and females. B-mode and Doppler imaging are used to examine the reproductive tract, bladder and large intestine. As well as imaging through the skin, transrectal and transvaginal approaches using specialized transducers are frequently employed to assess the prostate and rectum (transrectal), and the cervix, ovaries and uterus (transvaginal). Other clinical uses for ultrasonography in the pelvis include monitoring catheter placement as well as assessing the position of an intrauterine contraceptive device.

Transvaginal scanning in the clinic is often the preferred technique for assessing the uterus and ovaries. Examples of pelvic pathologies that can be identified using ultrasound include ovarian and tubal cysts and swellings, benign or malignant tumors, endometrial thickening and polyps.

Ultrasound is also employed to assess enlargement of the viscera, a common example being enlargement of the prostate in patients with benign prostatic hyperplasia.

During pregnancy, transabdominal B-mode ultrasound imaging is considered the gold standard for assessing fetal growth and gestational age (Fig. 4.19). It can also be used to assess placental implantation, as well as to diagnose developmental structural abnormalities, such as anencephaly, hydrocephalus, spina bifida, heart abnormalities, and cleft palates and lips. During the first trimester of pregnancy, ultrasound is routinely employed to measure fetal nuchal translucency (fluid accumulation in the posterior neck region) as a way of screening for trisomy 21, more commonly known as Down syndrome. Table 4.2 provides an overview of some of the pelvic conditions that can be diagnosed or monitored by ultrasound.

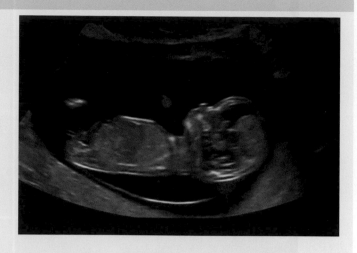

Fig. 4.19 Ultrasound image of pregnancy at 12 weeks.

Table 4.2 Examples of pelvic pathologies that are routinely diagnosed by ultrasound

Viscera	Pathology
Bladder	Ischuria (urinary retention), vesical calculus (bladder stones)
Prostate	Benign prostatic hyperplasia, prostate cancer
Testes	Testicular cancer, hydrocele testis, testicular torsion
Uterus	Endometrial polyps, endometrial carcinoma, fibroids
Ovaries	Ovarian cysts, polycystic ovaries
Uterine tubes	Ectopic pregnancy, hydrosalpinges and pyosalpinx associated with pelvic inflammatory disease
Cervix	Cervical cancer, nabothian follicles

Summary Checklist

- Surface projections of the bones of the pelvis
- Surface projections of the pelvic viscera
- Surface projections of the female genitalia
- Surface projections of the male genitalia
- Ultrasound imaging of the male pelvis
- Ultrasound imaging of the female pelvis

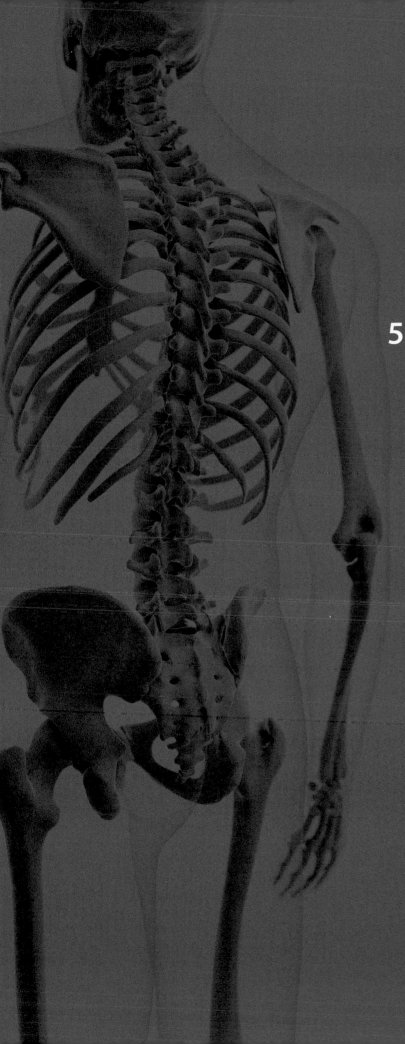

5 Back

Conceptual overview

The back forms the posterior aspect of the trunk and includes the vertebral column. Attached to the vertebral column are the pectoral and pelvic girdles by which the upper and lower limbs are connected. Also articulating with the vertebral column are the ribs and the base of the skull. The back can be divided into five regions: cervical, thoracic, lumbar, sacral and coccygeal. The vertebral column includes the vertebral canal which contains the spinal cord and the cauda equina. The back consists of musculoskeletal and nervous systems. Clinically the back is easily accessible to palpate and examine, and forms a key part of a physical examination for a range of conditions, which include back pain and disc herniation.

Surface anatomy

CURVATURES

The back gives support to the body by distributing weight through the vertebral column to the lower limbs. Support of body weight is facilitated by virtue of primary and secondary spinal curvatures. The curvatures are known as kyphosis and lordosis respectively (Fig. 5.1). The primary curvature of the vertebral column is oriented so that the concavity of the curve faces anteriorly. This shape first develops in embryonic life and this concavity becomes the curves of the thoracic region and the sacrum. The secondary curvatures develop as the individual learns to lift their head and to sit upright. The secondary curvatures have their concavities facing posteriorly in the lumbar and cervical regions. The net effect of the curvatures is to bring the line of gravity onto a vertical plane. In the normal vertebral column there should be no lateral deviation. The muscle groups on each side of the midline furrow should be of equal proportions. When lateral bending of the vertebral column is observed it is known as a scoliosis. Accentuated forward bending, usually associated with the thoracic region, is referred to as hyperkyphosis. Accentuated excessive lumbar curvature is called a hyperlordosis. In the elderly the height of the vertebral column reduces mainly because of bone loss and reduction of water content in the intervertebral discs.

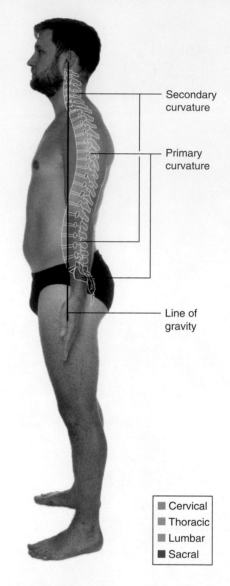

Fig. 5.1 Normal curvatures of the spine.

Secondary curvature

Primary curvature

Line of gravity

■ Cervical
■ Thoracic
■ Lumbar
■ Sacral

BONES

The bones of the vertebral column are important for the protection of the spinal cord. The 33 vertebrae are comprised of 7 cervical, 12 thoracic, 5 lumbar, 5 sacral (fused) and 3–4 coccygeal vertebrae. Vertebrae are classified as being typical and atypical. Typical vertebrae (Fig. 5.2) have a vertebral body and a vertebral arch. Together, the vertebral arch and body surround the spinal cord to provide protection. The vertebral body is the major weight bearing structure of the column. The vertebral bodies increase in size from cervical to lumbar regions, reflecting the cumulative increase in weight of the trunk. The arch consists of a pedicle that connects the body to the transverse process. The laminae are continuous with the transverse processes and come together to project posteriorly as the spinous process. The spinous processes are easily palpated in the midline of

---

To Do (Fig. 5.1)

Lateral aspect of the back:
• Observe the primary and secondary curvatures

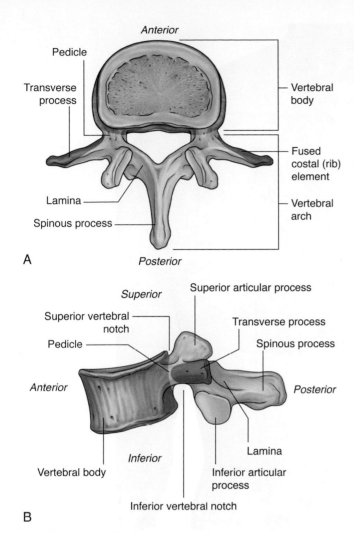

It is held in position by the transverse ligament of the atlas. The joint between the atlas and the occipital condyles (the atlanto-occipital joints) allows nodding movement of the head, while the atlanto-axial joint facilitates rotation, as in responding no.

Cervical vertebrae are the smallest, with relatively small bodies. In each transverse process there is a foramen which transmits the vertebral artery. Their spinous processes are bifid and may be palpated.

Thoracic vertebrae have bodies that increase in size from superior to inferior as superincumbent weight increases. The most distinguishing feature are their superior and inferior facets on the vertebral bodies and the facets on the transverse processes for articulation with the ribs. The spinous processes of the thoracic vertebrae are easily palpated.

Lumbar vertebrae have the largest bodies because body weight transmission is greatest in the lumbar region. The transverse and spinous processes are relatively short and stout. These vertebrae form the support for the posterior abdominal wall. The spinous processes can be palpated but this may be difficult because of the lumbar curvature. Therefore, patients may be asked to bend forward, flexing the lumbar vertebral column, so that the spinous processes can be more easily palpated (Fig. 5.3).

The five sacral elements are fused. There are anterior and posterior sacral foramina through which the anterior and posterior rami of the spinal nerves emerge.

Fig. 5.2 A typical vertebra. A, Superior view. B, Lateral view. *(From Drake, RL, Gray's Anatomy for Students, 3rd ed, 2015, Churchill Livingstone, Elsevier.)*

the back, especially with the vertebral column flexed. The transverse processes are harder to palpate in the thoracic region. The transverse processes of the lumbar region may be palpated 3–4 cm lateral from the midline. As the vertebrae stack on top of each other they create a space on each side for the paired spinal nerves to leave the column, known as intervertebral foramina. The atypical vertebrae include the first two cervical vertebrae, the atlas and axis, the sacrum and the coccygeal vertebrae.

Within each region, vertebrae have specialized features.

The atlas articulates with the base of the skull at the atlanto-occipital joints. It has no body, and so it has no intervertebral disc associated with it. The atlas forms a complete circle of bone with anterior and posterior arches. The transverse processes of the atlas are easily palpated inferior to the mastoid process. Projecting into the circle of bone is the dens of the second cervical vertebra, the axis.

LIGAMENTS

The vertebrae are bound together by numerous ligaments (Fig. 5.4). The long axis of the column is bound together by the anterior and posterior longitudinal ligaments. The anterior longitudinal ligament is attached from the base of the skull to the sacrum, to the anterior surface of the vertebral bodies and their intervening intervertebral discs. The posterior longitudinal ligament lies on the inside of the vertebral canal and lines the posterior surface of the vertebral bodies. The ligamenta flava lies between adjacent laminae to limit separation of adjacent vertebrae in flexion. The supraspinous ligament lies along the tips of the spinous processes from C7 to the sacrum and can be palpated. More superiorly, the ligament fans out and becomes known as the ligamentum nuchae. This part of the ligament is triangular in shape in the sagittal plane, and is attached to the base of the skull and the tips of the spinous processes of each cervical vertebra. It resists flexion of the neck and provides attachment sites for adjacent musculature. Lying between the spinous processes are interspinous ligaments, which merge with the supraspinous ligament and the ligamenta flava.

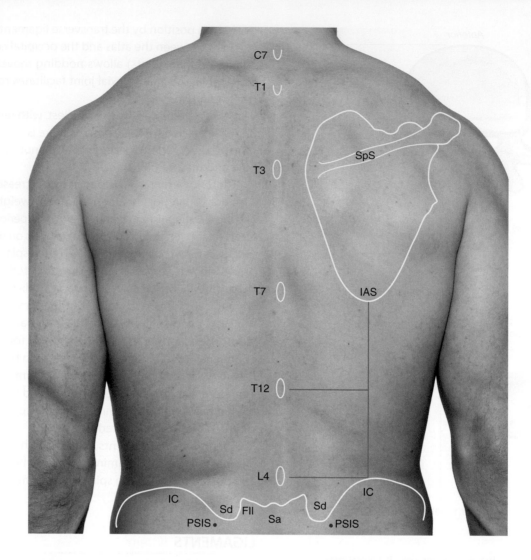

Fig. 5.3 Surface projections of the osteology of the back. *FII*, fascia iliaca; *IAS*, inferior angle of scapula; *IC*, iliac crest; *PSIS*, posterior superior iliac spine; *Sa*, sacrum; *Sd*, sacral dimple; *SpS*, spine of scapula.

To Do (Fig. 5.3)

Back:

Palpate the spinous processes:

- Cervical Region: Start at the base of the skull and move inferiorly as far as C7. Feel for the spinous process of the axis, about 1–2 cm below the occiput. It is the largest palpable spinous process in the upper cervical area. The small tubercle representing the spinous process of the atlas is usually too deep to be palpable. Locate C7, which is a very important landmark clinically and is the most prominent cervical spinous process. C7 may be easily palpated when the neck is flexed.
- Thoracic Region: T1 can be palpated below C7; the next palpable spinous processes depends on the amount of subcutaneous tissue. T3 is at the level of the spine of the scapula. T7 is at the level of the

inferior angle of the scapula. T12 can be located by drawing a line from the inferior angle of the scapula and the iliac crest, T12 is at the midpoint of this line. It may be possible to trace a rib laterally from the vertebrae.
- Lumbar Region: The highest point of the iliac crest is at the level of L4. From here it is possible to palpate the spinous processes of L3, L4 and L5.
- Sacral Region: The spinous process of S2 is located at the level of the sacral dimples and the posterior superior iliac spines.
- Coccygeal Region: The coccyx is palpable at the base of the sacrum in the intergluteal cleft.

Ligaments:

- Palpate the supraspinous ligament that runs between the tips of the spinous processes.
- Palpate the ligamentum nuchae in the cervical region by undertaking flexion of the cervical spine.

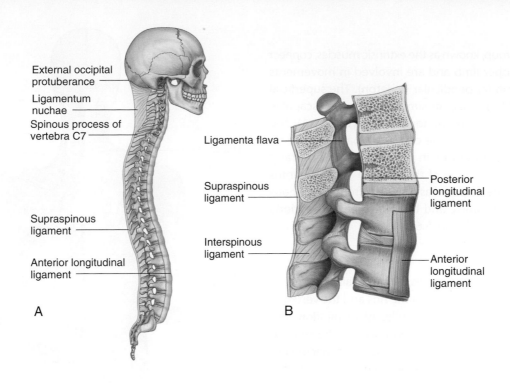

Fig. 5.4 A, Overview of the ligaments of the spine. B, Zoomed area showing ligaments. *(Modified from Drake, RL, Gray's Anatomy for Students, 3rd ed, 2015, Churchill Livingstone, Elsevier.)*

JOINTS

The vertebral column consists of five groups of joints: joints of the vertebral bodies, joints of the vertebral arches, craniovertebral joints, costovertebral joints and sacroiliac joints. The joints of the vertebral bodies are the intervertebral joints and the uncovertebral joints (cervical vertebrae only). The intervertebral joints are secondary cartilaginous and consist of an intervertebral disc (Fig. 5.5). The disc is formed of an outer anulus fibrosus and an inner 'jelly like' nucleus pulposus. During locomotion, they act as shock absorbers. While the discs cannot be palpated they are important clinically as a prolapsed disc (a prolapse of the nucleus pulposus through a tear in the anulus fibrosus) may place pressure on the spinal cord or nerve roots. The joints of the vertebral arches are the zygapophyseal joints (facet joints), which occur between the superior and inferior articular processes (Fig. 5.5). Zygapophyseal joints are of clinical relevance in back pain. The craniovertebral joints consist of two joints, namely the atlanto-occipital and atlanto-axial joints. The costovertebral joints occur between the heads of the ribs and the bodies of the thoracic vertebrae. The costotransverse joints occur between the tubercles of the rib and the transverse processes of the vertebrae. The sacroiliac joint occurs between the sacrum and the ilium of the pelvis.

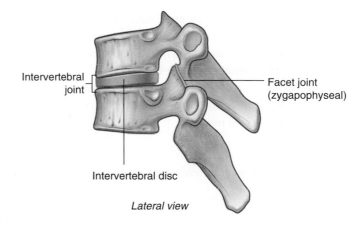

Fig. 5.5 Joints between thoracic vertebrae. *(From Drake, RL, Gray's Anatomy for Students, 3rd ed, 2015, Churchill Livingstone, Elsevier.)*

MUSCLES

There are three groups of muscles in the back: superficial, intermediate and deep. These muscles are important in movement and support of the appendicular and axial skeleton. Some of these muscles are covered posteriorly by thoracolumbar fascia.

Superficial

The superficial group, known as the extrinsic muscles, connect the back and upper limb and are involved in movements of the upper limb (appendicular skeleton). The superficial muscles include trapezius, latissimus dorsi, levator scapulae and rhomboid major and minor muscles (Table 5.1). The fibers of the trapezius muscle can be palpated sweeping from the spinous processes in the cervical and thoracic regions towards the spine of the scapula. The latissimus dorsi muscle can be palpated as it sweeps from the spinous processes in the thoracic and lumbar regions superiorly towards the upper limb (Fig. 5.6).

Intermediate

The intermediate group of muscles, which are also considered extrinsic muscles, are attached to the ribs and the vertebral column. These are accessory muscles of respiration. The intermediate group consists of two muscles: the serratus posterior superior muscle and the serratus posterior inferior muscle. It is not possible to palpate either muscle (Table 5.2 and Fig. 5.7).

Deep

The deep muscles, known as intrinsic muscles, are responsible for movements of the vertebral column and, importantly, maintain posture and provide stability for the vertebral column, as well as the neck and head. The deep muscles comprise of three main groups. From superficial to deep these are the spinotransversales muscles, the erector spinae muscles and the transversospinales muscles (Table 5.3). Deep to these muscles are several groups of smaller segmental muscles, the levatores costarum muscles and the interspinales and intertransversarii muscles.

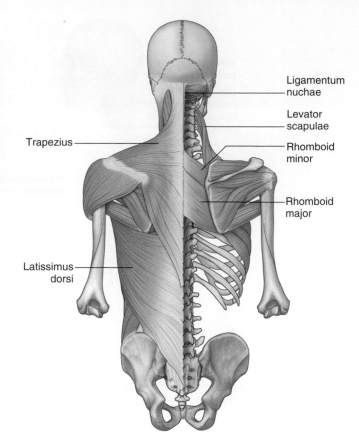

Fig. 5.6 Superficial group of back muscles—trapezius and latissimus dorsi—with rhomboid major, rhomboid minor and levator scapulae located deep to trapezius in the superior part of the back. *(From Drake, RL, Gray's Anatomy for Students, 3rd ed, 2015, Churchill Livingstone, Elsevier.)*

Table 5.1 Superficial (appendicular) group of back muscles

Muscle	Origin	Insertion	Innervation	Function
Trapezius	External occipital protuberance, spinous processes of C7–T12	Clavicle, acromion, spine of scapula	Motor—accessory nerve [11]; proprioception—C3, C4	Assists in rotating the scapula: upper fibers elevate, middle fibers adduct, and lower fibers depress scapula
Latissimus dorsi	Spinous processes of T7–L5 and sacrum, iliac crest, ribs 10–12	Floor of intertubercular sulcus of humerus	Thoracodorsal nerve (C6–C8)	Extends, adducts, and medially rotates humerus
Levator scapulae	Transverse processes of C1–C4	Upper portion medial border of scapula	C3–C4 and dorsal scapular nerve (C4, C5)	Elevates scapula
Rhomboid major	Spinous processes of T2–T5	Medial border of scapula	Dorsal scapular nerve (C4, C5)	Retracts (adducts) and elevates scapula
Rhomboid minor	Ligamentum nuchae, spinous processes of C7 and T1	Medial border of scapula at spine of scapula	Dorsal scapular nerve (C4, C5)	Retracts (adducts) and elevates scapula

Modified from Drake, RL, Gray's Anatomy for Students, 3rd ed, 2015, Churchill Livingstone, Elsevier.

Table 5.2 Intermediate (respiratory) group of back muscles

Muscle	Origin	Insertion	Innervation	Function
Serratus posterior superior	Spinous processes of C7–T3 and supraspinous ligaments	Upper border of ribs 2–5	Anterior rami of upper thoracic nerves (T2–T5)	Elevates ribs 2–5
Serratus posterior inferior	Spinous processes of T11–L3 and supraspinous ligaments	Lower border of ribs 9–12	Anterior rami of lower thoracic nerves (T9–T12)	Depresses ribs 9–11

Modified from Drake, RL, Gray's Anatomy for Students, 3rd ed, 2015, Churchill Livingstone, Elsevier.

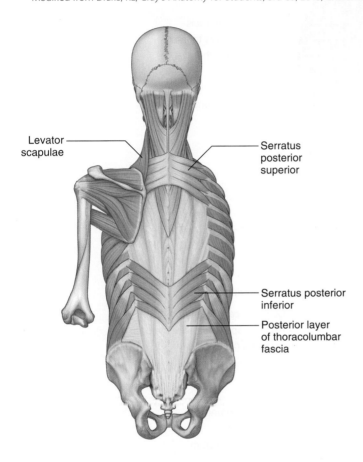

Fig. 5.7 Intermediate group of back muscles.
(From Drake, RL, Gray's Anatomy for Students, 3rd ed, 2015, Churchill Livingstone, Elsevier.)

The spinotransversales group of muscles are relatively superficial, and it is possible to palpate the splenius capitis muscle in the neck with gentle flexion. The erector spinae muscles can be palpated in the midline, especially the iliocostalis and longissimus muscles. It is not possible to palpate all of the deeper muscles; the multifidus muscle may be palpated in the lumbar region (Figs. 5.8 and 5.9).

The suboccipital triangle

The suboccipital muscles are a group of small muscles lying in the suboccipital triangle of the neck that are attached between the atlas and axis and skull base (Fig. 5.10). The group consists of rectus capitis posterior major, rectus capitis posterior minor, obliquus capitis inferior and obliquus capitis superior muscles. The suboccipital triangle is bordered medially by the rectus capitis posterior major muscle, laterally by the obliquus capitis superior muscle and inferiorly by the obliquus capitis inferior muscle. Within the triangle there are a number of structures, including the vertebral artery, the suboccipital venous plexus and the posterior ramus of C1 (the suboccipital nerve) (Table 5.4 and Fig. 5.11).

MOVEMENTS

Movements of the vertebral column are flexion and extension (in a sagittal plane), lateral flexion (in a coronal plane) and rotation. The movement between individual vertebrae is determined mainly by the shape and orientation of the zygapophyseal joints. In the cervical region, the upward slope of the joint permits flexion and extension, rotation and lateral flexion. In the thoracic region, the near vertical slope limits flexion and extension but permits lateral flexion and rotation. In the lumbar region, the shape of the joint limits rotational movement, although there is some degree of flexion and extension. Movements between individual vertebrae are small, but over the entire length of the column these individual differences are magnified. In the cervical region especially, a wide range of movement occurs. Cervical flexion and extension is greatest at the atlanto-occipital joints, whereas cervical rotation is greatest at the atlanto-axial joints. Between C2 and C7, the range of flexion increases towards C4–C5 level, after which it decreases.

VERTEBRAL CANAL AND SPINAL NERVES

The space enclosed by the vertebrae collectively forms a canal running the length of the column that contains the spinal cord and cauda equina. The spinal cord begins at the foramen magnum as a continuation of the medulla oblongata. The spinal cord exhibits enlargements in the cervical and lumbar regions. These correspond to areas of the cord that supply the limbs. In the adult, the spinal cord typically terminates as the conus medullaris near the intervertebral disc between L1 and L2 vertebrae (Fig. 5.12). From this point the dorsal and ventral roots of the lower lumbar, sacral and coccygeal cord segments leave the cord to form the cauda equina within the subarachnoid space. The dorsal and ventral roots merge to form spinal nerves that exit at their corresponding intervertebral foramina.

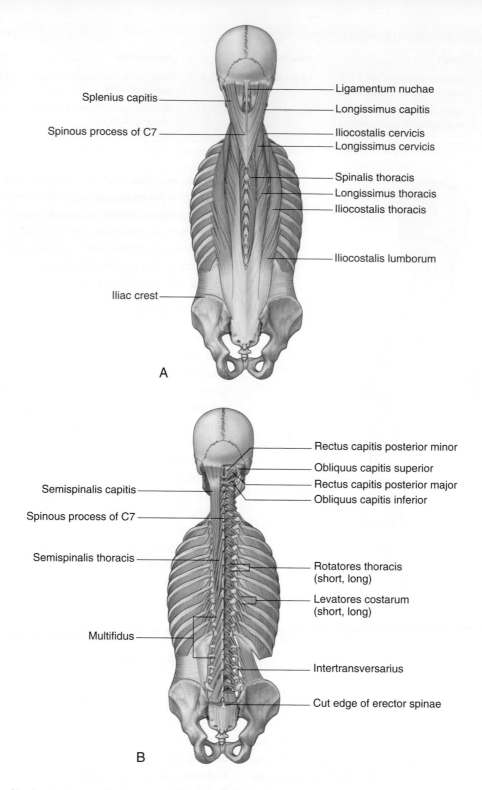

Splenius capitis

Spinous process of C7

Iliac crest

Ligamentum nuchae

Longissimus capitis

Iliocostalis cervicis

Longissimus cervicis

Spinalis thoracis

Longissimus thoracis

Iliocostalis thoracis

Iliocostalis lumborum

A

Semispinalis capitis

Spinous process of C7

Semispinalis thoracis

Multifidus

Rectus capitis posterior minor

Obliquus capitis superior

Rectus capitis posterior major

Obliquus capitis inferior

Rotatores thoracis
(short, long)

Levatores costarum
(short, long)

Intertransversarius

Cut edge of erector spinae

B

Fig. 5.8 Deep group of back muscles. A, Erector spinae muscles. B, Transversospinales and segmental muscles.
(From Drake, RL, Gray's Anatomy for Students, 3rd ed, 2015, Churchill Livingstone, Elsevier.)

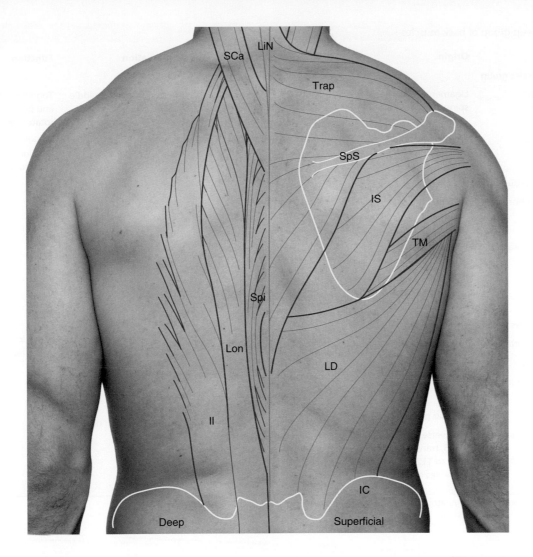

Fig. 5.9 Surface projections of back muscles. *IC*, iliac crest; *II*, iliocostalis; *IS*, infraspinatus; *LD*, latissimus dorsi; *LiN*, ligamentum nuchae, *Lon*, longissimus; *SCa,* semispinalis capitis; *Spi*, spinalis; *SpS*, spine of scapula; *TM*, teres major; *Trap*, trapezius.

To Do (Fig. 5.9)

Back:

- On the right side, draw the trapezius muscle. Starting at the external occipital protuberance, draw a line inferiorly in the midline to the level of the T12 spinous process. At T12, draw a line in a lateral and superior direction up to the insertion points on the spine of the scapula and acromion. Then continue the line in a superior and medial direction back to 2–3 cm lateral to the external occipital protuberance.
- On the right side, draw the latissimus dorsi muscle. Starting at T5 spinous process draw a line in a superior lateral direction, to the intertubercular sulcus of the humerus. Extend the line inferiorly to the iliac crest.
- On the left side, draw the splenius capitis muscle. In the neck region, palpate the splenius capitis muscle 5 cm lateral to the midline. To begin drawing, start at the external occipital protuberance. Move 5 cm laterally and trace this muscle inferiorly towards the midline to T4.
- On the left side, draw the erector spinae muscles. Starting in the midline immediately lateral to the spinous processes, draw in the spinalis muscle. Lateral to spinalis, add in longissimus and then the iliocostalis muscles at the level of the angles of the ribs.

Table 5.3 Deep group of back muscles

Muscle	Origin	Insertion	Innervation	Function
Spinotransversales group				
Splenius capitis	Ligamentum nuchae, spinous processes of C7–T4	Mastoid process, skull below superior nuchal line	Posterior rami of middle cervical nerves	Together—extend head and neck; individually—rotate head to one side
Splenius cervicis	Spinous processes of T3–T6	Transverse processes of C1–C3	Posterior rami of lower cervical nerves	Together—extend neck; individually—rotate head to one side
Erector spinae group				
Iliocostalis (lumborum, thoracis, cervicis)	Sacrum Angles of ribs	Angles of ribs Transverse processes of C4 to C7		
Longissimus (thoracis, cervicis, capitis)	Transverse processes of T1 to L5, articular processes of C4 to C7	Transverse processes of C2 to C6	Posterior rami of respective spinal nerves	
Spinalis (thoracis, cervicis, capitis)	Spinous processes of T10–L2	Spinous processes of T1 to T8 and C2		
Transversospinales group				
Semispinalis (thoracis, cervicis, capitis)	Transverse processes of C7–T10	Spinous processes of C2–T4		Extension, side flexion and rotation
Multifidus	Sacrum, mammillary process of L1–L5, transverse processes of T1–T12, articular process of C4–C7	Spinous processes of C2–L5	Posterior rami of respective spinal nerves	
Rotatores (thoracis)	Transverse process of L1–L5, transverse processes of T1 to T12, articular processes of C1 to C7	Spinous processes of thoracic vertebrae		

Modified from Drake, RL, Gray's Anatomy for Students, 3rd ed, 2015, Churchill Livingstone, Elsevier.

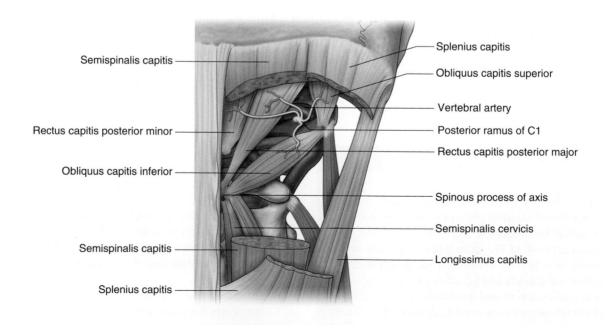

Fig. 5.10 Suboccipital triangle.
(From Drake, RL, Gray's Anatomy for Students, 3rd ed, 2015, Churchill Livingstone, Elsevier.)

Table 5.4   Suboccipital group of back muscles

Muscle	Origin	Insertion	Innervation	Function
Rectus capitis posterior major	Spinous process of axis (C2)	Lateral portion of occipital bone below inferior nuchal line		Extension of head; rotation of face to same side as muscle
Rectus capitis posterior minor	Posterior tubercle of atlas (C1)	Medial portion of occipital bone below inferior nuchal line		Extension of head
Obliquus capitis superior	Transverse process of atlas (C1)	Occipital bone	Posterior ramus of C1	Extension of head and bends it to same side
Obliquus capitis inferior	Spinous process of axis (C2)	Transverse process of atlas (C1)		Rotation of face to same side

Modified from Drake, RL, Gray's Anatomy for Students, 3rd ed, 2015, Churchill Livingstone, Elsevier.

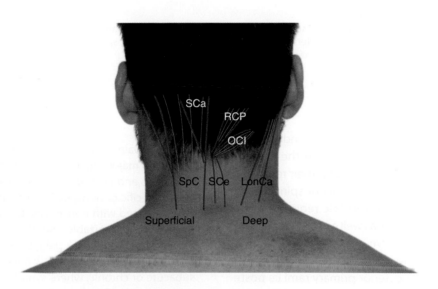

Fig. 5.11 Surface projections of the muscles of the posterior aspect of the neck. *LonCa*, longissimus capitis; *OCI*, obliquus capitis inferior; *RCP*, rectus capitis posterior; *SCa*, semispinalis capitis; *SCe*, semispinalis cervicis; *SpC*, splenius capitis.

To Do (Fig. 5.11)

Posterior neck:
- Palpate the occiput (the posterior aspect of the skull). Moving laterally, palpate the external occipital protuberance, and then across the nuchal areas to the mastoid process.
- Palpate the cervical facet joints, which are located about 2 cm lateral to each spinous process. These are small domelike projections beneath the trapezius muscle.

To Do (Fig. 5.11)

Test the range of cervical movement:
- First test extension and flexion by asking the subject to raise and lower their chin as far as possible without shoulder movement.
- Rotation is tested by asking the subject to turn their nose as far as possible to the right and left but with no shoulder movement.
- Lateral flexion is tested by asking the subject to touch each ear on the respective shoulder with no shoulder movement. About a 45° tilt should normally be observed.

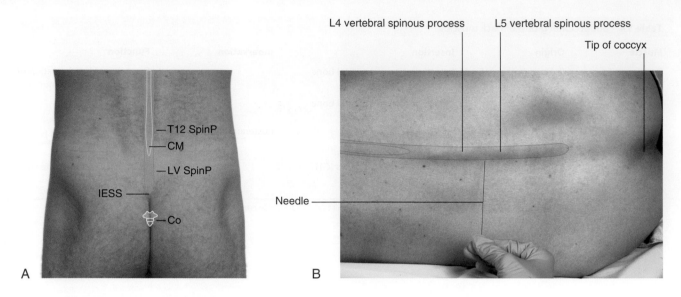

Fig. 5.12 Surface projections of the spinal cord and subarachnoid space indicated. A, In a man. B, Showing the position of a lumbar puncture. *CM*, conus medullaris; *Co*, Coccyx; *IESS*, inferior end of subarachnoid space; *SpinP*, spinous process.
(Modified from Drake, RL, Gray's Anatomy for Students, 3rd ed, 2015, Churchill Livingstone, Elsevier.)

There are 31 pairs of spinal nerves corresponding to the segmental arrangement of development in the embryo. Each pair is transmitted bilaterally through their respective intervertebral foramina. There are 8 pairs of spinal nerves in the cervical region, 12 in the thoracic region, 5 in the lumbar and 5 in the sacral region, as well as 1 in the coccygeal region (Fig. 5.13). After the nerve exits its respective intervertebral foramen it divides into anterior and posterior primary rami. The smaller posterior primary rami lie posteriorly and supply the deep back muscles as well as skin overlying that region. Medial branches from the posterior rami also supply the zygapophyseal joints. The larger anterior rami pass anteriorly, curving around the trunk, to supply body wall muscles and the limb plexuses.

In the Clinic

The surface features of the back may be used in the determination of thoracic and abdominal organ location as well as the positioning of spinal nerves for spinal nerve blocks (local or regional anesthesia). Surface features are also important for determining the termination level of the spinal cord for lumbar puncture.

Low back pain is a complex clinical condition that has become a major socio-economic problem due to lost work days and healthcare costs. It can be classified as either specific or nonspecific. The majority of patients are diagnosed with nonspecific low back pain, where there is no recognizable underlying cause. In many of these patients, low back pain is probably caused by muscle strain. Nonspecific low back pain can be acute, subacute or chronic, where symptoms persist for longer than 3 months. For the majority of patients, symptoms are acute and persist for less than 2 weeks. A specific cause can be determined in only 10% of patients with low back pain, for example, mechanical compression of a nerve, inflammation, infection, tumors, rheumatoid arthritis or osteoporosis. Mechanical compression of spinal nerves or nerve roots is usually caused by herniation of the nucleus pulposus, spinal stenosis (a narrowing of the spinal canal) and spondylolisthesis (movement of the vertebra in an anterior or posterior direction). Typically, patients will describe radiating pain into the lower limb (known as sciatica), as well as weakness and numbness. For the majority of these patients, symptoms will be chronic, persisting for longer than 3 months. Accurate assessment and diagnosis of low back pain is dependent on being able to perform a thorough examination of the vertebral column and lower limb. This will include an examination of joint motion, muscle tenderness, muscle strength, pulse points, dermatomes and cutaneous nerve mapping, all of which rely on a knowledge of surface anatomy.

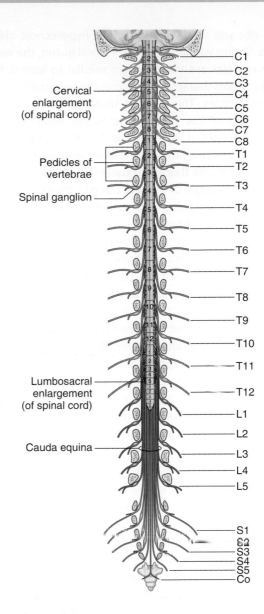

Cervical enlargement (of spinal cord)

Pedicles of vertebrae

Spinal ganglion

Lumbosacral enlargement (of spinal cord)

Cauda equina

C1
C2
C3
C4
C5
C6
C7
C8
T1
T2
T3
T4
T5
T6
T7
T8
T9
T10
T11
T12
L1
L2
L3
L4
L5
S1
S2
S3
S4
S5
Co

Fig. 5.13 Course of spinal nerves in the vertebral canal. *(From Drake, RL, Gray's Anatomy for Students, 3rd ed, 2015, Churchill Livingstone, Elsevier.)*

Ultrasound

Subject position

Imaging is performed with the subject sitting on a stool with their back to the operator, or lying prone. Flexion of the back will allow visualization of the space between the laminae and vertebral canal.

Transducer

Use either a linear or curved array transducer. The type of transducer used will depend upon the region of the back to be imaged and the muscle thickness. The curved array transducer can be used to image deeper structures. Set the depth setting to between 2–6 cm (linear array transducer), or 6–12 cm (curved array transducer).

Transducer position

Position the transducer immediately lateral to the spinous processes in the transverse plane for short-axis views or the sagittal plane for long-axis views. Scan either cranially or caudally along the vertebral column. To image the space between the lamina and spinal canal, the transducer is best positioned in a sagittal plane over the lamina and angled medially. Alternatively, the spinal canal can be imaged in transverse plane.

Image features

Cervical

In the transverse plane, the hyperechoic posterior surfaces of the cervical vertebrae can be inspected (Fig. 5.14). Prominent features include the bifid spinous processes of C2–C7 and lamina. Overlying the spinous processes, the ligamentum nuchae appears as a thick hyperechoic band spanning the length of the cervical region. Laterally the short transverse processes can be identified. Scanning cranially from the level of the C7 vertebra towards the atlas, several muscle layers can be inspected. Superficially, the upper fibers of the trapezius muscle will be visible. This muscle layer becomes thinner towards the occiput. Deep to the trapezius muscle, the splenius capitis muscle will be in view, and deep to this muscle, the semispinalis capitis and semispinalis cervicis muscles. Each of these muscles are surrounded by a clearly defined hyperechoic myofascial plane. Sitting adjacent to the lamina, between the spinous process and the articulating process, the multifidus muscle will be in view.

Thoracic

With the transducer in the transverse plane lateral to the mid thoracic spinous processes (T3–T6), the posterior surfaces of the thoracic vertebrae and the medial border of the scapula can be inspected (Fig. 5.15A). Between these bony landmarks, the trapezius (superficial) and rhomboid (deep) muscles are visible. With the transducer over the intercostal spaces, the intercostal muscles can also be examined. Deep to the intercostal muscles, the surface of the pleura appears as a mid-gray colored line. The lung tissue is anechoic, although horizontal reverberation lines may be present. In the sagittal plane, the outer surfaces of the ribs appear as a series of hyperechoic arcs (Fig. 5.15B).

With the transducer in the transverse plane immediately lateral to the lower thoracic spinous processes, the posterior of the ribs will be in view as bright hyperechoic oblique streaks. Sitting within the paravertebral gutter, the erector spinae muscles are visible. From medial to lateral, these are the spinales thoracis, longissimus thoracis and iliocostalis thoracis muscles. The spinales thoracis muscle, which is the smallest of the three muscles, lies adjacent to the spinous processes of the vertebrae. The longissimus thoracis muscle lies in close proximity to the transverse processes, and the iliocostalis thoracis muscle lies over the posterior surfaces of the angle of the ribs. Deep to the erector spinae muscles, the multifidus muscle can be seen against the lamina of the vertebrae.

With the transducer positioned in the sagittal plane over the lamina and angled medially, the space between the lamina and spinal canal can be visualized (Fig. 5.16B). In this view, the laminae appear as a series of hyperechoic curves. In between the laminae, several horizontal streaks should be visible. These are the ligamenta flava, posterior dura and anterior longitudinal ligament. The ligamenta flava may appear as a slightly thickened band. The epidural space is seen as a narrow hypoechoic gap between the ligamenta flava and posterior dura. The spinal cord sits between the posterior dura and anterior longitudinal ligament, although there is very little detail on ultrasound.

Lumbar

In the transverse plane, the posterior surfaces of the lumbar vertebrae will be in view (Fig. 5.17A). The supraspinous ligament can be seen superficial to the spinous processes. Superficial to the transverse processes, the deep back musculature can be inspected. Medially, the multifidus muscle is visible. It is at its thickest within the lumbar region and has a characteristic triangular shape. Lateral to the multifidus muscle, the erector spinae muscles can be observed. The most prominent are the longissimus thoracis muscle, which lies adjacent to the transverse processes, and the iliocostalis lumborum muscle, which lies over the ribs. With the probe positioned in the sagittal plane over a lamina and angled medially, the space between the lamina and spinal canal can be visualized (Fig. 5.17B). In this view, the image is similar to the thoracic region. In between the hyperechoic laminae, the ligamenta flava, posterior dura and anterior longitudinal ligament appear as a series of longitudinal streaks. The epidural space is seen as a narrow hypoechoic gap between the ligamenta flava and posterior dura.

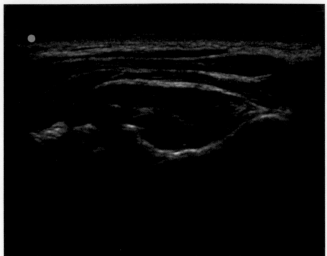

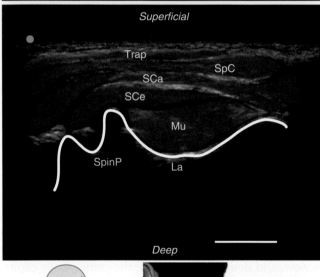

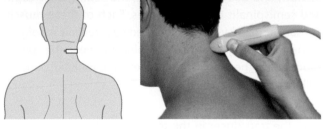

Fig. 5.14 Ultrasound of the right cervical region of the back at the level of the C5 vertebra. *La*, lamina; *Mu*, multifidus; *SCa*, semispinalis capitus; *SCe*, semispinalis cervicis; *SpC*, splenius capitis; *SpinP*, spinous process; *Trap*, trapezius. Scale bar = 1 cm.

surfaces of the thoracic vertebrae will be in view (Fig. 5.16A). The supraspinous ligament, which is a continuation of the ligamentum nuchae, can be seen as a hyperechoic arc superficial to the spinous processes. Lateral to the transverse processes, the posterior surfaces of the angle

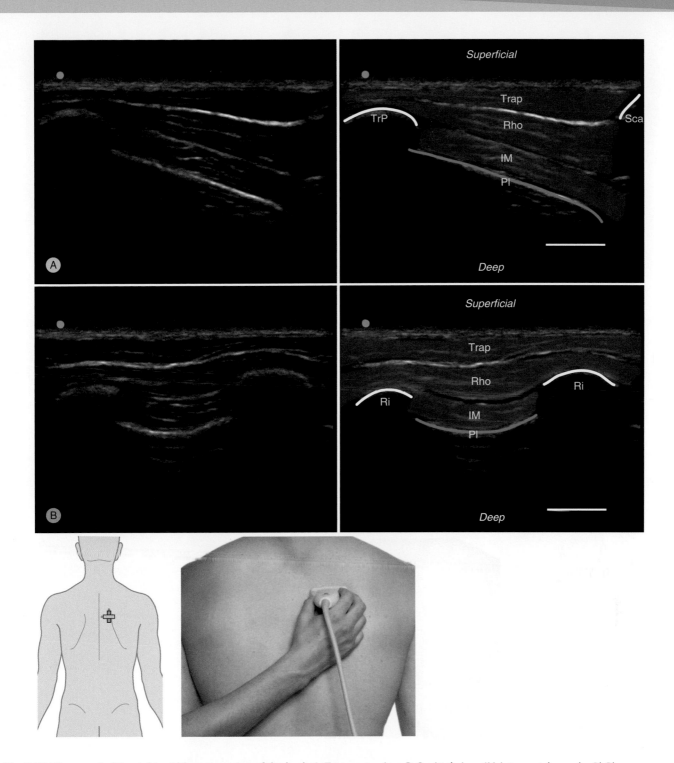

Fig. 5.15 Ultrasound of the right midthoracic region of the back. A, Transverse view. B, Sagittal view. *IM*, intercostal muscle; *Pl*, Pleura; *Rho*, rhomboid; *Ri*, rib; *Sca*, scapula; *Trap*, trapezius; *TrP*, transverse process. Scale bar = 1 cm.

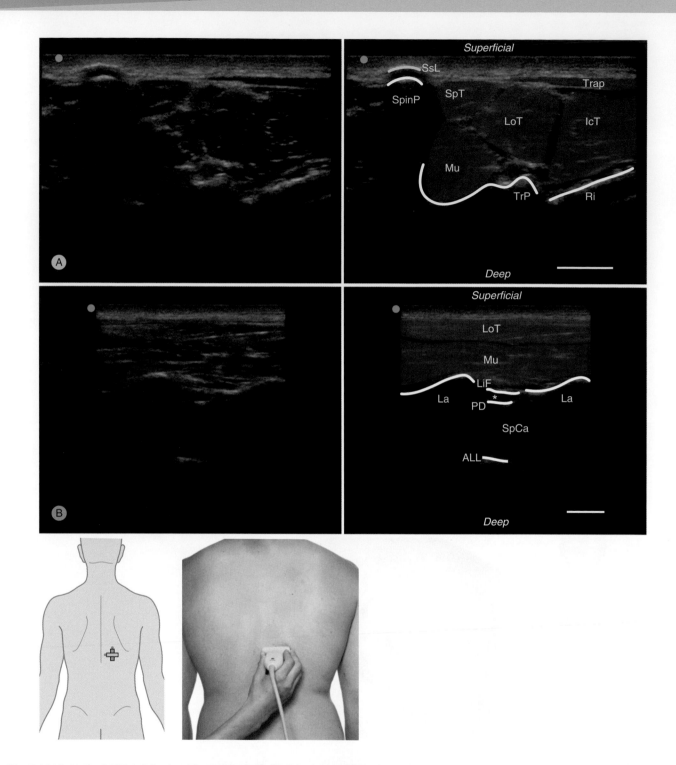

Fig. 5.16 Ultrasound of the right thoracic region of the back at the level of T10 vertebra. A, Transverse view. B, Sagittal view. *, epidural space; *ALL*, anterior longitudinal ligament; *IcT*, iliocostalis thoracis; *La*, lamina; *LiF*, ligamentum flava; *LoT*, longissimus thoracis; *Mu*, multifidus; *PD*, posterior dura; *Ri*, rib; *SpCa*, spinal canal; *SpinP*, spinous process; *SpT*, spinalis thoracis; *SsL*, supraspinous ligament; *Trap*, trapezius; *TrP*, transverse process. Scale bar = 1 cm.

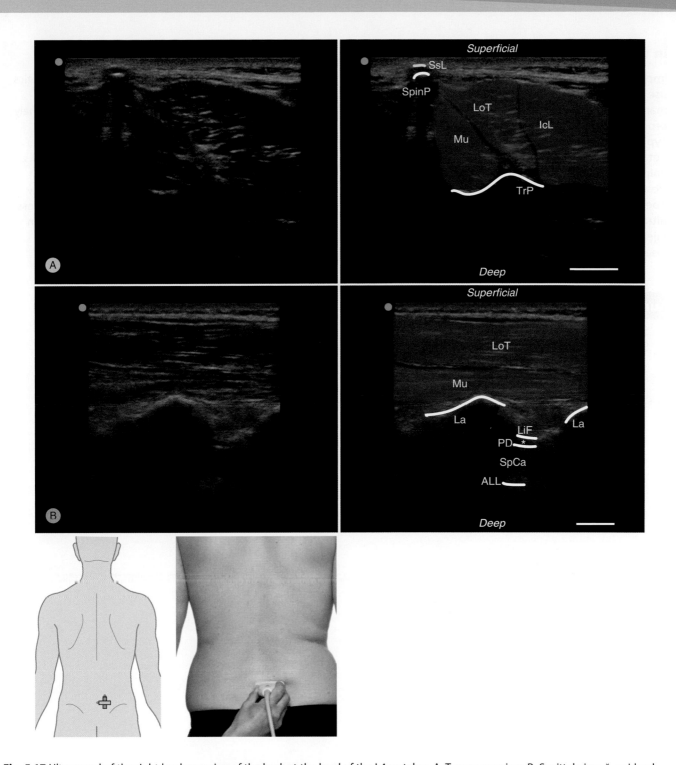

Fig. 5.17 Ultrasound of the right lumbar region of the back at the level of the L4 vertebra. A, Transverse view. B, Sagittal view. *, epidural space; *ALL*, anterior longitudinal ligament; *IcL*, iliocostalis lumborum; *La*, lamina; *LiF*, ligamentum flava; *LoT*, longissimus thoracis; *Mu*, multifidus; *PD*, posterior dura; *SpCa*, spinal canal; *SpinP*, spinous process; *SsL*, supraspinous ligament; *TrP*, transverse process. Scale bar = 1 cm.

In the Clinic

Improvements in image quality have led to the growing use of ultrasound in the field of anesthesiology and pain management, where it is used to guide neuraxial procedures, such as epidural and intrathecal injections. Typically, neuraxial drug administration relies on a detailed knowledge of surface anatomy and the ability to palpate bony features, such as the spinous processes. However, in some patients, including those who are obese, bony landmarks can be difficult to identify. Thus, ultrasound has become an important tool to guide injections into the epidural space, as well as for the insertion of epidural catheters. This approach is particularly important for the administration of anesthetics for pain relief during labor, abdominal surgery or the management of radicular pain. Ultrasound is also routinely used to guide injections around facet joints for the treatment of back pain as well as lumbar punctures in patients where it is difficult to identify surface landmarks. Importantly, the use of ultrasound has been shown to reduce the number of puncture attempts. More recently, ultrasound has been used to identify changes in thickness of the deep back muscles in patients with low back pain and as a tool to assess scoliosis (lateral deviation of the curve of the spine).

Summary Checklist

- Surface projections of the bones related to the back
- Surface projections of the muscles of the back
- Curvatures of the back
- Movement of the back
- Ultrasound imaging of the back muscles

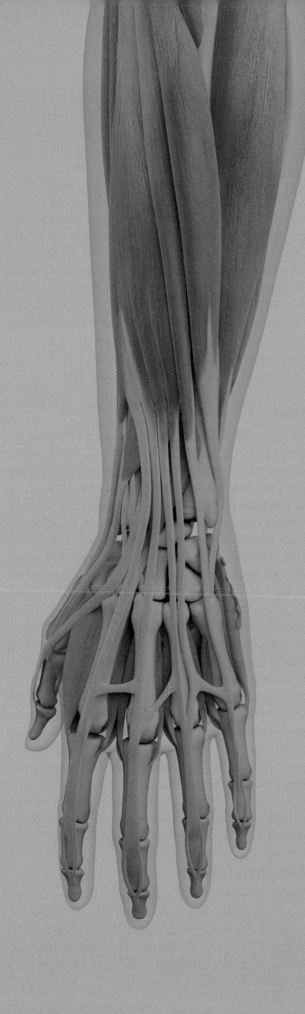

6 Upper limb

Conceptual overview

The upper limbs articulate with the pectoral girdle at the glenohumeral joint. The main function of the upper limbs is to enable the mechanical manipulation of objects. The surface contours of the upper limb are defined by its musculature, bony points, superficial tissues and the prominence of certain blood vessels, particularly superficial veins. The bones of the upper limb are the scapula, clavicle, humerus, radius, ulna, carpals, metacarpals and phalanges. The upper limb is divided into four regions: the shoulder, arm, forearm and hand. The arm and forearm are further divided into compartments that are separated by fascial septa. Each compartment is occupied by a group of functionally related muscles. Knowledge of the surface markings of the structures of the upper limb is important in the management and treatment of fractures, peripheral nerve injuries and sports injuries.

Surface anatomy

SHOULDER

Bones

The bones of the shoulder are the scapula, clavicle and humerus. The clavicle and scapula form the pectoral girdle. The pectoral girdle is attached to the trunk by the superficial back muscles, which extend from the vertebral column to the scapula and humerus.

The clavicle is an S-shaped bone that has a forward-facing convex curve medially and a concave curve laterally, both of which can be palpated. It articulates at its medial end with the sternum to form the sternoclavicular joint, and at its lateral end with the acromion to form the acromioclavicular joint (Fig. 6.1). Both joints can be palpated. The clavicle is essential in supporting the limb on the trunk via the coracoclavicular ligament, which cannot be palpated.

The scapula is a flat triangle-shaped bone on the posterior surface of the thoracic cage. The body of the scapula has a clearly defined lateral, medial and superior borders, and a superior and inferior angle at either pole. The lateral and medial borders can be easily palpated, whereas the superior border is more difficult to identify. On the superior border is a hooklike projection, the coracoid process, which can be felt inferior to the lateral end of the clavicle. Running across the dorsal surface of the scapula is a ridge called the spine, which terminates laterally as the acromion. The spine can be easily palpated on the posterior surface of the thorax. The acromion can be palpated superior to the glenohumeral

joint. The region above the spine of the scapula is the supraspinous fossa, and below is the infraspinous fossa (Fig. 6.2). The coracoacromial ligament extends between the coracoid and acromion to form the coracoacromial arch. This arch is palpable between these bony points.

The major joint in the shoulder region is the glenohumeral joint, which is an articulation between the glenoid fossa of the scapula and the head of the humerus (see glenohumeral joint, p 86). The round contour of the shoulder is provided by the greater tubercle of the humerus and the overlying deltoid muscle. With the arm by the side, the greater tubercle can be palpated. Medial to the greater tubercle, on the anterior surface, the lesser tubercle can be felt with the arm laterally rotated. The intertubercular sulcus (or bicipital groove) lies between the tubercles, inferior to the acromioclavicular joint when the arm is adducted (Fig. 6.3). The proximal part of this vertical groove is palpable.

Muscles

The most superficial muscles of the shoulder are the trapezius and deltoid muscles (Table 6.1 and Fig. 6.4). The trapezius muscle is a large sheetlike triangular-shaped muscle that sweeps from the spinous processes to the spine of the scapula and distal clavicle and is easily palpable. Similarly, the deltoid muscle is also easily palpated. Deep to the trapezius muscle are the levator scapulae and rhomboid muscles (Table 6.1 and Fig. 6.4). The rhomboid major muscle can be palpated between the lower fibers of the trapezius muscle and the most inferior part of the medial border of the scapula.

Surrounding the glenohumeral joint are the supraspinatus, infraspinatus, teres minor and subscapularis muscles. These are jointly known as the rotator cuff muscles (Table 6.2 and Fig. 6.5). The rotator cuff muscles originate from the scapula and insert into the greater or lesser tubercles of the humerus. The infraspinatus and teres minor muscles can be identified inferior to the spine of the scapula toward the lateral edge of the bone during a resisted lateral rotation of the arm. The other rotator cuff muscles cannot easily be observed. Inferior to the teres minor muscle is the teres major muscle. With the arm abducted and medially rotated, this muscle can be palpated between the lateral border of the scapula and the humerus.

Glenohumeral joint

The glenohumeral joint is a ball and socket joint with a wide range of movement, which includes flexion, extension, abduction, adduction, medial and lateral rotation and circumduction of the arm. This range of movement is mainly due to the large head of the humerus articulating on a shallow glenoid fossa.

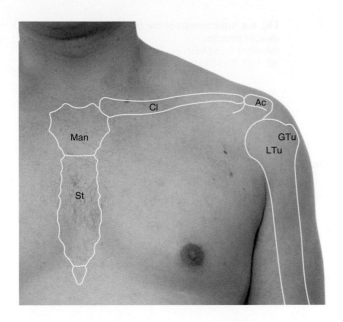

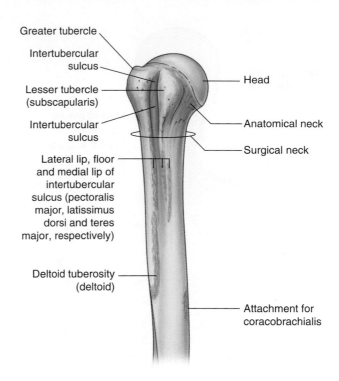

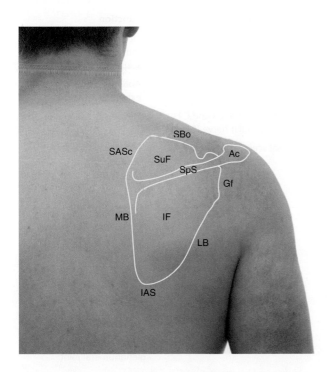

Fig. 6.1 Surface projections of the shoulder region. *Ac*, acromion; *Cl*, clavicle; *GTu*, greater tubercle; *Hu*, humerus; *LTu*, lesser tubercle; *Man*, manubrium; *St*, sternum.

Fig. 6.3 Proximal end of right humerus.
(From Drake, RL, Gray's Anatomy for Students, 3rd ed, 2015, Churchill Livingstone, Elsevier.)

Fig. 6.2 Surface projections of the scapula. *Ac*, acromion; *Gf*, glenoid fossa; *IAS*, inferior angle of scapula; *IF*, infraspinous fossa; *LB*, lateral border; *MB*, medial border; *SASc*, superior angle of scapula; *SBo*, superior border; *SpS*, spine of scapula; *SuF*, supraspinous fossa.

To Do (Figs. 6.1 and 6.2)

Lateral aspect:
- Start by palpating the lesser tubercle which is more anterior. You may find palpation easier when the arm is by the side and laterally rotated.
- Examine the distal half of the shaft of the humerus. The proximal part is surrounded by the deltoid muscle and so it is not palpable.

Anterior aspect of the thorax:
- Palpate the length of the clavicle.
- At the medial end of the clavicle, palpate the sternoclavicular joint. To appreciate movement at this joint, try elevating (shrugging) and depressing or protracting and retracting your shoulders.
- At the lateral end of the clavicle, palpate the acromioclavicular joint. To appreciate movement at this joint, try abducting your arm above your head.
- Palpate the acromion and coracoid process. The coracoid process lies inferior to the lateral end of the clavicle.

Posterior aspect of the thorax:
- Locate the inferior angle of the scapula at the level of the seventh rib and make a dot. Palpate the medial border and continue up to the superior angle, which lies level with the second rib, and make another dot. Join the two dots by drawing a line along the medial border.
- Palpate the spine of the scapula, which ends close to the midline at the medial border of the scapula at the level of the T3 vertebra. Draw a line following the spine of the scapula.

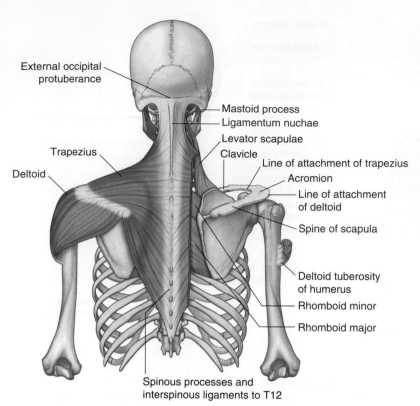

External occipital protuberance

Mastoid process
Ligamentum nuchae
Levator scapulae
Clavicle
Line of attachment of trapezius
Acromion
Line of attachment of deltoid
Spine of scapula

Trapezius

Deltoid

Deltoid tuberosity of humerus
Rhomboid minor
Rhomboid major

Spinous processes and interspinous ligaments to T12

Fig. 6.4 Attachments of the trapezius and deltoid muscles.
(Modified from Drake, RL, Gray's Anatomy for Students, 3rd ed, 2015, Churchill Livingstone, Elsevier.)

Table 6.1 Muscles of the shoulder

Muscle	Origin	Insertion	Innervation	Function
Trapezius	External occipital protuberance, nuchal ligament and spinous processes of C7 to T12 vertebrae	Spine of the scapula, acromion, and lateral one-third of clavicle	Accessory nerve and anterior rami of C3 and C4	Elevates, depresses, retracts and rotates scapula
Deltoid	Spine of the scapula, acromion and lateral one-third of clavicle	Deltoid tuberosity of humerus	Axillary nerve (C5, C6)	Abducts, flexes and extends arm
Levator scapulae	Transverse processes of C1 to C4 vertebrae	Superior angle of the scapula	Anterior rami of C3 and C4 and dorsal scapular nerve (C5)	Elevates the scapula
Rhomboid minor	Spinous processes of C7 and T1 vertebrae	Medial border of scapula	Dorsal scapular nerve (C4, C5)	Elevates and retracts the scapula
Rhomboid major	Spinous processes of T2 to T5 vertebrae			

Modified from Drake, RL, Gray's Anatomy for Students, 3rd ed, 2015, Churchill Livingstone, Elsevier.

Table 6.2 Muscles of the scapular region

Muscle	Origin	Insertion	Innervation	Function
Supraspinatus	Supraspinous fossa of the scapula	Superior facet on the greater tubercle of the humerus	Suprascapular nerve (C5, C6)	Initiates abduction of arm to 15° at glenohumeral joint
Infraspinatus	Infraspinous fossa of the scapula	Middle facet on the greater tubercle of the humerus		Lateral rotation of arm at glenohumeral joint
Teres minor	Lateral border of the scapula	Inferior facet on the greater tubercle of the humerus	Axillary nerve (C5, C6)	
Teres major	Inferior angle of the scapula	Medial lip of the intertubercular sulcus on the humerus	Inferior subscapular nerve (C5, C6, C7)	Medial rotation and extension of the arm at the glenohumeral joint
Subscapularis	Subscapular fossa of the scapula	Lesser tubercle of the humerus	Upper and lower subscapular nerves (C5, C6, C7)	Medial rotation of arm at glenohumeral joint

Modified from Drake, RL, Gray's Anatomy for Students, 3rd ed, 2015, Churchill Livingstone, Elsevier.

Due to the shape of the glenoid cavity and the presence of the surrounding ligaments, the arm can only be abducted to 90 degrees (Figs. 6.6 and 6.7). To position the upper limb above the head, further degrees of abduction are possible by rotating the scapula, thus rotating the angle of the glenoid cavity superiorly. As the scapula is rotated, its positional change may be verified by palpation of the spine or inferior angle of the scapula.

AXILLA

The axilla is a gateway for structures entering or leaving the upper limb from the neck and thorax. It is formed by an apex, base (floor) and four walls. The muscles, bony features and skin folds that form the boundaries can be palpated. The main structures passing through the axilla are the axillary artery and vein and various components of the brachial plexus.

The triangular inlet of the axilla is formed anteriorly by the clavicle, medially by the first rib and posteriorly by the superior border of the scapula. Each of these bony features can be palpated. The first rib can be felt at the lateral margin of the trapezius muscle at the base of the neck, as well as posteroinferior to the clavicle. The superior border of the scapula can be located by tracing along the medial edge toward the superior angle. The base of the axilla is formed by skin and subcutaneous tissue, which creates the axillary fossa (armpit). The anterior axillary wall is formed by the pectoralis major and minor muscles. The posterior wall is formed by the teres major, latissimus dorsi and subscapularis muscles. The medial wall of the axilla is formed by serratus anterior muscle. Each of these muscles is palpable. Laterally, the axilla is bordered by the shaft of the humerus (Figs. 6.8 and 6.9).

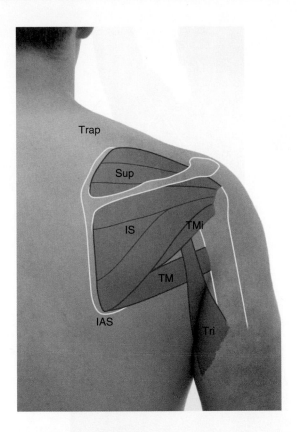

Fig. 6.5 Surface projections of muscles of the shoulder. *IAS*, inferior angle of scapula; *IS*, infraspinatus; *Sup*, supraspinatus; *TM*, teres major; *TMi*, teres minor; *Trap*, trapezius; *Tri*, triceps.

To Do (Fig. 6.5)

Posterior aspect:
- With your thumb on the medial border of the scapula and your index and middle fingers on the lateral border, examine the rotation of the scapula during abduction of the arm.
- Locate the infraspinatus muscle immediately inferior to the spine of the scapula. Also, palpate the teres major and minor muscles.
- Using the landmarks of the scapula already marked out, draw in the teres minor muscle extending from lateral border of the scapula.
- Add in the teres major muscle as it arises from the inferior angle and sweeps superiorly and laterally to the medial lip of the intertubercular sulcus.
- Add in the supraspinatus, infraspinatus and teres minor muscles as they pass laterally to the greater tubercle of the humerus.

To Do (Fig. 6.5)

Anterior aspect:
- Palpate the axillary inlet, which is bordered anteriorly by the clavicle, medially by the first rib, and posteriorly by the superior border of the scapula.
- Locate the pectoralis major muscle as it forms the anterior axillary wall. It is possible to grasp the anterior axillary fold between your finger and thumb.
- Locate the latissimus dorsi and teres major muscles as they form the posterior axillary wall.

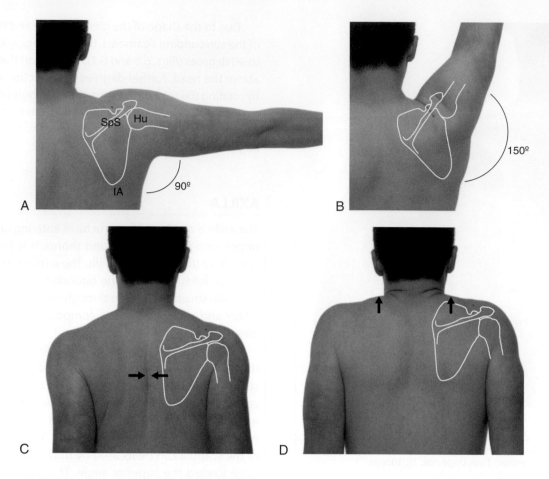

A

B

C

D

Fig. 6.6 Movement of the scapula. A, 90-degree abduction. B, 150-degree abduction. C, Retraction. D, Elevation. *Hu*, humerus; *IA*, inferior angle; *SpS*, spine of scapula.

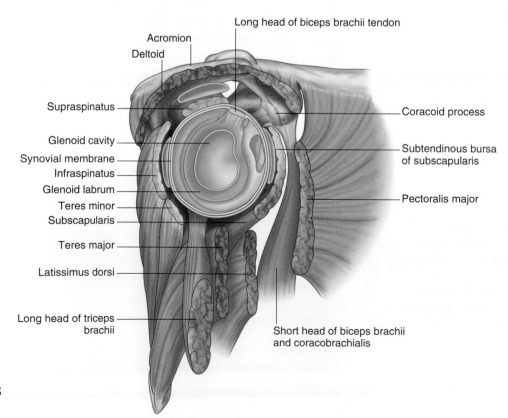

Long head of biceps brachii tendon

Acromion

Deltoid

Supraspinatus

Glenoid cavity

Synovial membrane

Infraspinatus

Glenoid labrum

Teres minor

Subscapularis

Teres major

Latissimus dorsi

Long head of triceps brachii

Coracoid process

Subtendinous bursa of subscapularis

Pectoralis major

Short head of biceps brachii and coracobrachialis

Fig. 6.7 Lateral view of right glenohumeral joint and surrounding muscles with proximal end of humerus removed.
(From Drake, RL, Gray's Anatomy for Students, 3rd ed, 2015, Churchill Livingstone, Elsevier.)

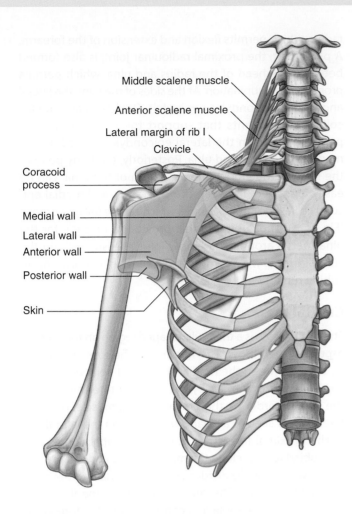

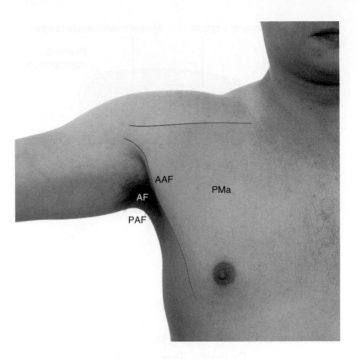

Fig. 6.9 Surface projections of the axilla. *AAF*, anterior axillary fold; *AF*, axillary fossa; *PAF*, posterior axillary fold; *PMa*, pectoralis major.

Muscles

Anterior compartment

The anterior compartment contains the biceps brachii, coracobrachialis and brachialis muscles (Table 6.3). The biceps brachii muscle forms a bulge on the anterior aspect of the arm, particularly when it is contracted during flexion of the forearm (Figs. 6.11 and 6.12). With the arm abducted and laterally rotated, the coracobrachialis muscle sits along an oblique line that extends from the coracoid to the shaft of the humerus. The brachialis muscle lies deep to the biceps brachii muscle. Immediately proximal to the elbow, this flat muscle can be palpated on either side of the biceps brachii muscle.

Posterior compartment

The only muscle of the posterior compartment of the arm is the triceps brachii muscle (Table 6.3 and Figs. 6.11 and 6.12). With the arm abducted and laterally rotated, each of the three heads can be observed. The long head can be observed extending from its origin on the scapula. Both lateral and medial heads are palpable on the posterolateral and posteromedial aspects of the arm, respectively. The tendon of the triceps brachii muscle can be tracked to its insertion into the olecranon of the ulna.

Elbow joint

The elbow joint involves three separate articulations (Fig. 6.13). A hinge joint is formed between the trochlea of the humerus and ulna and the capitulum of the humerus and

Fig. 6.8 The axilla. Walls and transition between neck and arm. *(From Drake, RL, Gray's Anatomy for Students, 3rd ed, 2015, Churchill Livingstone, Elsevier.)*

Middle scalene muscle
Anterior scalene muscle
Lateral margin of rib I
Clavicle
Coracoid process
Medial wall
Lateral wall
Anterior wall
Posterior wall
Skin

ARM

Bones

The bone of the arm is called the humerus. The head and greater and lesser tubercles have already been described (Fig. 6.3). Immediately inferior to the greater and lesser tubercles, which are both palpable, is the surgical neck of the humerus. The shaft of the humerus is triangular in cross section and can be palpated along much of its length. On the posterior surface is the radial groove for the radial nerve and profunda brachii artery, which cannot be felt. Since the shaft lies along the middle of the arm, together with fascia, it creates a division of the region into the anterior and posterior compartments. At the distal aspect, the lateral epicondyle and more prominent medial epicondyle can be identified on either side of the elbow joint. Similarly, the bony ridges immediately superior to the epicondyles, called the lateral and medial supraepicondylar ridges, can be felt. The condyle has two articular parts, the capitulum (lateral) and the trochlea (medial), which are not easily palpable (Fig. 6.10).

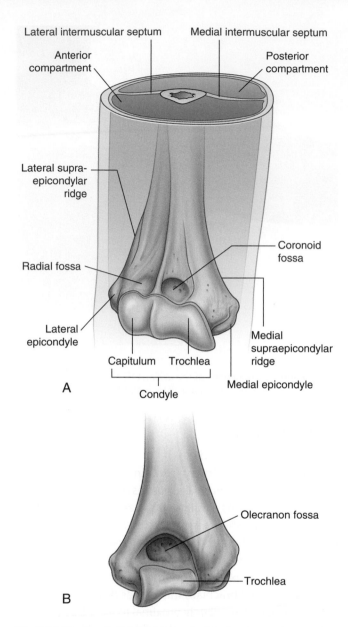

Fig. 6.10 Distal end of the humerus. A, Anterior aspect. B, Posterior aspect.
(From Drake, RL, Gray's Anatomy for Students, 3rd ed, 2015, Churchill Livingstone, Elsevier.)

radius, which permits flexion and extension of the forearm. A pivot joint, the proximal radioulnar joint, is also formed between the head of the radius and ulna, which permits pronation and supination. At the sides of the joint, the lateral and medial epicondyles can be felt. The lateral and medial collateral ligaments that support the joint can also be palpated between the lateral epicondyle and radius and medial epicondyle and ulna. Posteriorly, the bony point at the back of the elbow, the olecranon of the ulna, can be easily identified. Between the olecranon and medial epicondyle lies the cubital tunnel, which can be felt as a groove (Fig. 6.14). The cubital tunnel provides a passage for the ulnar nerve around the elbow joint. Pressure within the cubital tunnel may compress the ulnar nerve, leading to cubital tunnel syndrome.

Cubital fossa

The cubital fossa is a triangular-shaped region on the anterior aspect of the elbow. The midline of the fossa is marked by a line between the medial and lateral epicondyles. The medial border is formed by the pronator teres muscle and the lateral border by the brachioradialis muscle, pronator teres can be seen as a clear prominence on the lateral side of the proximal forearm (Fig. 6.15). Principal contents of the cubital fossa include the median nerve and the brachial artery, which usually divides within the fossa into the radial and ulnar arteries. The median nerve lies medial to the ulnar artery in the fossa and continues into the forearm to supply the anterior compartment. When the elbow joint is flexed, the biceps tendon is palpable as it descends to its insertion on the radial tuberosity. In most individuals, the median cubital vein can be observed coursing obliquely across the cubital fossa. This vein connects the basilic vein, on the medial side of the limb, with the cephalic vein, on the lateral side. The median cubital vein is an important site for venepuncture.

Table 6.3 Muscles of the anterior and posterior compartment of the arm

Muscle	Origin	Insertion	Innervation	Function
Coracobrachialis	Coracoid process	Midshaft of humerus	Musculocutaneous nerve (C5, C6, C7)	Flexor of the arm at the glenohumeral joint
Biceps brachii	Long head—supraglenoid tubercle of scapula; short head—coracoid process	Radial tuberosity	Musculocutaneous nerve (C5, C6)	Flexor and supinator of the forearm; flexor of the arm at the glenohumeral joint
Brachialis	Anterior surface of humerus	Tuberosity of the ulna	Musculocutaneous nerve (C5, C6)	Flexor of the forearm at the elbow joint
Triceps brachii	Long head—infraglenoid tubercle of scapula; medial and lateral heads—posterior surface of humerus	Olecranon of the ulna	Radial nerve (C6, C7, C8)	Extension of the arm at the glenohumeral joint and forearm at the elbow joint

Modified from Drake, RL, Gray's Anatomy for Students, 3rd ed, 2015, Churchill Livingstone, Elsevier.

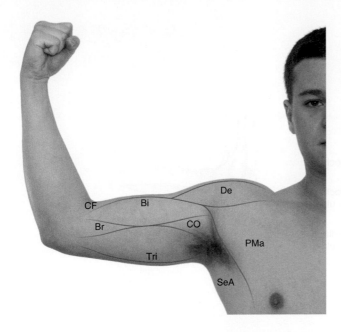

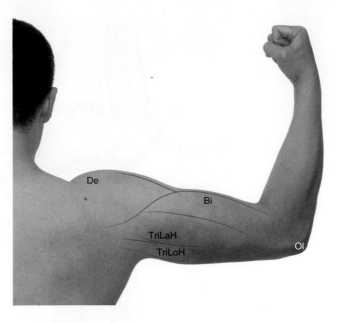

Fig. 6.11 Surface projections of the anterior aspect of the arm. *Bi*, biceps; *Br*, brachialis; *CF*, cubital fossa; *CO*, coracobrachialis; *De*, deltoid; *PMa*, pectoralis major; *SeA*, serratus anterior; *Tri*, triceps.

Fig. 6.12 Surface projections of the posterior aspect of the arm. *Bi*, biceps; *De*, deltoid; *Ol*, olecranon; *TriLaH*, triceps lateral head; *TriLoH*, triceps long head.

To Do (Figs. 6.11 and 6.12)

- Palpate the deltoid muscle during abduction of the arm.
- Palpate the biceps brachii and brachialis muscles during an isometric contraction of these muscles. This can be performed by asking the subject to flex their forearm against resistance.
- Palpate the triceps brachii muscle during an isometric contraction of this muscle. This can be performed by asking the subject to extend their forearm against resistance. Locate the long, lateral and medial heads of this muscle.
- Palpate the tendon of triceps as it attaches to the olecranon. This superficial point gives good access for testing the tendon reflex.

FOREARM

Bones

The bones of the forearm are the ulna and radius (Fig. 6.16). In the anatomical position, the radius is on the lateral side and the ulna on the medial side. Distally, the radius has a large expansion that articulates with the proximal carpal bones to form the radiocarpal, or wrist, joint. The proximal shaft of the radius is surrounded by muscle and is therefore not palpable, but it is possible to palpate the radius in the distal forearm. Immediately proximal to the

wrist joint, the radial styloid process can be easily felt on the lateral side of the forearm. The radial styloid process is relatively easily fractured, typically caused by a fall onto an outstretched hand. In contrast to the radius, the ulna has a large expansion proximally at the elbow joint, the olecranon. The olecranon and the shaft of the ulna can be easily palpated. At the distal end of the ulna, the ulnar styloid process is the palpable bony point projecting distally. There are two articulations between the radius and ulna, namely the proximal and distal radioulnar joints. Both joints allow the radius to move over the ulna during pronation and supination (Fig. 6.17). During this movement, the ulna remains stationary.

Muscles

Anterior compartment

There are three layers of muscles in the anterior compartment of the forearm: superficial, intermediate and deep (Table 6.4). These muscles are responsible for flexion, abduction and adduction of the hand at the wrist joint, and flexion of the digits and pronation of the forearm.

In the superficial layer there are four muscles, which are, from lateral to medial, pronator teres, flexor carpi radialis, palmaris longus and flexor carpi ulnaris muscles (Figs. 6.18, 6.19A and Table 6.4). The weak palmaris longus muscle is vestigial and is absent from approximately 15% of the population. These superficial muscles arise from the common flexor origin, which is the medial epicondyle of the humerus. Each muscle can be easily palpated in the forearm. Resisted

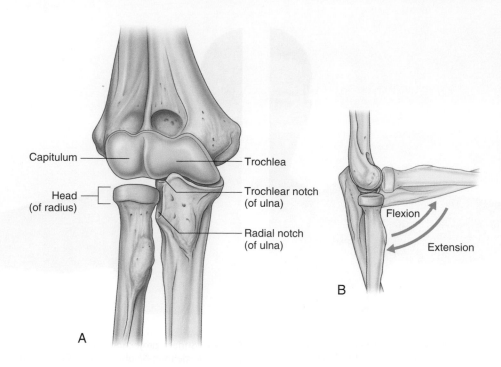

Capitulum

Head
(of radius)

Trochlea

Trochlear notch
(of ulna)

Radial notch
(of ulna)

Flexion

Extension

B

A

Fig. 6.13 Components and movements of the elbow joint. A, Bones and joint surfaces. B, Flexion and extension.
(From Drake, RL, Gray's Anatomy for Students, 3rd ed, 2015, Churchill Livingstone, Elsevier.)

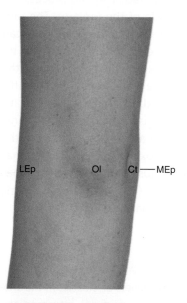

LEp   Ol   Ct —— MEp

Fig. 6.14 Surface projections of the posterior aspect of the elbow joint. *Ct,* cubital tunnel; *LEp,* lateral epicondyle; *MEp,* medial epicondyle; *Ol,* olecranon.

To Do (Figs. 6.13 and 6.14)
• Locate the medial and lateral epicondyles of the humerus, which are the bony protuberances at the sides of the elbow joint.
• On the posterolateral side of the elbow, locate the head of the radius. With the forearm extended, its position is indicated by a depression in the skin that can be observed between the bulge formed by the brachioradialis muscle and the olecranon.
• Palpate the head of the radius during pronation and supination of the forearm.
• Posteriorly, palpate the olecranon of the ulna.

pronation will allow identification of the pronator teres muscle, which can be seen following an oblique course toward the midshaft of the radius. With resisted flexion and abduction of the wrist, the flexor carpi radialis muscle and its large tendon can be observed passing toward the second and third metacarpal. To observe the tendon of the palmaris longus muscle, bring digits 1 and 5 together while flexing the wrist against resistance. If present, the tendon can be seen protruding proximal to the distal wrist crease toward the middle of the wrist. With resisted flexion and adduction of the wrist, the flexor carpi ulnaris muscle can be palpated on the medial side of the forearm. Clinically, identifying these tendons can help with locating the radial and ulnar arteries, and the median and ulnar nerves.

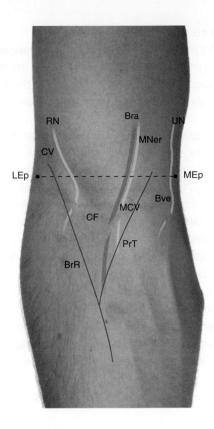

Fig. 6.15 Surface projections of the cubital fossa. *Bra*, brachial artery; *BrR*, brachioradialis; *Bve*, basilic vein; *CF*, cubital fossa; *CV*, cephalic vein; *LEp*, lateral epicondyle; *MCV*, median cubital vein; *MEp*, medial epicondyle; *Mner*, median nerve; *PrT*, pronator teres; *RN*, radial nerve; *UN*, ulnar nerve.

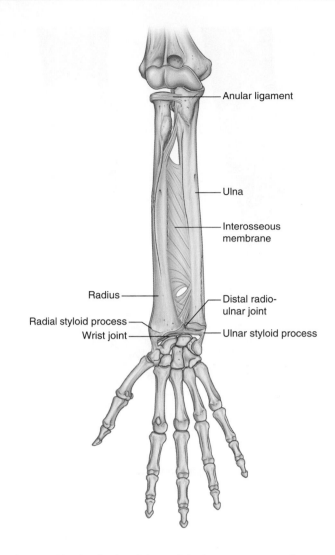

Fig. 6.16 Distal radioulnar joint and the interosseous membrane. *(Modified from Drake, RL, Gray's Anatomy for Students, 3rd ed, 2015, Churchill Livingstone, Elsevier.)*

To Do (Fig. 6.15)

With the arm in the anatomical position:

- Identify the borders of the cubital fossa. For the superior border, draw a line between the medial and lateral epicondyles. For the medial border, draw a line over the pronator teres muscles. For the lateral border, draw a line over the brachioradialis muscle.
- Apply a tourniquet (or grasp with a hand if not available) halfway between the shoulder and elbow, and palpate the cephalic, basilic and median cubital veins. The median cubital vein crosses the midline joining the cephalic and basilic veins.
- With the elbow partly flexed, palpate the biceps tendon within the cubital fossa.

To Do (Figs. 6.16 and 6.17)

- Palpate the shaft of the ulna and the ulnar styloid process.
- Palpate the shaft of the radius and radial styloid process.
- Examine the movement of the radius during pronation and supination of the forearm.

In the intermediate layer there is only one muscle, the flexor digitorum superficialis muscle (Fig. 6.19B and Table 6.4). This muscle gives off four tendons that insert into the middle phalanx of digits 2–5. During resisted flexion of the wrist, it may be possible to identify some of the tendons of flexor digitorum superficialis sitting below the superficial group.

In the deep layer there are three muscles: the flexor digitorum profundus, flexor pollicis longus and pronator quadratus muscles. The deep muscles and their tendons cannot be observed from the surface (Fig. 6.19C and Table 6.4).

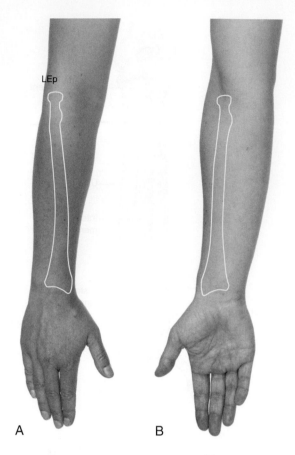

Fig. 6.17 A, Pronation. B, Supination. *LEp,* lateral epicondyle.

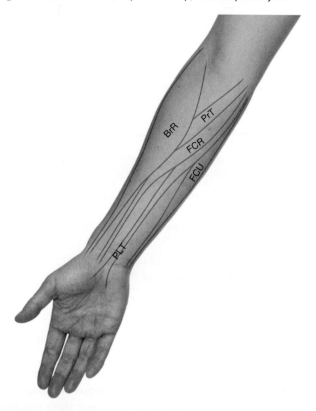

Fig. 6.18 Surface projections muscles of the anterior compartment of the forearm. *BrR,* brachioradialis; *FCR,* flexor carpi radialis; *FCU,* flexor carpi ulnaris; *PLT,* palmaris longus tendon; *PrT,* pronator teres.

Posterior compartment

The muscles in the posterior compartment are arranged in a superficial and a deep layer. These muscles are responsible for extension, abduction and adduction of the hand at the wrist joint, extension of the digits and supination of the forearm.

In the superficial layer there are seven muscles: the brachioradialis, extensor carpi radialis longus, extensor carpi radialis brevis, extensor digitorum, extensor digiti minimi, extensor carpi ulnaris and anconeus muscles (Table 6.5).

The brachioradialis muscle forms a prominent bulge on the lateral side of the anterolateral surface of the forearm, where proximally it forms the lateral boundary of the cubital fossa. The extensor carpi radialis longus and brevis muscles lie deep to brachioradialis muscle and can be palpated on the posterolateral side of the forearm during resisted extension and abduction of the wrist (Fig. 6.20).

The main extensor of digits 2–5 is the extensor digitorum muscle. During extension of the hand at the wrist joint, the muscle bellies are palpable over the posterior forearm. On the dorsum of the hand, the four tendons of the extensor digitorum muscle can be observed as they pass toward their

---

To Do (Fig. 6.18)

- Identify the pronator teres muscle during an isometric contraction of the muscle. This can be performed by asking the subject to pronate their forearm against resistance.
- Identify the flexor carpi radialis muscle during an isometric contraction of the muscle. This can be performed by asking the subject to flex and abduct their hand at the wrist joint against resistance. Palpate the tendon of the flexor carpi radialis proximal to the wrist.
- Palpate the flexor carpi ulnaris muscle on the medial side of the forearm.
- Immediately proximal to the wrist, identify the tendons of the flexor digitorum superficialis muscle. Its tendons lie deep to the tendon of the flexor carpi radialis muscle.
- Beginning at the medial epicondyle, draw in the pronator teres muscle toward its insertion on the radius.
- Draw in the flexor carpi radialis muscle as it crosses the forearm to insert into the base of the metacarpals 2 and 3.
- Draw in the palmaris longus muscle as a small muscle belly with its tendon heading toward the palmar aponeurosis of the hand.
- Draw in the flexor carpi ulnaris muscle toward the pisiform bone.

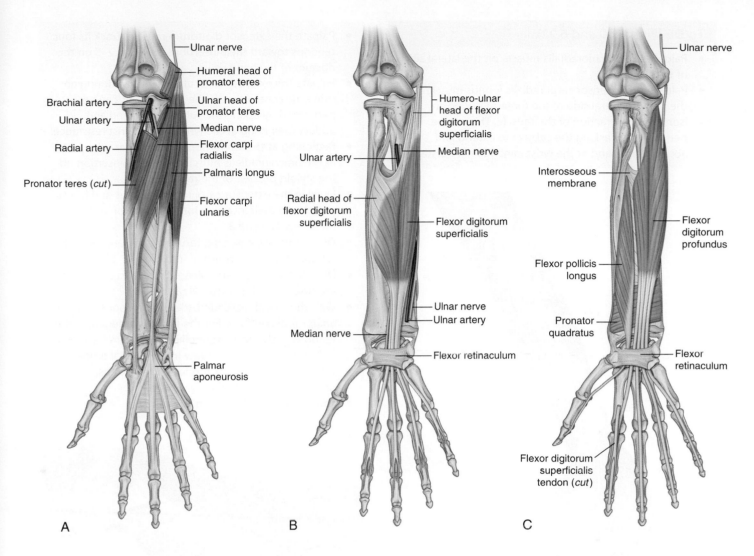

Fig. 6.19 A, Superficial layer of forearm muscles. B, Intermediate layer of forearm muscles. C, Deep layer of forearm muscles.
(From Drake, RI., Gray's Anatomy for Students, 3rd ed, 2015, Churchill Livingstone, Elsevier.)

insertions on the middle and distal phalanges of digits 2–5 (Fig. 6.21). The extensor digiti minimi muscle is not easy to identify. However, over the dorsum of the hand, on the medial side, it is possible to palpate two tendons projecting to digit five. The tendon of the extensor digiti minimi muscle is the more lateral tendon. The extensor carpi ulnaris muscle can be palpated on the posteromedial side of the forearm during resisted extension and adduction of the wrist (Fig. 6.20). The anconeus muscle is a short muscle that lies in the anconeus triangle, the borders of which are a line between the radial head, lateral epicondyle and tip of the olecranon. This muscle is easily palpable and provides a landmark for aspiration of the elbow joint.

There are five muscles in the deep layer of the posterior compartment: the supinator, abductor pollicis longus,

extensor pollicis brevis, extensor pollicis longus and extensor indicis muscles. Although the muscles themselves cannot be identified from the surface, the tendons of the extensor pollicis brevis and longus and abductor pollicis longus muscles, also known as the 'outcropping muscles', can be observed. These tendons emerge from between the extensor digitorum and extensor carpi radialis brevis muscles to form the boundaries of the anatomical snuffbox (Fig. 6.22). The boundaries of the snuffbox can be more easily identified with the thumb extended. In the anatomical position, the lateral border is formed by the tendons of the abductor pollicis longus and extensor pollicis brevis muscles. The medial border is formed by the large tendon of the extensor pollicis longus muscle, which can be observed as it passes toward the distal phalanx of digit 1 (the thumb).

To Do (Figs. 6.20 and 6.22)

- Palpate the brachioradialis muscle on the lateral side of the forearm.
- Palpate the extensor carpi radialis longus muscle on the posterolateral side of the forearm during an isometric contraction of the muscle. This can be performed by asking the subject to extend and abduct their hand at the wrist joint against resistance.

- Palpate the extensor digitorum muscle. Track its four tendons toward their insertions on digits 2–5 on the dorsum of the hand.
- Palpate the extensor carpi ulnaris muscle during an isometric contraction of the muscle. This can be performed by asking the subject to extend and adduct their hand at the wrist joint against resistance.
- Beginning at the lateral supraepicondylar ridge, draw in the brachioradialis muscle toward its insertion on the styloid process of the radius.
- Draw in the extensor carpi radialis longus and brevis muscles to their insertion into the base of metacarpals 2 and 3.
- Draw in the extensor digitorum muscle and its four tendons into their insertion into digits 2–5.
- Draw in the flexor carpi ulnaris muscle to its insertion into the base of metacarpal 5.
- With the thumb extended, identify the borders of the anatomical snuffbox. For the lateral border, draw the tendons of the abductor pollicis longus and extensor pollicis brevis muscles. Draw in the medial border, which is formed by the tendon of the extensor pollicis longus muscle.
- Palpate the radial artery in the snuffbox.

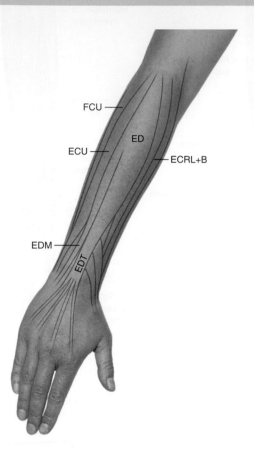

Fig. 6.20 Surface projections of muscles of the posterior of the forearm. *ECRL+B*, extensor carpi radialis longus and brevis; *ECU*, extensor carpi ulnaris; *ED*, extensor digitorum; *EDM*, extensor digiti minimi; *EDT*, extensor digitorum tendon; *FCU*, flexor carpi ulnaris.

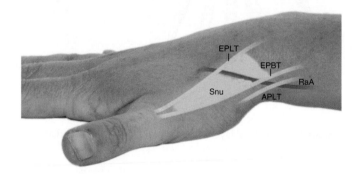

Fig. 6.22 Surface projections anatomical snuffbox. *APLT*, abductor pollicis longus tendon; *EPBT*, extensor pollicis brevis tendon; *EPLT*, extensor pollicis longus tendon; *RaA*, radial artery; *Snu,* snuffbox.

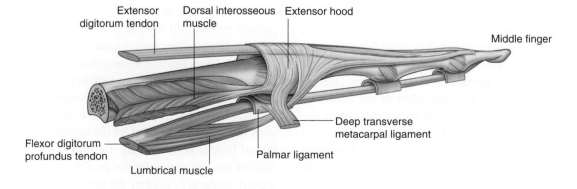

Fig. 6.21 Extensor hood.

(From Drake, RL, Gray's Anatomy for Students, 3rd ed, 2015, Churchill Livingstone, Elsevier.)

Table 6.4 Layers of muscles in the anterior compartment of the forearm

Muscle	Origin	Insertion	Innervation	Function
Superficial layer				
Flexor carpi ulnaris	Medial epicondyle of humerus	Pisiform bone, hamate and base of metacarpal 5	Ulnar nerve (C7, C8, T1)	Flexes and adducts the wrist joint
Palmaris longus		Palmar aponeurosis of hand	Median nerve (C7, C8)	Flexes wrist joint
Flexor carpi radialis		Metacarpals 2 and 3		Flexes and abducts the wrist joint
Pronator teres	Medial epicondyle of humerus and coronoid process of ulna	Midshaft of radius	Median nerve (C6, C7)	Pronation
Intermediate layer				
Flexor digitorum superficialis	Medial epicondyle of humerus, coronoid process of ulna, and radius	Middle phalanges of medial four fingers	Median nerve (C8, T1)	Flexes metacarpophalangeal joints and proximal interphalangeal joints of medial four fingers; flexes the wrist joint
Deep layer				
Flexor digitorum profundus	Ulna and interosseous membrane	Distal phalanges of medial four fingers	Lateral half by median nerve (anterior interosseous nerve); medial half by ulnar nerve (C8, T1)	Flexes metacarpophalangeal joints and proximal and distal interphalangeal joints of the medial four fingers; flexes the wrist joint
Flexor pollicis longus	Radius and interosseous membrane	Distal phalanx of thumb	Median nerve (anterior interosseous nerve) (C7, C8)	Flexes metacarpophalangeal and interphalangeal joint of the thumb
Pronator quadratus	Distal anterior surface of ulna	Distal anterior surface of radius	Median nerve (anterior interosseous nerve) (C7, C8)	Pronation

Modified from Drake, RL, Gray's Anatomy for Students, 3rd ed, 2015, Churchill Livingstone, Elsevier

Table 6.5 Layers of muscles in the posterior compartment of the forearm

Muscle	Origin	Insertion	Innervation	Function
Superficial layer				
Brachioradialis	Lateral supraepicondylar ridge of humerus	Distal end of radius	Radial nerve (C5, C6)	Flexor of elbow joint when forearm is midpronated
Extensor carpi radialis longus		Metacarpal 2	Radial nerve (C6, C7)	Extends and abducts the wrist
Extensor carpi radialis brevis		Metacarpals 2 and 3	Deep branch of radial nerve (C7, C8)	
Extensor digitorum	Lateral epicondyle of humerus	Middle and distal phalanges of medial four fingers via extensor hoods	Posterior interosseous nerve (C7, C8)	Extends medial four fingers; extends the wrist joint
Extensor digiti minimi		Extensor hood of the little finger		Extends the little finger
Extensor carpi ulnaris	Lateral epicondyle of humerus and ulna	Metacarpal 5		Extends and adducts the wrist joint
Anconeus	Lateral epicondyle of humerus	Olecranon of the ulna	Radial nerve (C6, C7, C8)	Abduction of the ulna in pronation

Continued

Table 6.5 Layers of muscles in the posterior compartment of the forearm—cont'd

Muscle	Origin	Insertion	Innervation	Function
Deep layer				
Supinator	Lateral epicondyle of humerus and ulna	Lateral surface of radius	Posterior interosseous nerve (C6, C7)	Supination
Abductor pollicis longus	Ulna, radius and intervening interosseous membrane	Metacarpal I		Abducts carpometacarpal joint of thumb
Extensor pollicis brevis	Radius and interosseous membrane	Proximal phalanx of the thumb	Posterior interosseous nerve (C7, C8)	Extends carpometacarpal and metacarpophalangeal joints of the thumb
Extensor pollicis longus	Ulna and interosseous membrane	Distal phalanx of thumb		Extends carpometacarpal, metacarpophalangeal and interphalangeal joints of the thumb
Extensor indicis		Extensor hood of index finger		Extends index finger

Modified from Drake, RL, Gray's Anatomy for Students, 3rd ed, 2015, Churchill Livingstone, Elsevier.

HAND

Bones

The bones of the hand include 8 carpal bones (scaphoid, lunate, triquetrum, pisiform, trapezium, trapezoid, capitate and hamate), 5 metacarpal bones and 15 phalanges (Fig. 6.23). All of the carpal bones can all be examined at the wrist. The pisiform can be palpated on the medial palmar surface within the tendon of the flexor carpi ulnaris muscle. The triquetrum can be palpated on the medial side of the hand when the wrist is abducted. The scaphoid can be palpated in the floor of the anatomical snuffbox, distal to the radial styloid process. The tubercle of the scaphoid is palpable as a bony prominence at the distal wrist crease, immediately lateral to the tendon of the flexor carpi radialis muscle. The hook of hamate is palpable on the medial palmar surface, immediately distal of the pisiform bone. The trapezium can be palpated in the anatomical snuffbox at the base of the first metacarpal. The lunate, capitate and trapezoid are more difficult to identify. The lunate and capitate can be felt from the dorsal surface, proximal to the base of the third metacarpal. The trapezoid sits lateral to the capitate. The metacarpals and phalanges are all palpable on the dorsum of the hand. On the palmar side, they are covered by muscle and tendons, although the lateral surfaces of the first and second metacarpals and medial surface of the fifth can be readily palpated.

The joints of the hand are the wrist joint, intercarpal joints, carpometacarpal joints, metacarpophalangeal joints and interphalangeal joints. The wrist joint (or radiocarpal joint) is an articulation between the distal end of the radius and an articular disc at the distal end of the ulna, and the scaphoid, lunate and triquetrum. It enables a wide range of movement, including flexion, extension, abduction, adduction and circumduction of the hand. The intercarpal joints have limited movement. The carpometacarpal joints between the distal row of carpal bones and the metacarpals also have limited movement, except for the articulation between the trapezium and the first metacarpal. This saddle joint is responsible for the wide range of movements that the thumb can perform. The metacarpophalangeal joints between the metacarpals and the phalanges are condyloid joints that permit flexion, extension, abduction and adduction of the digits. They are visible as prominences on the dorsum of the hand, particularly when the digits are flexed. The interphalangeal joints are hinge joints that allow flexion and extension.

Carpal tunnel

The carpal tunnel is formed by the arch of the carpal bones and the overlying flexor retinaculum (or transverse carpal ligament; Fig. 6.23). The contents of the carpal tunnel include the tendons of the flexor digitorum superficialis, flexor digitorum profundus and flexor pollicis longus muscles and the median nerve. The carpal tunnel is an important clinical landmark as the median nerve may become compressed at this location. The flexor retinaculum can be palpated

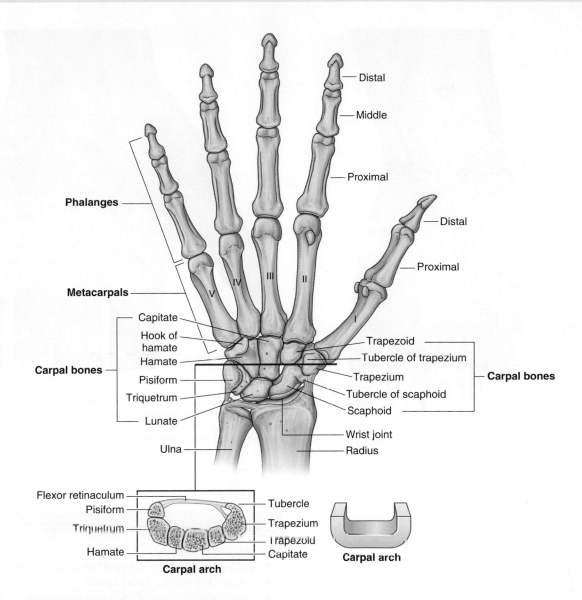

Distal

Middle

Proximal

Distal

Proximal

Phalanges

III

II

IV

V

I

Metacarpals

Capitate

Hook of hamate

Hamate

Carpal bones

Pisiform

Triquetrum

Lunate

Ulna

Trapezoid

Tubercle of trapezium

Trapezium **Carpal bones**

Tubercle of scaphoid

Scaphoid

Wrist joint

Radius

Flexor retinaculum

Pisiform

Triquetrum

Hamate

Tubercle

Trapezium

Trapezoid

Capitate

Carpal arch

Carpal arch

Fig. 6.23 Bones of the wrist and hand.
(Modified from Drake, RL, Gray's Anatomy for Students, 3rd ed, 2015, Churchill Livingstone, Elsevier.)

To Do (Figs. 6.23 and 6.24)

- Locate the pisiform within the tendon of the flexor carpi ulnaris muscle on the medial side of the palmar surface. It lies approximately 1 cm distal to the end of the ulna.
- Locate the hook of hamate on the medial side of the hand. It can be palpated distal and medial to the pisiform bone.
- Locate the tuberosity of the scaphoid on the palmar surface, which lies immediately lateral to the tendon of the flexor carpi radialis muscle.
- Locate the styloid process of the radius, the scaphoid, the trapezium and the base of

the first metacarpal within the anatomical snuffbox.

- Draw a line between the pisiform bone and the scaphoid bone, which indicates the proximal margin of the flexor retinaculum. Demarcate the distal margin of the retinaculum, which lies approximately deep to where the thenar and hypothenar eminences meet on the palmar surface of the hand.
- Demonstrate the location of the wrist joint by drawing a convex line between the styloid processes of the radius and ulna, with the apex of the curve about 1 cm superior to the center of a horizontal line between the two processes.

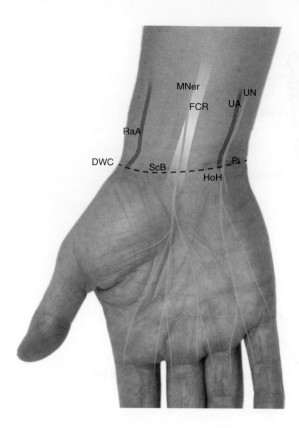

Fig. 6.24 Surface projections of the carpal tunnel. *DWC*, distal wrist crease; *FCR*, flexor carpi radialis; *HoH*, hook of Hamate; *MNer*, median nerve; *Pi*, pisiform bone; *RaA*, radial artery; *ScB*, scaphoid bone; *UA*, ulnar artery; *UN*, ulnar nerve.

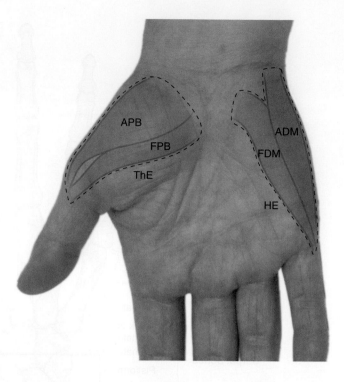

Fig. 6.25 Surface projections of the palmar surface of the hand. *ADM*, adductor digiti minimi; *APB*, abductor pollicis brevis; *FDM*, flexor digiti minimi; *FPB*, flexor pollicis brevis; *HE*, hypothenar eminence; *ThE*, thenar eminence.

between the pisiform, hook of hamate and the tubercle on the scaphoid bone. Immediately proximal to the carpal tunnel, there is a prominent skin crease, called the distal wrist crease. The median nerve can be located proximal to this crease, medial to the tendon of the flexor carpi radialis muscle (Fig. 6.24).

Muscles

Intrinsic muscles of the hand are summarized in Table 6.6. There are two observable prominences on the palmar surface of the hand. These are the thenar eminence, which is located at the base of digit 1 (the thumb) and the hypothenar eminence, which is located at the base of digit 5 (the little finger) (Fig. 6.25). These two eminences are raised by the underlying muscles. The muscles of the thenar eminence are the flexor pollicis brevis and abductor pollicis brevis muscles, beneath which is the opponens pollicis muscle. The muscles of the hypothenar eminence are the abductor digiti minimi, flexor digiti minimi brevis and opponens digiti minimi muscles.

> **To Do** (Fig. 6.25)
>
> On the palmar side:
> - Locate the thenar and hypothenar eminence.
> - Palpate the palmar aponeurosis.
> - Locate the tendons of the flexor digitorum superficialis muscle as they pass to their insertions on digits 2–5. These are best palpated with the digits flexed at the metacarpophalangeal joints.
>
> On the dorsal side:
> - Locate the tendons of the extensor digitorum muscle as they pass to their insertions on digits 2–5. These are best palpated with the digits extended.
> - Identify the dorsal interossei muscles. These are easiest to palpate with the digits abducted.

Overlying the long flexor tendons is a large triangular aponeurosis, called the palmar aponeurosis. This protective thickening of deep fascia can be easily palpated (Fig. 6.26). Deep to the palmar aponeurosis, the tendons of the flexor digitorum superficialis muscle are palpable over the metacarpals as they project toward their insertions on the

Table 6.6 Intrinsic muscles of the hand

Muscle	Origin	Insertion	Innervation	Function
Dorsal interossei	Metacarpals 1–5	Extensor hood of index, middle and ring fingers	Deep branch of ulnar nerve (C8, T1)	Abducts index, middle and ring fingers
Palmar interossei	Metacarpals 1, 2 and 5	Extensor hoods of index, ring and little fingers		Adducts index, ring and little fingers
Adductor pollicis	Transverse head—metacarpal 3; oblique head—capitate and metacarpals 2 and 3	Proximal phalanx of thumb		Adducts thumb
Lumbricals	Tendons of flexor digitorum profundus	Extensor hoods of fingers 2–5	Medial two by the deep branch of the ulnar nerve; lateral two by digital branches of the median nerve	Flex metacarpophalangeal joints while extending interphalangeal joints
Thenar muscles				
Opponens pollicis	Trapezium and flexor retinaculum	Metacarpal 1		Medially rotates thumb
Abductor pollicis brevis	Scaphoid and trapezium and flexor retinaculum	Proximal phalanx of the thumb	Recurrent branch of median nerve (C8, T1)	Abducts thumb at metacarpophalangeal joint
Flexor pollicis brevis	Trapezium and flexor retinaculum			Flexes thumb at metacarpophalangeal joint
Hypothenar muscles				
Opponens digiti minimi	Hook of hamate and flexor retinaculum	Medial aspect of metacarpal 5		Laterally rotates metacarpal V
Abductor digiti minimi	Pisiform and tendon of flexor carpi ulnaris	Proximal phalanx of little finger	Deep branch of ulnar nerve (C8, T1)	Abducts little finger
Flexor digiti minimi brevis	Hook of the hamate and flexor retinaculum			Flexes little finger

Modified from Drake, RL, Gray's Anatomy for Students, 3rd ed, 2015, Churchill Livingstone, Elsevier.

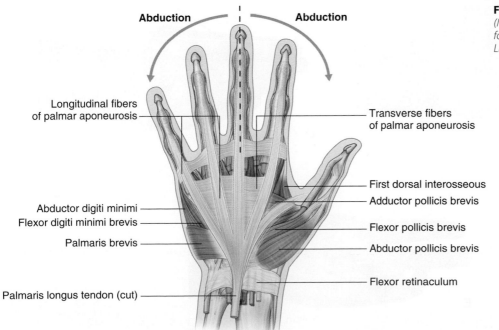

Fig. 6.26 Muscles of the hand. *(Modified from Drake, RL, Gray's Anatomy for Students, 3rd ed, 2015, Churchill Livingstone, Elsevier.)*

phalanges of digits 2–5. They are most prominent during flexion and extension of the digits at the metacarpophalangeal joints. Between the long flexor tendons are the lumbrical muscles. These intrinsic muscles, which extend the interphalangeal joints and flex the metacarpophalangeal joints, can be palpated with 90 degree flexion at the metacarpophalangeal joints.

On the dorsum of the hand, the tendons of the extensor digitorum muscle can be observed, especially with the digits extended. Lying between the metacarpals are the dorsal interossei muscles, which abduct digits 2, 3 and 4 at the metacarpophalangeal joints. These muscles can be easily palpated with the digits abducted. Deep to the dorsal interossei muscles are the palmar interossei muscles, which

can be palpated from the palmar surface during abduction and adduction of the digits.

Movements of the thumb

Movements of the thumb are extension, flexion, abduction, adduction, opposition and reposition. The orientation of the thumb is at right angles to the other digits in the anatomical position; hence in flexion the thumb lies across the palm of the hand, and with extension the thumb points laterally. In abduction, it moves away from the other digits to point anteriorly. Uniquely, the thumb may be brought into opposition to the rest of the digits. Thus, the pad of the thumb is brought into a position facing the pads of the other digits, essential for a precision grip (Fig. 6.27).

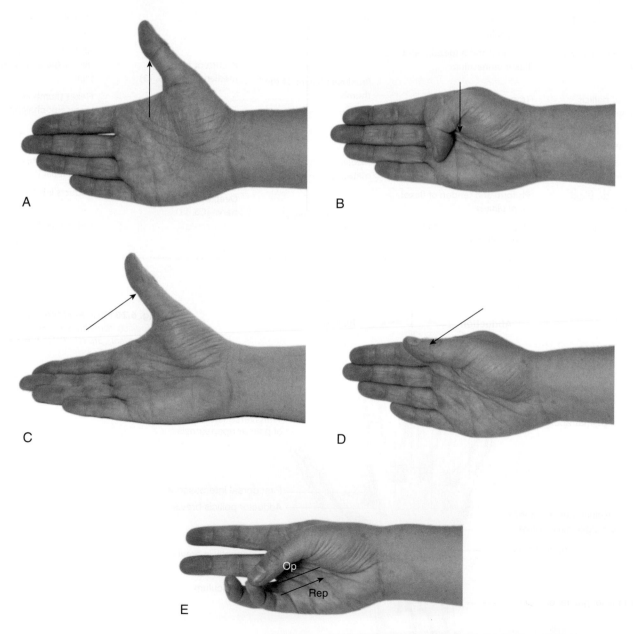

Fig. 6.27 Movements of the thumb. A, Extension. B, Flexion. C, Abduction. D, Adduction. E, Opposition (Op)/reposition (Rep).

Grip

From the position at rest, three key grips can be undertaken (Fig. 6.28).

- power grip
- hook grip
- precision grip

NEUROVASCULAR STRUCTURES

Vasculature

The main arterial supply to the upper limb is the brachial artery (Fig. 6.29), which is a continuation of the axillary artery, a continuation of the subclavian artery. The subclavian artery becomes the axillary artery at the lateral margin of the first rib. As its name suggests, the axillary artery is located within the axilla. At the inferior border of the teres major muscle, the axillary artery becomes the brachial artery. The first major branch of the brachial artery is the profunda brachii artery. This artery crosses posterior to the humerus, at the level of the deltoid tuberosity, to supply the posterior compartment of the arm.

The brachial artery bifurcates in the cubital fossa to become the radial and ulnar arteries. The radial artery descends to the wrist under the brachioradialis muscle. It continues dorsally through the anatomical snuffbox and pierces the first dorsal interosseous muscle to reach the palmar side of the hand. At this point, it forms the deep palmar arch, which lies deep to the long flexor tendons. The ulnar artery descends to the hand under the flexor carpi ulnaris muscle to form the superficial palmar arch, which is superficial to the long flexor tendons (Fig. 6.29). When the thumb is fully extended, the deep palmar arch

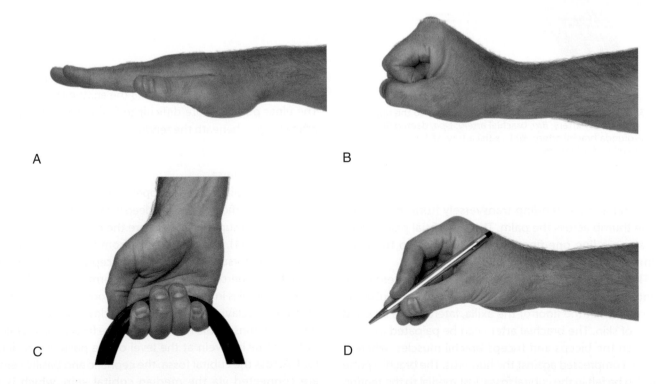

A B

C D

Fig. 6.28 Different grips. A, Resting. B, Power grip. C, Hook grip. D, Precision grip.

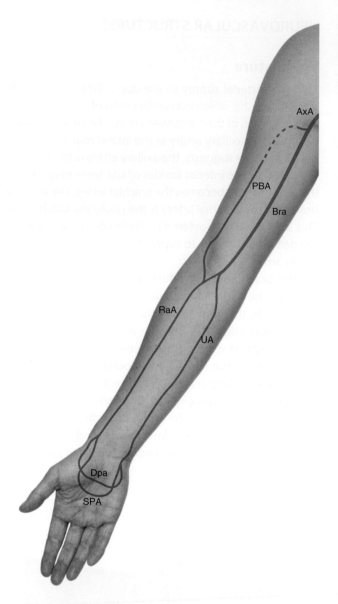

Fig. 6.29 Surface projections of the arterial supply to the upper limb. *AxA*, axillary artery; *Bra*, brachial artery; *Dpa*, deep palmar arch; *PBA*, profunda brachii artery; *RaA*, radial artery; *SPA*, superficial palmar arch; *UA*, ulnar artery.

To Do (Fig. 6.29)

- To represent the course of the axillary artery, with the arm abducted to 90 degrees, draw a line from the midclavicular point to where the tendon of the pectoralis major muscle crosses the coracobrachialis muscle.
- To represent the course of the brachial artery, continue the line on the medial side of the arm, between the triceps and biceps brachii muscles, toward the cubital fossa.
- To represent the course of the radial artery, with the forearm supinated, continue a line laterally from the cubital fossa to the medial side of the styloid process of the radius. Continue this line dorsally, through the anatomical snuffbox to the first dorsal interosseous muscle. Continue an arch medially across the palm of the hand, at the level of the dorsum of the thumb when fully extended. This represents the deep palmar arch.
- To represent the course of the ulnar artery, draw a second line medially from the cubital fossa to the pisiform. Continue an arch laterally across the palm of the hand, a finger's breadth distal to the deep palmar arch. This represents the superficial palmar arch.
- Identify the axillary, brachial and radial pulse points on a volunteer.

lies along a line extending transversely from the dorsum of the thumb across the palm. The superficial palmar arch lies along a line one finger's breadth distal to the deep palmar arch.

There are six locations in the upper limb where pulse points can be determined (Fig. 6.30). The axillary pulse can be palpated in the floor of the axilla, lateral to its inverted dome of skin. The brachial artery can be palpated as it lies between the biceps and triceps brachii muscles, where it may be compressed against the humerus. The brachial pulse can also be felt in the cubital fossa, just medial to the tendon of the biceps brachii muscle. The radial pulse can be palpated lateral to the tendon of the flexor carpi radialis muscle. It can also be palpated in the floor of the anatomical snuffbox. The ulnar pulse is more difficult to feel because the ulnar artery lies just beneath the tendon of the flexor carpi ulnaris muscle.

Venous drainage

The venous drainage of the upper limb is provided by both deep and superficial veins. The deep veins follow the arteries. The two main superficial veins are the cephalic and basilic veins (Fig. 6.31). Both veins arise from the dorsal venous arch on the dorsum of the hand. The cephalic vein runs up the lateral side of the forearm and arm. Proximally, the cephalic vein lies in the deltopectoral groove before it drains into the subclavian vein at the infraclavicular fossa. The basilic vein runs up the medial side of the forearm and drains into the brachial vein at the level of the posterior axillary fold. Across the cubital fossa, the cephalic and basilic veins are connected via the median cubital vein, which is a common site for venepuncture.

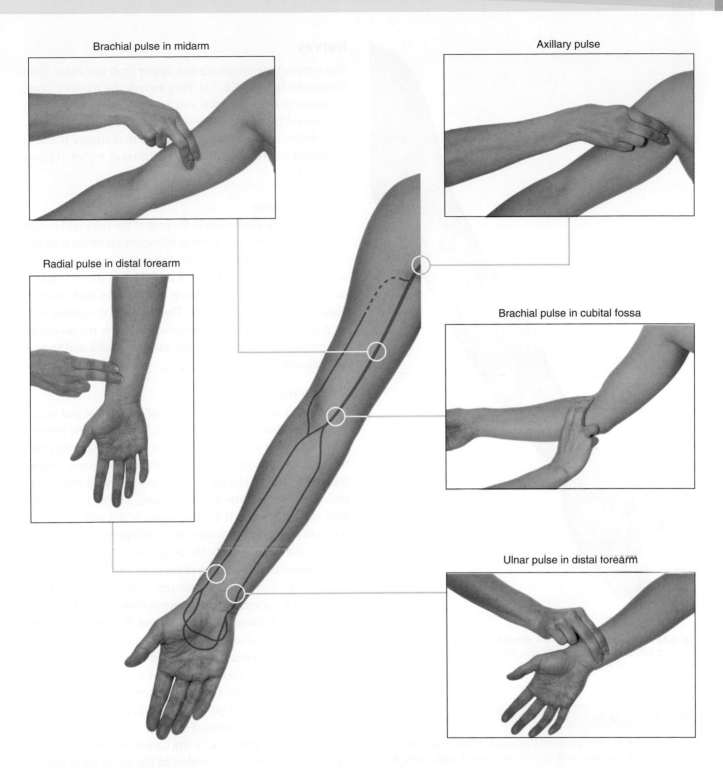

Brachial pulse in midarm

Axillary pulse

Radial pulse in distal forearm

Brachial pulse in cubital fossa

Ulnar pulse in distal forearm

Fig. 6.30 Upper limb pulse points.

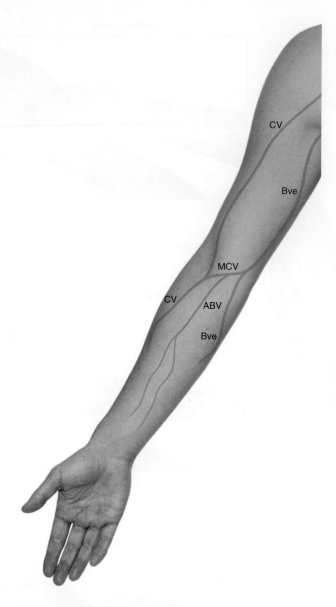

Fig. 6.31 Surface projections of the upper limb veins. *ABV*, antibrachial vein; *Bve*, basilic vein; *CV*, cephalic vein; *MCV*, median cubital vein.

To Do (Fig. 6.31)

- To draw out the veins of the upper limb, begin with the cephalic vein as it lies on the lateral side. Trace it superiorly in the delto-pectoral groove.
- The basilic vein can be drawn in on the medial side running up the limb to the posterior axillary fold.
- Join the basilic and cephalic vein in a V-shape in the midline of the cubital fossa. The antebrachial vein extends inferiorly from the median cubital vein in the midline.

Nerves

The nerves that innervate the upper limb originate from the brachial plexus (C5–T1). They include the median, ulnar, musculocutaneous, radial and axillary nerves. In addition to innervating muscles, these nerves also supply the skin. Knowledge of the cutaneous nerves that supply the skin is important for testing for peripheral nerve lesions (Fig. 6.32).

Brachial plexus

The brachial plexus begins in the root of the neck and passes through the axilla. Its terminal branches continue into the arm. The plexus is derived from the anterior rami of cervical spinal nerves C5, C6, C7 and C8 and the first thoracic spinal nerve, T1. The brachial plexus is divided into roots, trunks, divisions and cords (Fig. 6.33). The trunks of the plexus may be palpated in the supraclavicular fossa; the remainder of the plexus lies deep within the fat-filled axilla and thus is not palpable.

Median nerve

The median nerve is a termination of the medial and lateral cords of the brachial plexus (C5–T1). In the arm, the median nerve lies lateral to the brachial artery within the medial inter-muscular septum. In the distal arm, the median nerve crosses the brachial artery to be situated medially. The nerve then enters the anterior compartment of the forearm, anterior to the elbow joint, to pass through the cubital fossa. At this point, it can be palpated medial to the tendon of the biceps muscle.

The median nerve descends between the two heads of the pronator teres muscle to sit between the flexor digitorum superficialis and flexor digitorum profundus muscles. It supplies the superficial and intermediate layers of muscles in the anterior compartment, except for the flexor carpi ulnaris muscle. It also gives rise to the anterior interosseous nerve, which supplies the deep layer of muscles (except for the medial two bellies of the flexor digitorum profundus muscle), and the palmar cutaneous nerve, which innervates the skin of the lateral palm. The median nerve enters the hand via the carpal tunnel (Fig. 6.34).

Immediately proximal to the carpal tunnel, the median nerve lies medial to the tendon of the flexor carpi radialis muscle. At this location, it can be easily palpated. Within the hand, it terminates as the recurrent branch, which supplies the thenar muscles, and the common and proper palmar digital nerves that supply the palmar surface and fingertips of the lateral three and a half digits. This branch also supplies the lateral two lumbrical muscles.

Ulnar nerve

The ulnar nerve is a termination of the medial cord of the brachial plexus (C8–T1). It passes within the medial

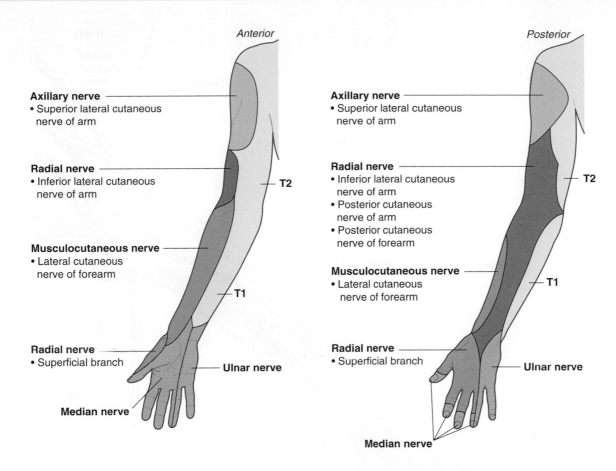

Fig. 6.32 Anterior and posterior areas of skin innervated by major peripheral nerves in the arm and forearm (see Fig. 1.7). *(From Drake, RL, Gray's Anatomy for Students, 3rd ed, 2015, Churchill Livingstone, Elsevier.)*

To Do (Fig. 6.32)

- Using the tips of your index and middle fingers, palpate the median nerve proximal to the carpal tunnel. It lies immediately medial to the tendon of the flexor carpi radialis muscle.
- With the forearm partly flexed, palpate the ulnar nerve immediately proximal to the cubital fossa.
- To represent the course of the median nerve, draw a line on the medial side of the arm, between the triceps and biceps brachii muscles, toward the cubital fossa. At the cubital fossa, continue the line down the middle of the anterior compartment of the forearm toward the carpal tunnel. At this point, the line should be medial to the tendon of the flexor carpi radialis muscle.
- To represent the course of the ulnar nerve, draw a line down the medial side of the arm, between the triceps and biceps brachii muscles, toward the cubital tunnel. In the arm, the ulnar nerve lies just posterior to the median nerve. From the cubital tunnel, continue the line down the medial side of the arm toward the wrist. At this point, the line should be between the pisiform and the hook of hamate.

- To represent the course of the radial nerve, draw a line from the posterior axillary wall to the postero lateral side of the mid shaft of the humerus. Continue the line down the posterior compartment of the arm toward the lateral epicondyle of the humerus. At this point, continue the line along the lateral side of the anterior compartment of the forearm toward the dorsolateral aspect of the hand to represent the superficial radial nerve.

intermuscular septum of the arm, posterior to the median nerve. At the elbow, it lies posterior to the medial epicondyle to enter the cubital tunnel, where it can be easily palpated.

Within the forearm, the ulnar nerve sits under the flexor digitorum ulnaris muscle with the ulnar artery to supply this muscle and the medial two bellies of the flexor digitorum profundus muscle. It also gives off a palmar and dorsal branch, which supply the skin on the medial palm and dorsum of the hand. At the wrist, the ulnar nerve lies superficial to the flexor retinaculum (Fig. 6.32).

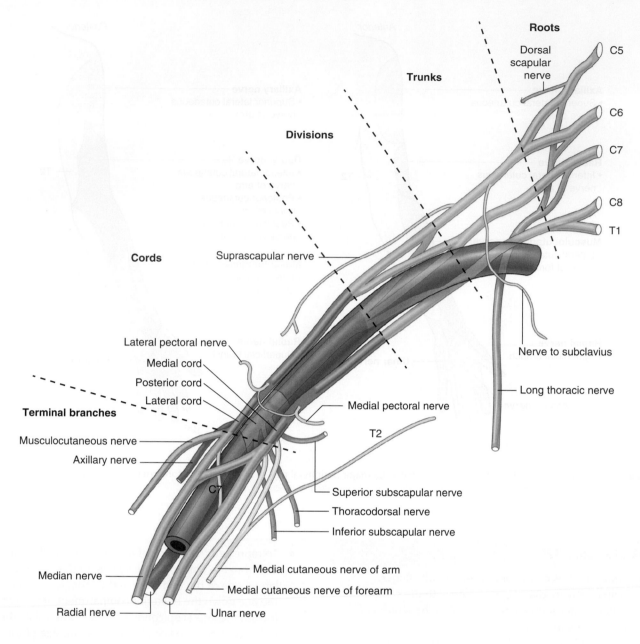

Fig. 6.33 Brachial plexus.
(From Drake, RL, Gray's Anatomy for Students, 3rd ed, 2015, Churchill Livingstone, Elsevier.)

It enters the hand via the ulnar (or Guyon's) canal, which is formed between the pisiform bone and hook of hamate, where it can also be palpated. Within the hand, the ulnar nerve terminates as a deep branch, which supplies some intrinsic muscles, and a superficial branch that divides into common and proper palmar digital nerves to supply the skin over the medial half of digit 4 and digit 5.

Musculocutaneous nerve

The musculocutaneous nerve is a termination of the lateral cord of the brachial plexus (C5, C6 and C7). The nerve exits

the axilla, piercing the coracobrachialis muscle. It then passes between the biceps brachii and brachialis muscles. It supplies all anterior muscles of the arm. Lateral to the biceps tendon, the nerve continues as the lateral cutaneous nerve of the forearm, emerging from the deep fascia close to the cephalic vein.

Axillary nerve

The axillary nerve is a termination of the posterior cord of the brachial plexus (C5–C6). It lies posterior to the axillary artery and anterior to the subscapularis muscle. It exits the axilla via the quadrangular space, accompanied by the supinator muscle to enter the posterior compartment of the forearm as the posterior interosseous nerve, where it supplies the posterior compartment muscles. The superficial branch sits under the brachioradialis muscle with the radial artery to supply the skin on the dorsal lateral aspect of the hand.

In the Clinic

Carpal tunnel syndrome

Carpal tunnel syndrome is caused by compression of the median nerve in the carpal tunnel. It leads to pain, paresthesia, numbness and muscle weakness in the hand. Symptoms occur in the distribution of the median nerve. Typically, patients experience altered sensation over the thumb, index finger, middle finger, and radial half of the ring finger, as well as weakness of the thenar muscles. In more severe cases, wasting of the muscles of the thenar eminence will be evident on inspection. Causes of increased pressure within the carpal tunnel, which can lead to median nerve compression, include pregnancy, diabetes, hypothyroidism, rheumatoid arthritis and tenosynovitis.

Ultrasound

SCALENE TRIANGLE

Subject position

Imaging is performed with the subject sitting, facing the operator.

Transducer

Use a linear array transducer. Set the depth setting to 2–5 cm.

Transducer position

Position the transducer in the transverse plane, immediately superior to the midpoint of the clavicle. The probe should be orientated so that the beam is directed 30–45 degrees inferiorly.

Image features

Superficially, the sternocleidomastoid muscle can be observed (Fig. 6.35). Approximately 1 cm below the surface, the subclavian artery will be visible as an anechoic circle. Sitting anterolateral to the artery, the brachial plexus can be seen. The roots or trunks (depending upon the location

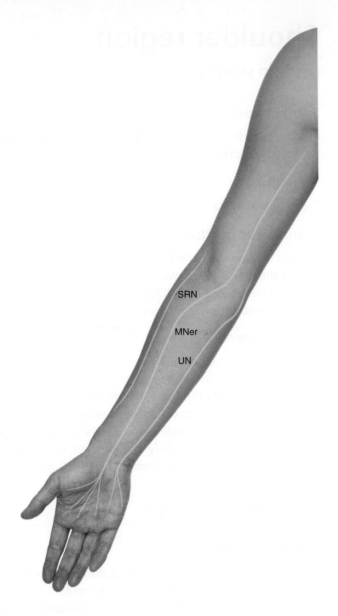

Fig. 6.34 Surface projections of nerves in the upper limb. *MNer*, median nerve; *SRN*, superficial radial nerve; *UN*, ulnar nerve.

posterior circumflex humeral artery. The axillary nerve supplies the deltoid and teres minor muscles and skin over the inferior part of the deltoid muscle.

Radial nerve

The radial nerve is a termination of the posterior cord of the brachial plexus (C5–T1). The nerve passes posteriorly in the arm to lie within the radial groove on the posterior shaft of the humerus with the profunda brachii artery. In the arm it supplies the triceps muscle.

The radial nerve passes laterally at the elbow, where it can be palpated, to enter the forearm under the brachioradialis muscle. At this point, it divides into deep and superficial branches. The deep branch pierces the

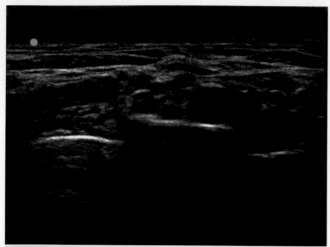

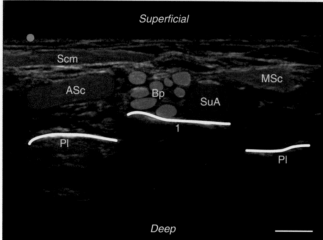

Superficial

Scm

ASc   Bp   MSc
            SuA

            1

Pl

        Pl

Deep

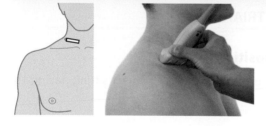

Fig. 6.35 Ultrasound of the right brachial plexus. *ASc*, anterior scalene; *Bp*, brachial plexus (roots and trunks); *1*, first rib; *MSc*, middle scalene; *Pl*, pleura; *Scm*, sternocleidomastoid; *SuA*, subclavian artery. Scale bar = 1 cm.

and orientation of the beam) appear as several small heterogeneous textured circles of mid-gray color. The artery and brachial plexus lie superiorly to the surface of the first rib, which is seen as a curved hyperechoic line. Either side of this neurovascular bundle, the anterior (lateral) and middle (medial) scalene muscles can be observed. These muscles form the walls of the scalene triangle. Medial to the anterior scalen muscle, the subclavian vein will be in view. Deep to the first rib, the pleura can be seen as hyperechoic horizontal streaks. These will appear to move during breathing.

Shoulder region

DELTOID MUSCLE

Subject position

Imaging is performed with the subject sitting with their arm by the side, facing sideways to the operator.

Transducer

Use a linear array transducer. Set the depth setting to 3–6 cm.

Transducer position

Position the transducer on the lateral aspect of the proximal third of the arm in the transverse plane for short-axis views of the deltoid muscle (Fig. 6.36). Scan in either an anterior or posterior direction to inspect the three heads.

Image features

In the transverse plane, the hyperechoic lateral surface of the humerus will be in view toward the bottom of the image (Fig. 6.36). Overlying this bone, the deltoid muscle can be seen. The anterior, intermediate and posterior parts of the deltoid muscle can be delineated by their surrounding myofascia. Scanning anteriorly, the cephalic vein may be visible between the anterior border of the deltoid muscle and the pectoralis major muscle.

ROTATOR CUFF MUSCLES

Subject position

Imaging is performed with the subject sitting, either facing the operator (for the supraspinatus or subscapularis muscles) or with their back to the operator (for the infraspinatus and teres minor muscles). For the supraspinatus muscle, position the arm behind the back as if reaching into a back pocket (i.e. medially rotated). For the infraspinatus or teres minor muscles, position the arm across the chest toward the opposite shoulder. For subscapularis, the arm should be laterally rotated.

Transducer

Use a linear array transducer. Set the depth setting to 2–5 cm.

Transducer position

The rotator cuff muscles are best viewed in their long axis. For the supraspinatus muscle, position the transducer in a coronal plane, anterosuperior to the glenohumeral joint with the proximal end of the probe on or anterior to the acromion (Fig. 6.37). The orientation marker should point cephalically. For the infraspinatus muscle, position the transducer in a transverse plane, posterior to the glenohumeral joint, immediately inferior to the spine of the scapula. From this location, scan

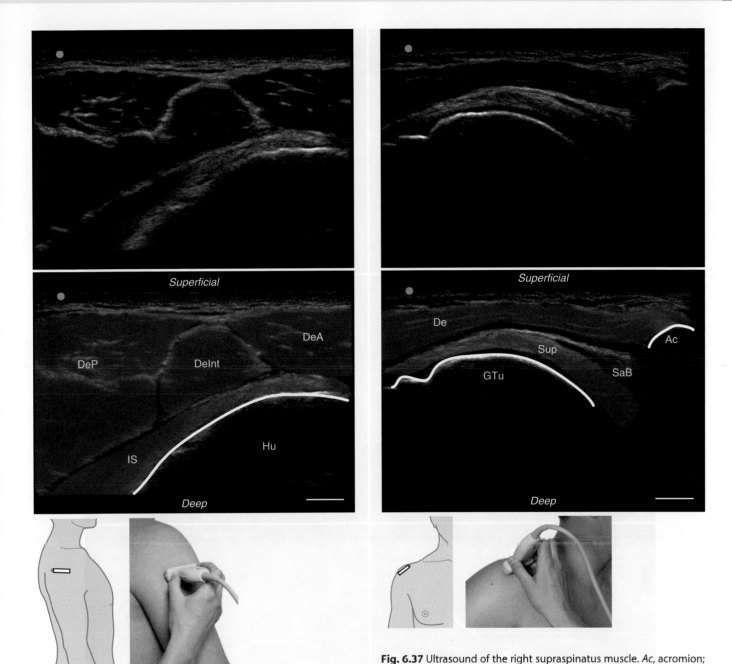

Fig. 6.37 Ultrasound of the right supraspinatus muscle. *Ac*, acromion; *De*, deltoid; *GTu*, greater tubercle; *SaB*, subacromial bursa; *Sup*, supraspinatus. Scale bar = 1 cm.

Fig. 6.36 Ultrasound of the right deltoid muscle. *DeA*, deltoid anterior fibers; *DeInt*, deltoid intermediate fibers; *DeP*, deltoid posterior fibers; *Hu*, humerus; *IS*, infraspinatus. Scale bar = 1 cm.

anterolaterally to see the tendon of the infraspinatus insert into the greater tuberosity, just inferior of the supraspinatus. Track in an inferior direction to locate the teres minor muscle. For the subscapularis muscle, position the transducer in a transverse plane, anterior to the glenohumeral joint (Fig. 6.38).

Image features

Supraspinatus muscle

The surface of the anterior facet of the greater tubercle will be in view (Fig. 6.37). The tendon of the supraspinatus muscle appears as a dense curved band with a mid-gray appearance lying over the humerus. The tendon tapers at its distal insertion into the anterior facet. Towards the medial side of the image, the acromion will be in view as a short hyperechoic streak. The supraspinatus tendon or muscle can be inspected as it descends below the acromion, under the coracoacromial arch. Lying between the acromion and supraspinatus tendon, it may be possible to see the sub-acromial bursa, which appears as a narrow anechoic sac. The deltoid muscle can be observed passing over the top of the supraspinatus tendon.

111

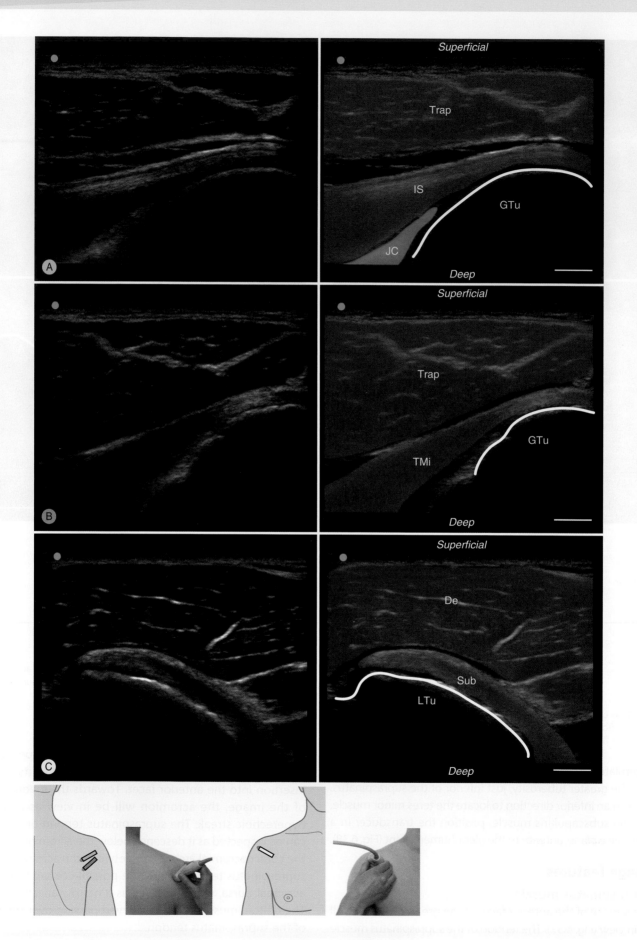

Fig. 6.38 Ultrasound of the right A, infraspinatus, B, teres minor and C, subscapularis muscles. *De*, deltoid; *GTu*, greater tubercle; *IS*, infraspinatus; *JC*, joint capsule; *LTu*, lesser tubercle; *Sub*, subscapularis; *TMi*, teres minor; *Trap*, trapezius. Scale bar = 1 cm.

Infraspinatus muscle

The surface of the middle facet of the greater tubercle will be in view (Fig. 6.38A). The curved tendon of the infraspinatus muscle appears similar to the supraspinatus muscle (mid-gray color) as it follows the contours of the bone. Inferior to the tendon, at the bottom of the image, the glenohumeral joint capsule may be in view. Scanning medially, the relatively thick hypoechoic infraspinatus muscle is seen arising from the infraspinous fossa of the scapula. The trapezius muscle can be observed passing over the top of the infraspinatus tendon.

Teres minor muscle

The surface of the posterior facet of the greater tubercle will be in view (Fig. 6.38B). The narrow tendon of the teres minor muscle is seen inserting onto the posterior facet inferior to the tendon of the infraspinatus muscle. Superficial to the teres minor muscle, the trapezius muscle can be observed.

Subscapularis muscle

The surface of the lesser tubercle will be in view (Fig. 6.38C). The curved tendon of subscapularis muscle can be seen as it passes toward its attachment on the lesser tubercle. Lying superficial to the subscapularis muscle, the deltoid muscle is visible.

ANTERIOR ARM

Subject position

Imaging is performed with the subject sitting, facing the operator. The arm should be abducted to 30–40 degrees, or laterally rotated, so that the medial side can be more easily imaged. It may be more comfortable to rest the elbow on a table.

Transducer

Use a linear array transducer. Set the depth setting to 2–8 cm.

Transducer position

To examine the long tendon of the biceps brachii muscle within the bicipital groove, position the transducer in the transverse plane for short-axis views over the anterior of the arm, immediately inferior to the head of the humerus (Figs. 6.39 and 6.40). From the medial aspect of the arm, the brachial artery and the median and ulnar nerves can be inspected, as well as the biceps brachii, coracobrachialis and brachialis muscles.

Image features

With the transducer oriented in the transverse plane over the proximal end of the anterior humerus, the bicipital groove will be in view (Fig. 6.39). It appears as a curved indent on

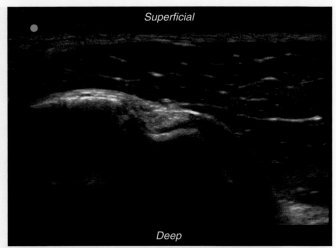

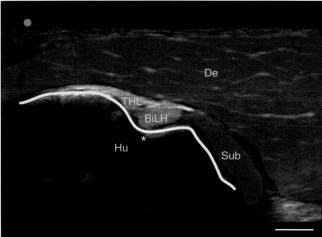

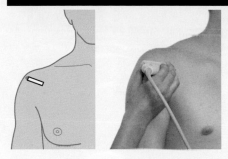

Fig. 6.39 Ultrasound of the right bicipital groove. *, bicipital groove. *BiLH*, biceps long head; *De*, deltoid; *Hu*, humerus; *Sub*, subscapularis; *THL*, transverse humeral ligament. Scale bar = 1 cm.

the anterior surface of the bone. Sitting within the groove, the long tendon of the biceps brachii muscle can be seen, which has the appearance of a small medium-gray oval. Forming a roof over the bicipital groove, the hyperechoic transverse ligament should be visible.

With the transducer positioned in the transverse plane on the medial aspect of the proximal third of the arm, the coracobrachialis, biceps and brachialis muscles of the arm and their associated neurovascular structures can be seen (Fig. 6.40A). Toward the bottom of the image,

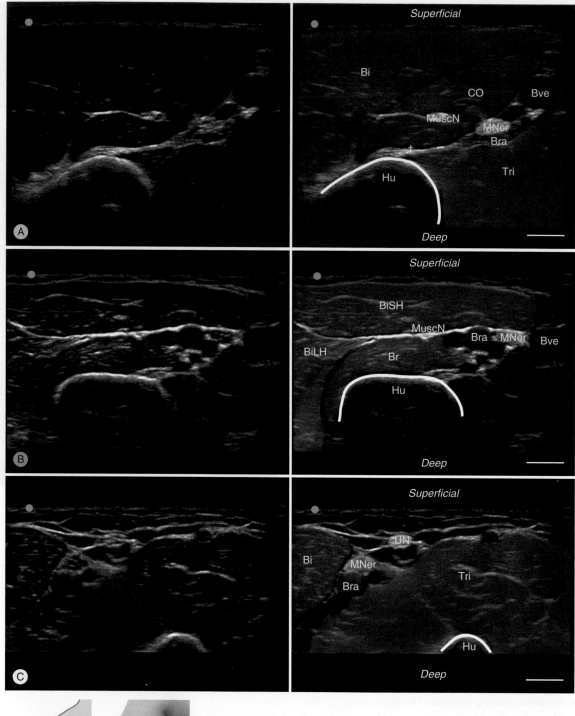

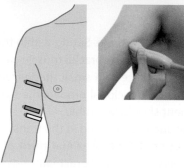

Fig. 6.40 Ultrasound of the right anterior compartment of the arm. A, Proximal arm. B, Midshaft of humerus. C, Immediately posterior to midshaft of humerus. †, medial intermuscular septum; *Bi*, biceps; *BiLH*, biceps long head; *BiSH*, biceps short head; *Br*, brachialis; *Bra*, brachial artery; *Bve*, basilic vein; *CO*, coracobrachialis; *Hu*, humerus; *MNer*, median nerve; *MuscN*, musculocutaneous nerve; *Tri*, triceps; *UN*, ulnar nerve. Scale bar = 1 cm.

the surface of the humerus will be visible. The fascia of the medial intermuscular septum can be observed extending from the humerus to the skin. Within the septum, the brachial artery and paired veins are visible in transverse orientation. With reduced pressure on the skin, the large basilic vein can be observed immediately below the surface of the skin. Situated along the septum, between the brachial artery and basilic vein, the median nerve can be seen. Its medium-gray appearance contrasts with the anechoic appearance of the vessels.

Anterior to the medial intramuscular septum (left on image), the coracobrachialis muscle will be in view, which has a large oval appearance. Within the muscle, the musculocutaneous nerve can be inspected as it passes through the muscle. The biceps brachii muscle is visible anterior to the coracobrachialis muscle, and fills much of the image. The triceps brachii muscle will be in view posterior to the medial intermuscular septum.

Tracking distally along the medial intermuscular septum, the course of the brachial artery, paired veins and median nerve can be inspected (Fig. 6.40B). At approximately the level of the midshaft of the humerus, the origin of the brachialis muscle is seen wrapping anteriorly around the bone immediately anterior to the brachial vessels and median nerve. Superficial to the brachialis muscle, one or two of the heads of the biceps brachii muscle can be observed. The short head lies medial to the long head, and therefore with the transducer on the medial side of the arm, it can be seen close to the surface of the image. Both muscles are surrounded by a dense myofascia, which allows easy delineation from the surrounding structures. Sandwiched within the myofascia, between the brachialis and biceps brachii muscles, the musculocutaneous nerve can be observed.

Moving the transducer in a posterior direction from the medial intermuscular septum, the triceps brachii muscle comes in to view (Fig. 6.40C). The medial and long heads of the triceps brachii muscle fill much of the image. The ulnar nerve can also be seen sitting posterior to the median nerve, brachial artery and veins. It is relatively superficial in the image and appears smaller than the median nerve. With the transducer positioned in a transverse plane on the anterior aspect of the distal third of the arm, the biceps brachii (superficial) and brachialis (deep) muscles can be observed.

POSTERIOR ARM

Subject position

Imaging is performed with the subject sitting with their back to the operator. It may be more comfortable to rest the elbow on a table.

Transducer

Use a linear array transducer. Set the depth setting to 2–8 cm.

Transducer position

The triceps brachii muscle can be inspected by positioning the transducer in the transverse plane on the posterior aspect of the arm for short-axis views. For the radial nerve as it crosses the posterior surface of the humerus, position the transducer over the posterolateral or posterior of the arm, approximately midway along the length of the humerus (Fig. 6.41).

Image features

With the transducer positioned in the transverse plane on the posterior or posterolateral aspect or the arm, distal to the middle of the shaft of the humerus, the radial nerve can be seen as it winds though the spiral groove. The radial nerve appears as a fairly flattened medium gray colored structure sitting on the posterior surface of the humerus. Running with the nerve, the relatively small profunda brachii artery may be visible. Forming the walls of the spiral groove, the lateral and medial heads of triceps brachii muscle will be in view (Fig. 6.41A). Scanning distally toward the lateral side of the arm, the radial nerve and profunda brachii artery can be tracked toward the elbow (Fig. 6.41B). The structures are seen passing between the myofascial layers that separate the lateral head of the triceps brachii muscle from the brachialis muscle, which will be in view toward the bottom of the image. As the radial nerve is scanned over the elbow, it is seen sitting under the brachioradialis muscle on the lateral aspect of the arm.

ELBOW

Subject position

Imaging is best performed with the subject lying supine, although it can be performed with the subject sitting facing the operator. The elbow joint should be maintained in extension. The cubital tunnel can be imaged by abducting the arm or raising the arm above the head.

Transducer

Use a linear array transducer. Set the depth setting to 2–6 cm.

Transducer position

Position the transducer in the sagittal plane over the anterior of the joint for long-axis views (Fig. 6.42). The proximal end of the radius and ulna can be inspected by scanning in a lateral or medial direction, respectively. The cubital tunnel is best viewed by positioning the transducer in the transverse plane over the posteromedial aspect of the elbow, over the medial epicondyle and olecranon (Fig. 6.42C).

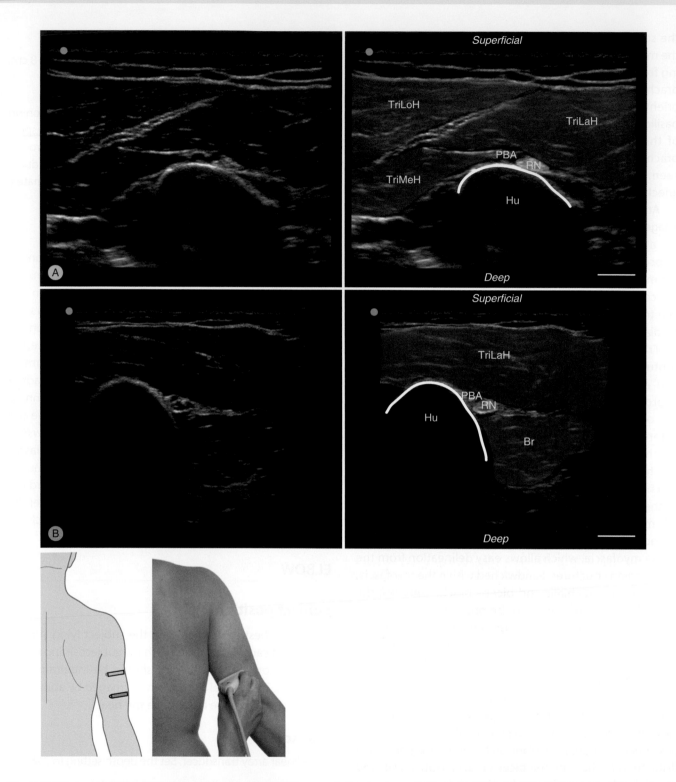

Fig. 6.41 Ultrasound of the right posterior compartment of the arm. A, Proximal arm. B, Distal arm. *Br*, brachialis; *Hu*, humerus; *PBA*, profunda brachii artery; *RN*, radial nerve; *TriLoH*, triceps long head; *TriLaH*, triceps lateral head; *TriMeH*, triceps medial head. Scale bar = 1 cm.

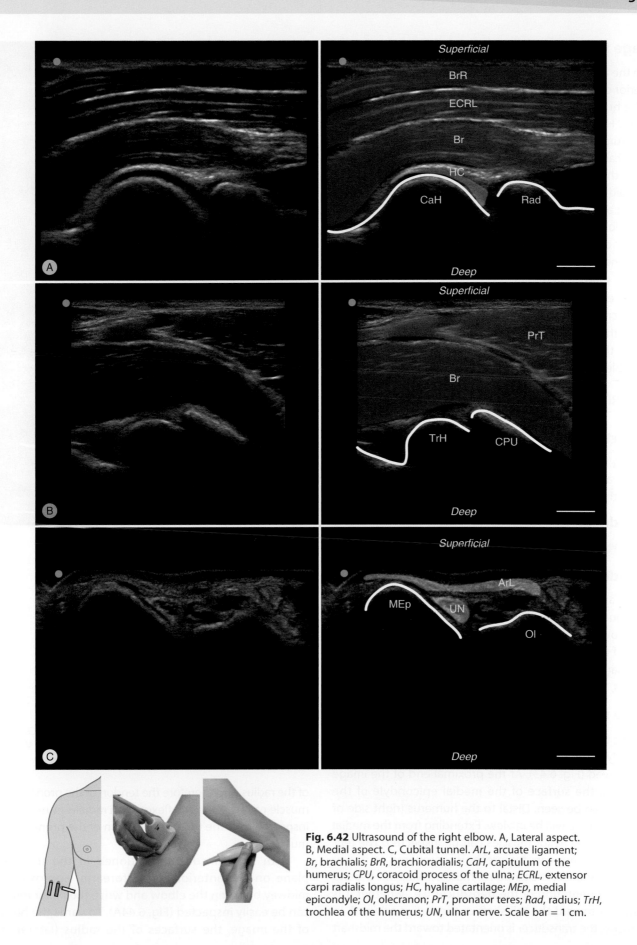

Fig. 6.42 Ultrasound of the right elbow. A, Lateral aspect. B, Medial aspect. C, Cubital tunnel. *ArL*, arcuate ligament; *Br*, brachialis; *BrR*, brachioradialis; *CaH*, capitulum of the humerus; *CPU*, coracoid process of the ulna; *ECRL*, extensor carpi radialis longus; *HC*, hyaline cartilage; *MEp*, medial epicondyle; *Ol*, olecranon; *PrT*, pronator teres; *Rad*, radius; *TrH*, trochlea of the humerus; *UN*, ulnar nerve. Scale bar = 1 cm.

Image features

With the transducer positioned in the sagittal plane over the anterior of the elbow toward the lateral side, the capitulum of the humerus and the radial head come into view (Fig. 6.42A). Hyaline cartilage can be observed overlying the capitulum. Within the joint recess, extrasynovial fat can be seen. Scanning toward the medial side of the anterior of the elbow, the surfaces of the trochlear of the humerus and the coronoid process of the ulna can be observed (Fig. 6.42B). Passing anteriorly over the joint, the brachialis muscle will be invisible. Superficial to the brachialis muscle, the superficial anterior compartment muscles of the forearm can be seen on the medial side, and the superficial posterior compartment muscles on the lateral side.

At the cubital tunnel, the surface of the medial epicondyle and olecranon will be in view (Fig. 6.42C). Sitting within the tunnel, the ulnar nerve can be seen in transverse orientation against the medial epicondyle. The arcuate ligament may be visible forming a roof over the tunnel.

ANTERIOR FOREARM

Subject position

Imaging is best performed with the subject sitting, facing the operator, elbow flexed to 90 degrees, forearm supinated and resting on a table.

Transducer

Use a linear array transducer. Set the depth setting to 2–6 cm.

Transducer position

For the anterior compartment muscles, position the transducer on the anteromedial side of the proximal forearm, at the elbow joint, and scan toward the wrist. For long-axis views of the muscles, the transducer should be positioned in the sagittal plane (Fig. 6.43), and short-axis views of the muscles, in the transverse plane (Fig. 6.44).

Image features

With the transducer aligned in the sagittal plane at the lateral epicondyle, the tendinous origin of the flexor muscles can be observed (Fig. 6.43). At the proximal end of the image (left side), the surface of the medial epicondyle of the humerus can be seen. Distal to the humerus (right side of image), the ulna will be in view. Extending from the medial epicondyle, the flexor muscles can be inspected. The tendinous origin appears hyperechoic, compared to darker hypoechoic muscle. The tendon or muscle in view will depend upon the orientation of the transducer (i.e., whether it is orientated toward the midshaft of the radius or wrist). In the image, the transducer is orientated toward the midshaft

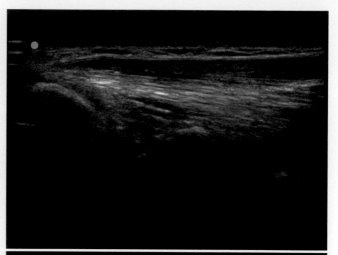

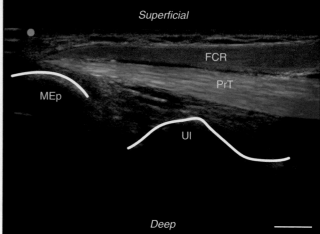

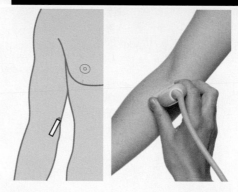

Fig. 6.43 Ultrasound of the right common flexor origin. *FCR*, flexor carpi radialis; *MEp*, medial epicondyle; *PrT*, pronator teres; *Ul*, ulna. Scale bar = 1 cm.

of the radius, and therefore the tendon of the pronator teres muscle can be seen. The flexor carpi radialis muscle can be inspected over the top of the tendon of the pronator teres muscle.

With the transducer positioned in the transverse plane on the anterior of the forearm, approximately midway between the elbow and wrist, the flexor muscles can be easily inspected (Fig. 6.44A). Towards the bottom of the image, the surfaces of the radius (lateral) and

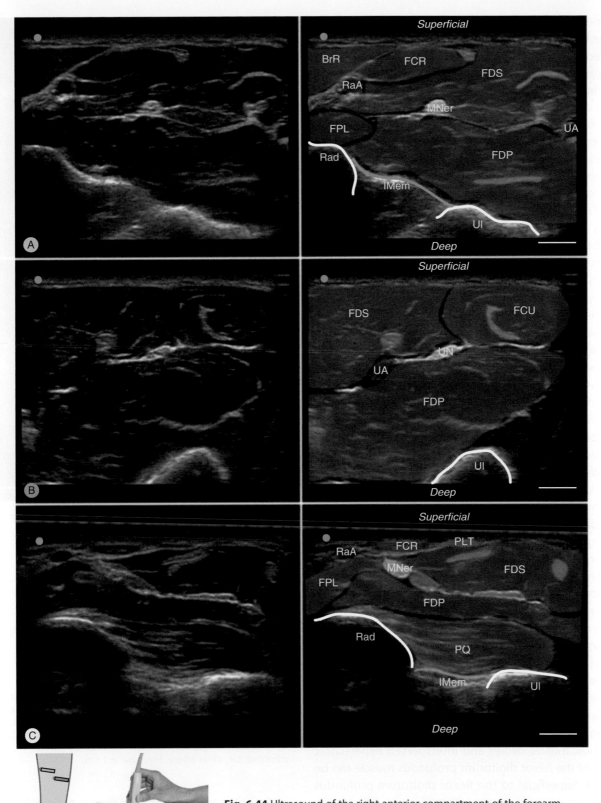

Fig. 6.44 Ultrasound of the right anterior compartment of the forearm. A, Mid forearm. B, Medial aspect. C, Distal forearm. *BrR*, brachioradialis; *FCR*, flexor carpi radialis; *FCU*, flexor carpi ulnaris; *FDP*, flexor digitorum profundus; *FDS*, flexor digitorum superficialis; *FPL*, flexor pollicis longus; *IMem*, interosseous membrane; *MNer*, median nerve; *PLT*, palmaris longus tendon; *PQ*, pronator quadratus; *RaA*, radial artery; *Rad*, radius; *UA*, ulnar artery; *Ul*, ulna; *UN*, ulnar nerve. Tendons are shown in green. Scale bar = 1 cm.

ulna (medial) will be in view. On the lateral side of the anterior forearm, the flexor pollicis longus muscle can be observed adjacent to the radius. Medial to this muscle, the muscle bellies of the flexor digitorum profundus muscle will be in view. By moving the distal interphalangeal joint of each digit in turn, it is possible to identify each of the muscle bellies.

Superficial to the flexor digitorum profundus muscle, the flexor digitorum superficialis muscle can be observed. The muscle bellies of flexor digitorum superficialis muscle can be identified by moving the proximal interphalangeal joints. The flexor digitorum profundus and superficialis muscles are separated by a dense hyperechoic myofascial plane that extends horizontally across the image. Located in approximately the middle of the image within this myofascia, the median nerve can be inspected. It appears relatively circular in its short axis and has a characteristic medium-gray heterogeneous texture.

Above the flexor digitorum superficialis muscle, the flexor carpi radialis muscle can be observed as a large flattened oval. On the radial side of the image, the brachioradialis muscle may also be in view. Sitting below the myofascia of the brachioradialis muscle, the radial artery will be visible in its short axis.

On the medial side of the anterior forearm, the medial bellies of the flexor digitorum profundus muscle can be inspected adjacent to the ulna (Fig. 6.44B). Superficial to the flexor digitorum profundus muscle, the flexor digitorum superficialis muscle can be seen. Medial to this muscle, the flexor carpi ulnaris muscle will be in view. The ulnar nerve can be observed within the myofascial plane between the flexor digitorum profundus muscle and the more superficial flexor carpi ulnaris and flexor digitorum superficialis muscles. The nerve appears flattened. Lateral to the ulnar nerve, the ulnar artery will appear within the same myofascial plane.

Scanning distally along the anterior forearm, the muscles become tendinous (Fig. 6.44C). With the transducer aligned transversely across the distal forearm, the hyperechoic contours of the radius and ulna, and the adjoining interosseous membrane, are visible toward the bottom of the image. Adjacent to these structures, the pronator quadratus muscle is seen extending between the ulna and radius.

Lying superficial to the pronator quadratus muscle, the hypoechoic muscle bellies and interspersed hyperechoic tendons of the flexor digitorum profundus muscle can be observed. Superficial to the flexor digitorum profundus muscle, above an obvious myofascial plane, the muscle bellies and tendons of the flexor digitorum superficialis muscle will be in view. By moving each digit in turn, it will be possible to identify each of the individual tendons. At the top of the image, directly below the skin, the flattened tendons, or muscular tendinous junction, of the flexor carpi radialis and palmaris longus muscles can be inspected.

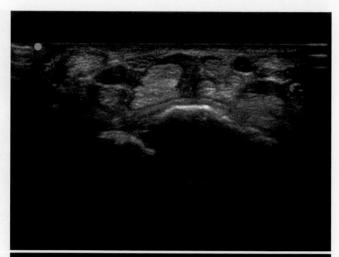

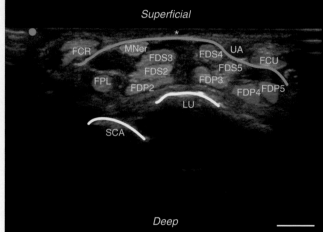

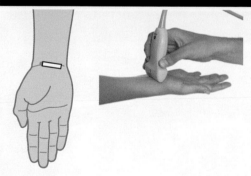

Fig. 6.45 Ultrasound of the right anterior wrist. The tendons to the individual digits have been numbered (2–5). *, transverse carpal ligament; *FCR*, flexor carpi radialis; *FCU*, flexor carpi ulnaris; *FDP*, flexor digitorum profundus; *FDS*, flexor digitorum superficialis; *FPL*, flexor pollicis longus; *LU*, lunate; *MNer*, median nerve; *SCA*, scaphoid; *UA*, ulnar artery. Scale bar = 1 cm.

Scanning toward the carpal tunnel, the proximal row of carpal bones comes into view (Fig. 6.45). With the transducer aligned transversely at the distal wrist crease, the curved anterior surface of the lunate bone appears a clearly identifiable feature. Superficial to the carpal bones, the flexor tendons can be observed. They appear relatively hyperechoic and are often surrounded by hypoechoic synovium. By moving each digit in turn, the individual tendons can be identified. The tendon of the flexor pollicis longus muscle sits within the deeper row of tendons on the lateral side of the image.

Medial to the tendon of the flexor pollicis longus muscle, the four tendons of the flexor digitorum profundus muscle can be inspected. Superficial to these structures, the four tendons of the flexor digitorum superficialis muscle will be in view. Forming the roof of the carpal tunnel, the flexor retinaculum muscle can be seen as a curved arching line across the image. Directly below the transverse carpal ligament, the median nerve will be visible. It appears as a flattened oval, with a medium-gray heterogeneous texture with a hyperechoic border. The tendons of the flexor carpi radialis and flexor carpi ulnaris muscles can be seen superficial to the transverse carpal ligament.

By rotating the transducer so that it is aligned longitudinally along the anterior forearm, the fascicles of individual flexor muscles and tendons can be inspected. In this view, muscle contraction can be easily visualized (Video 6.1).

POSTERIOR FOREARM

Subject position

Imaging is best performed either sitting or lying prone, with the elbow extended and forearm supinated.

Transducer

Use a linear array transducer. Set the depth setting to 2–6 cm.

Transducer position

For the posterior compartment muscles, position the transducer on the posterolateral side of the proximal forearm, at the elbow joint, and scan obliquely in a medial direction toward the wrist. For long-axis views of the muscles, the transducer should be positioned in the sagittal plane (e.g., Fig. 6.46A), and for short-axis views, in the transverse plane (Figs. 6.46B and C, 6.47).

Image features

With the transducer aligned in the sagittal plane at the lateral epicondyle, the common tendinous origin of the extensor muscles can be observed (Fig. 6.46A). At the proximal side of the image (left side), the surface of the lateral epicondyle of the humerus can be seen. Distal to the humerus (right side of image), the head of the radius will be in view. Extending from the lateral epicondyle, the tendinous origin of extensor carpi radialis brevis and/or extensor digitorum can be observed. Lying superficial to the common extensor origin, the extensor carpi radialis longus and brachioradialis muscles will be in view.

With the transducer positioned in the transverse plane on the lateral side of the proximal forearm adjacent to the elbow, the supinator muscle can be inspected (Fig. 6.46B). It has a characteristic crescent shape as it wraps around the surface of the radius. The radial nerve, or its superficial and deep branch, can be observed within the myofascial plane overlying the supinator muscle. It may be possible to observe the deep branch piercing through the supinator muscle. These nerves appear as small flattened ovals.

Superficial to the supinator muscle, the extensor carpi radialis longus and brevis muscles can be inspected. The extensor carpi radialis longus muscle lies over the top of the extensor carpi radialis brevis muscle. Both muscles have clearly defined myofascial planes surrounding them. Abduction and adduction of the wrist can be performed to confirm the identity of these muscles. Sitting superficially to these muscles, the brachioradialis muscle will be in view.

With the transducer positioned in the transverse plane at a midpoint along the posterior forearm, the extensor muscles can be seen (Fig. 6.46C). Towards the bottom of the image, the posterior surface of radius and ulnar will be in view. Bridging these bones, the interosseous membrane can be observed. Above these structures, two layers of muscles are seen. The muscles within the deep layer, from lateral to medial, are the abductor pollicis longus, extensor pollicis brevis, extensor pollicis longus and extensor indicis muscles. The muscles in view will depend upon proximity to the wrist. The abductor pollicis longus muscle has the most proximal origin and will tend to dominate the layer at more proximal locations.

In the superficial layer, from lateral to medial, the muscle bellies of the extensor digitorum muscle D2 to D5 and the extensor carpi ulnaris muscle can be seen. The extensor carpi ulnaris muscle is closely associated with the ulna. The muscle bellies of the extensor digitorum muscle can be identified by individually moving the digits. Hyperechoic tendons may be visible within these muscles.

Tracking distally, the extensor muscles can be seen forming tendons. At the wrist, the extensor retinaculum and its six compartments can be inspected (Fig. 6.47). The extensor retinaculum has a light-gray appearance and extends superficially across the wrist. The tendons appear as hyperechoic circles directly below the retinaculum, and are organized as follows (lateral to medial): abductor pollicis longus and extensor pollicis brevis in compartment one, extensor carpi radialis longus and brevis in compartment two, extensor pollicis longus in compartment three, extensor digitorum and extensor indicis in compartment four, extensor digiti minimi in compartment five and extensor carpi ulnaris in compartment six. Deep to the tendons, the surface of the radius (lateral) and ulna (medial) can be observed.

121

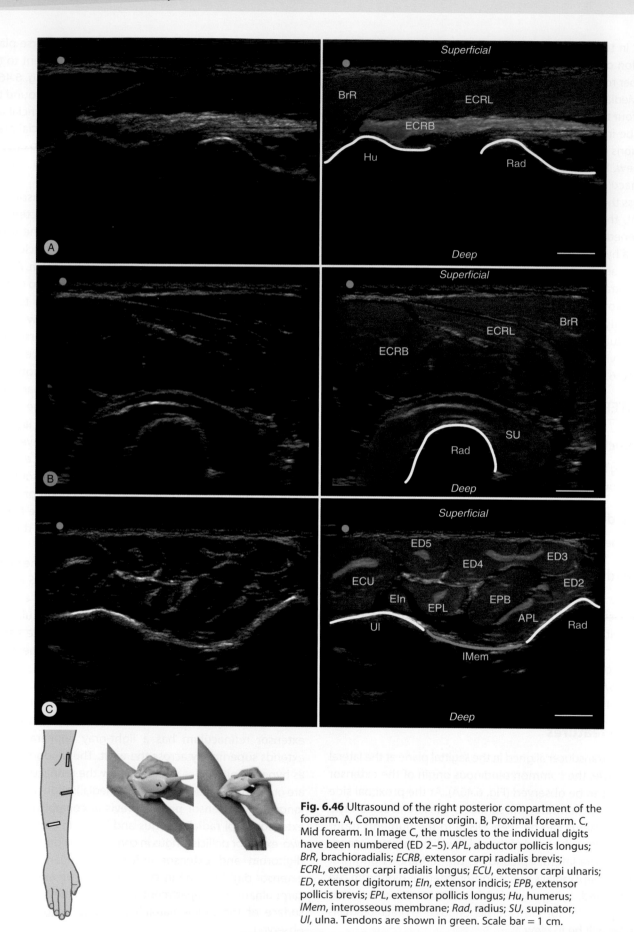

Fig. 6.46 Ultrasound of the right posterior compartment of the forearm. A, Common extensor origin. B, Proximal forearm. C, Mid forearm. In Image C, the muscles to the individual digits have been numbered (ED 2–5). *APL*, abductor pollicis longus; *BrR*, brachioradialis; *ECRB*, extensor carpi radialis brevis; *ECRL*, extensor carpi radialis longus; *ECU*, extensor carpi ulnaris; *ED*, extensor digitorum; *EIn*, extensor indicis; *EPB*, extensor pollicis brevis; *EPL*, extensor pollicis longus; *Hu*, humerus; *IMem*, interosseous membrane; *Rad*, radius; *SU*, supinator; *Ul*, ulna. Tendons are shown in green. Scale bar = 1 cm.

By rotating the transducer so that it is aligned longitudinally along the posterior arm, the fascicles of individual extensor muscles and tendons can be inspected. In this view, muscle contraction can be easily visualized.

HAND

Subject position

Imaging is performed with the subject sitting, facing the operator, elbow flexed and hand resting on a desk.

Transducer

Use a linear array transducer. Set the depth setting to 1–3 cm.

Transducer position

Position the transducer over the palm of the hand in the transverse plane for short-axis views of the tendons. For long-axis views of the digits, position the transducer in the sagittal plane on the anterior surface of the digit of interest (Fig. 6.48A).

Image features

With the transducer positioned in the transverse plane over the palm of the hand, the anterior surfaces of the metacarpals can be seen toward the bottom of the image (Fig. 6.48A). Within the space surrounding the metacarpals, the palmar and dorsal interossei muscles will be visible. By abducting and adducting the digits, the individual muscles can be identified. Directly superior to the interossei muscles, a dense hyperechoic horizontal fascial plane will be in view. Above this plane, the paired tendons of the flexor superficialis and profundus muscles can be seen as flattened hyperechoic circles. Adjacent to each pair of tendons, directly below the skin, the palmar digital arteries and nerves may be visible. Sitting between the pairs of flexor tendons, the relatively hypoechoic lumbrical muscles will be in view.

With the transducer positioned in the sagittal plane on the anterior surface of the digits, the metacarpophalangeal and interphalangeal joints can be inspected (Fig. 6.48B). The tendons of the flexor digitorum superficialis and profundus muscles will be in view superficial to the joints as they insert on the middle or distal phalanx, respectively. In this view, the linear arrangement of the fascicles can be observed.

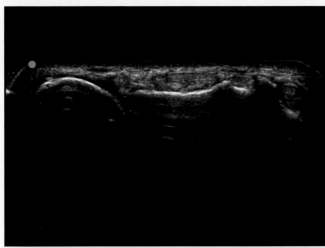

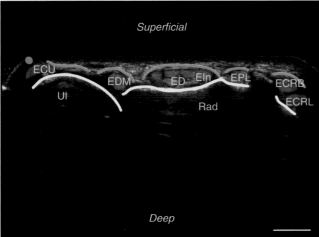

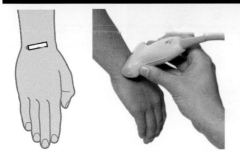

Fig. 6.47 Ultrasound of the right posterior wrist. *ECRB*, extensor carpi radialis brevis; *ECRL*, extensor carpi radialis longus; *ECU*, extensor carpi ulnaris; *ED*, extensor digitorum; *EDM*, extensor digiti minimi; *EIn*, extensor indicis; *EPL*, extensor pollicis longus; *Rad*, radius; *UI*, ulna. Scale bar = 1 cm.

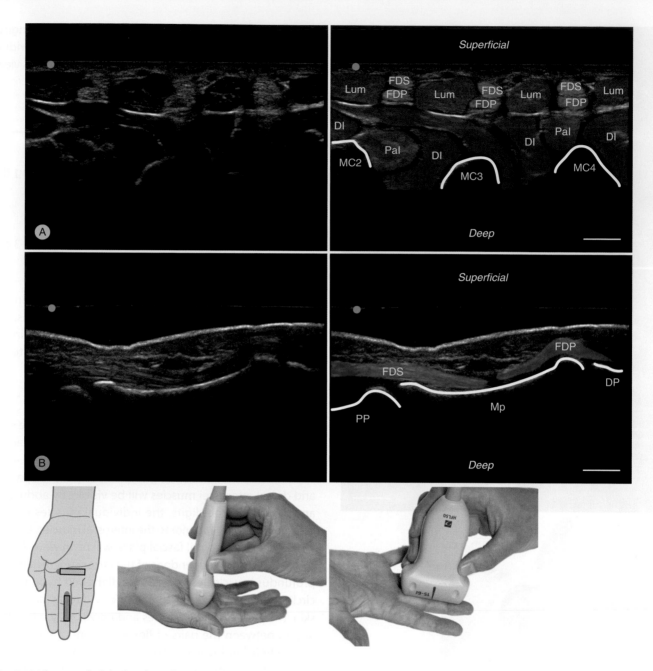

Fig. 6.48 Ultrasound of the hand. *DI*, dorsal interossei; *DP*, distal phalanx; *FDP*, flexor digitorum profundus; *FDS*, flexor digitorum superficialis; *Lum*, lumbricals; *MC2–MC4*, metacarpals 2–4; *Mp*, middle phalanx; *Pal*, palmar interossei; *PP*, proximal phalanx. Scale bar = 1 cm.

In the Clinic

The incorporation of ultrasound as a tool to aid the diagnosis of musculoskeletal conditions represents a major advancement in clinical practice. With the development of higher frequency linear array transducers, musculoskeletal structures can be observed with improved resolution. B-mode ultrasound can be employed to assess and monitor a range of musculoskeletal pathologies, which include muscle, tendon or ligament injury; synovitis; bursitis; hematomas; abscesses; edema; and masses such as ganglion cysts and lipomas. Doppler ultrasound is an important tool in the diagnosis of vascular and inflammatory pathologies within the limbs, in particular, deep vein thrombosis. Real-time imaging has meant that ultrasound is now the gold standard for performing guided peripheral nerve blocks as well as for the aspiration of joints. Real-time imaging has also become an important tool for examining joint biomechanics and stability. There has been substantial development in ultrasound elastography, which is a technique for measuring the 'stiffness' of tissues, potentially giving further diagnostic information of tissue pathology. This technique may prove a useful clinical tool for assessing musculoskeletal conditions that involve a change in mechanical properties, such as tendinopathy. Table 6.7 provides an overview of some of the upper limb musculoskeletal conditions that can be diagnosed or monitored by ultrasound.

Table 6.7 Examples of musculoskeletal pathologies that are diagnosed by ultrasound

Region	Pathology
Shoulder	Rotator cuff tendinopathy or tears
	Supraspinatus impingement
	Subacromial bursitis
	Acromioclavicular joint instability
	Shoulder joint effusion
	Glenohumeral joint effusions
	Acromioclavicular joint ganglia
Arm	Long head of biceps ruptures or subluxation
	Deep vein thrombosis
Forearm	Lateral epicondylitis
	Joint effusions
	Olecranon bursitis
	Tendon ruptures
	Ulnar nerve entrapment
Hand	Carpal tunnel syndrome
	Flexor or extensor tendinopathy
	Synovitis
	Ganglions

Summary Checklist

- Surface projections of the bones related to the upper limb
- Surface projections of the muscles of the upper limb
- Surface projections of the axilla
- Movement of the upper limb
- Ultrasound imaging of the shoulder region
- Ultrasound imaging of the arm
- Ultrasound imaging of the cubital fossa
- Ultrasound imaging of the forearm and hand

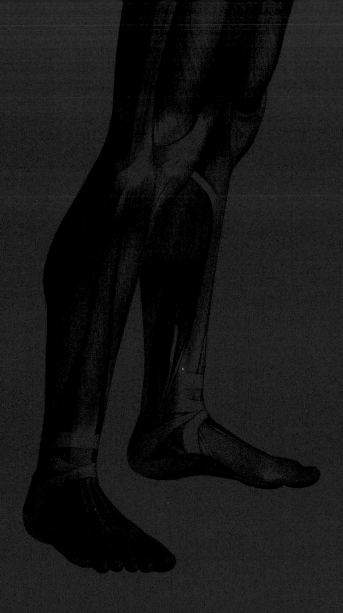

7 Lower limb

Conceptual overview

The lower limbs articulate with the pelvic girdle at the hip joint. The main function of the lower limbs is to provide support to the body, distribute body weight and participate in locomotion. The surface contours of the lower limb are defined by its musculature, bony points, superficial tissues and the prominence of certain blood vessels, particularly superficial veins. The bones of the lower limb are the femur, tibia, fibula, patella, tarsals, metatarsals and phalanges. The lower limb is divided into four regions: gluteal region, thigh, leg and foot. The thigh and leg are divided into compartments separated by fascial septa. Each compartment is occupied by a group of functionally related muscles. Knowledge of surface markings of the structures of the lower limb is important in management and treatment of fractures, peripheral nerve injuries and sports injuries.

Surface anatomy

GLUTEAL REGION

The gluteal region is located posterior to the pelvic girdle and connects the back to the lower limb. The gluteal region extends from the iliac crests superiorly, the greater trochanter of the femur laterally and the gluteal fold inferiorly. In the midline of the gluteal region is the intergluteal (natal) cleft, which separates the right and left buttocks (Fig. 7.1).

Bones

The bones of the gluteal region consist of the ilium, ischium, pubis and sacrum which together form the pelvis and articulate with the femur (Fig. 7.2). There are several bony features that can be palpated within this region. Laterally, the iliac crests can be palpated at the level of L4 as two horizontal bony ridges. At the most anterior aspect of the iliac crests are the anterior superior iliac spines which can be palpated. At the most posterior aspect of the iliac crests, the posterior superior iliac spines can be easily identified by slight depressions in the skin. These are located at vertebral level S2, lateral to the vertebral column. On the posterior surface in the midline is the sacrum. The lateral margins of the sacrum articulate with the ilium via the paired sacroiliac joints. Although the joints themselves cannot be easily palpated, the overlying posterior sacroiliac ligaments can be felt. Inferiorly, at the level of the gluteal fold, the bony prominences formed by the ischial tuberosity are easily palpable.

The major joint in the gluteal region is the hip joint, which is the articulation between the acetabulum of the ilium and the femur. The hip joint itself cannot be palpated, although both the greater trochanter and pubic tubercle are palpable. The greater trochanter is located on the lateral aspect of the hip, inferior to the iliac crest. The pubic tubercle (Chapter 4) can be identified on the superior pubic ramus, just lateral to the pubic symphysis.

Muscles

The buttock comprises of the gluteal muscles, and overlying subcutaneous fat and skin. The contours of the buttocks are defined by the gluteus maximus muscles inferiorly and the gluteus medius muscles superiorly. Located deep to the gluteus medius muscles are the gluteus minimus muscles (Table 7.1). The lateral rotators of the hip joint comprise a group of short muscles: the piriformis, superior and inferior gemelli, obturator internus and quadratus femoris muscles. The piriformis muscle is a clinical landmark for the underlying sciatic nerve, which usually emerges from the lower border of the muscle. However, particularly where there are variations in the relationship between the nerve and the piriformis muscle, compression of the nerve can lead to piriformis syndrome, with resultant pain and paresthesia. Emerging superior and inferior to the piriformis muscle are the superior and inferior gluteal nerves and blood vessels.

Injection sites

Intramuscular injections in the gluteal region must avoid damaging underlying structures, especially nerves. The gluteal region is divided into four quadrants: upper lateral, upper medial, lower lateral and lower medial (Fig. 7.3). The quadrants are created by a vertical line passing inferiorly from the highest point of the iliac crest, intersected by a horizontal line lying midway between the highest point of the iliac crest and the ischial tuberosity. The sciatic nerve passes between the greater trochanter and the ischial tuberosity in the lower medial quadrant. The superior gluteal nerve passes in the upper medial quadrant. The safe area for injections is the upper lateral quadrant.

THIGH

Bones

The bone of the thigh is the femur. The femur articulates superiorly with the acetabulum and inferiorly with the tibia at the knee joint (Fig. 7.4). The degree of adduction of the femur (or Q angle) is more pronounced in the female than male, which is due to a wider pelvis in females. Although the shaft of the femur cannot be palpated, there are a number of bony features that are palpable. The greater trochanter lies in the upper lateral part of the thigh and is easily palpated. In contrast, the lesser trochanter is not palpable. At the distal end of the femoral shaft are the medial and lateral femoral condyles. The lateral and medial epicondyles can be easily identified as the bony prominences on the

To Do (Fig. 7.1)

- Observe the two depressions on each side of the upper surface of the gluteal region at the level of S2, which correspond to the location of the posterior superior iliac spines. Alternatively, to locate these spines, rest your index finger on the top of the iliac crests. Your thumbs should naturally find these more medially located depressions.
- Palpate the ischial tuberosity.

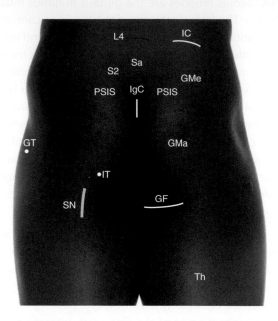

Fig. 7.1 Surface projections of the gluteal region. *GF*, gluteal fold; *GMa*, gluteus maximus; *GMe*, gluteus medius; *GT*, greater trochanter; *IC*; iliac crest; *IgC*, intergluteal cleft; *IT*, ischial tuberosity; *PSIS*, posterior superior iliac spine; *Sa*, sacrum; *SN*, sciatic nerve, *Th*, thigh.

To Do (Fig. 7.2)

- Palpate the greater trochanter of the femur by taking an approximate line from the pubic tubercle laterally.
- Locate the adductor tubercle on the medial side of the distal femur.
- Palpate the lateral and medial epicondyles of the femur.

To Do (Figs. 7.1, 7.2 and 7.3)

Posterior aspect:

- Observe the gluteal folds and the intergluteal cleft.
- Perform a contraction of the gluteus maximus muscle by standing. Palpate the gluteus maximus muscle.
- Palpate the gluteus medius muscle in the upper quadrants. It can be palpated immediately superior to the greater trochanter.
- Try walking a couple of steps while palpating the gluteus medius muscle. The gluteus medius muscle contracts to prevent pelvic drop when the opposite foot is raised off the ground (midstance).
- Trace the outlines of the gluteus maximus and minimus muscles on a volunteer.
- Demonstrate flexion, extension, abduction, adduction, medial rotation and lateral rotation of the lower limb at the hip joint.
- Draw gridlines that delineate the safe area in the gluteal region. To create the vertical line start at the highest point of the iliac crest and draw inferiorly to the level of the gluteal fold. To create the horizontal line, locate the midpoint between the iliac crest and the ischial tuberosity and draw a line laterally.

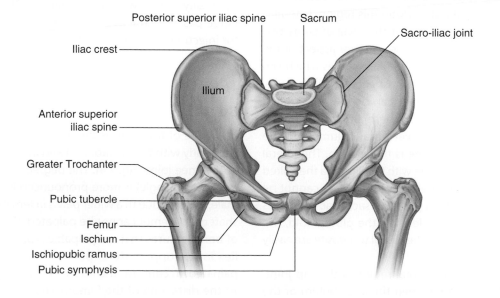

Fig. 7.2 Bones of the pelvis.
(Modified from Drake, RL, Gray's Anatomy for Students, 3rd ed, 2015, Churchill Livingstone, Elsevier.)

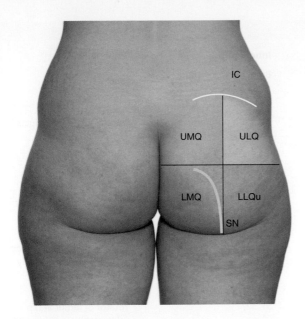

Fig. 7.3 Injection site in the gluteal region. *IC,* iliac crest; *LLQu,* lower lateral quadrant; *LMQ,* lower medial quadrant; *SN,* sciatic nerve; *ULQ,* upper lateral quadrant; *UMQ,* upper medial quadrant.

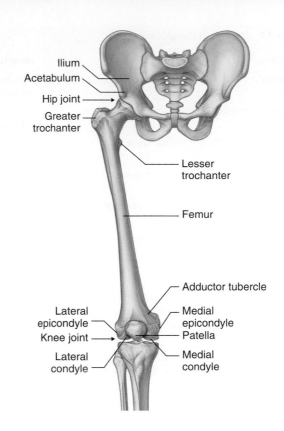

Fig. 7.4 Bones of the proximal lower limb.
(Modified from Drake, RL, Gray's Anatomy for Students, 3rd ed, 2015, Churchill Livingstone, Elsevier.)

sides of the knee. Deep on the medial side, the adductor tubercle may be palpated between the vastus medialis muscle and the distal insertion of the sartorius muscle. The patella is the sesamoid bone lying anterior to the knee joint, within the quadriceps femoris tendon. The anterior surface and margins of the patella are easily palpable. Extending inferiorly from the patella, the patellar ligament can be felt as a band passing from the patella to its inferior attachment on the tibial tuberosity.

Iliotibial tract

The thigh is encased in deep fascia known as the fascia lata. The fascia lata is thickened laterally to form a flat longitudinal band that passes along the lateral aspect of the thigh, known as the iliotibial tract. The tract (or band) is seen as a groove on the lateral thigh. It can be palpated along its length from the iliac crest to its insertion onto the lateral epicondyle of the tibia at Gerdy's tubercle. The iliotibial tract assists with knee stability and can be more easily observed when the knee is flexed. Iliotibial band syndrome is a common overuse injury in runners and cyclists, where the iliotibial tract rubs against the lateral femoral epicondyle. The tensor fasciae latae and gluteus maximus muscles tense the tract (Fig. 7.5). The tensor faciae latae muscle can be palpated immediately inferior to the anterior superior iliac spine.

Muscles

Anterior compartment

The muscles of the anterior compartment of the thigh are the quadriceps and sartorius muscles. The quadriceps muscles form the bulk of the anterior thigh and consist of the rectus femoris, vastus medialis, vastus lateralis and vastus intermedius muscles (Table 7.2). All but the vastus intermedius muscle, which lies deep to the rectus femoris muscle, can be palpated. In the midline, when contracted, the rectus femoris muscle appears raised along the length of the anterior thigh. On the medial side is the vastus medialis muscle. This muscle forms a particular bulge at its distal insertion point when contracted (Fig. 7.6). On the lateral side of the thigh is the vastus lateralis, which forms a less obvious bulge on the lateral side of the knee when contracted.

Lying superficial to the quadriceps muscles is the sartorius muscle (Table 7.2). This narrow straplike muscle passes from lateral to medial across the anterior surface of the thigh. The sartorius muscle can be palpated along its length when the knee is extended, the hip joint flexed and laterally rotated. The upper part of sartorius forms the lateral boundary of the femoral triangle. Lying deep to the sartorius muscle are the saphenous branch of the femoral nerve, the femoral artery and the femoral vein. These neurovascular structures pass through the adductor canal toward the medial side of the distal thigh. The saphenous nerve carries on into the leg to supply the skin on the medial side of the proximal part of the foot and ankle.

Table 7.1 Muscles of the gluteal region

Muscle	Origin	Insertion	Innervation	Function
Piriformis	Anterior surface of sacrum	Greater trochanter of femur	Branches from S1 and S2	
Obturator internus	True pelvis; obturator membrane	Greater trochanter of femur	Nerve to obturator internus (L5, S1)	Laterally rotates abducts femur at hip
Gemellus superior	Ischial spine	Greater trochanter of femur		
Gemellus inferior	Ischial tuberosity	Greater trochanter of femur	Nerve to quadratus femoris (L5, S1)	
Quadratus femoris	Lateral surface of ischium	Quadrate tubercle on femur		Laterally rotates femur at hip joint
Gluteus minimus	External surface of ilium	Greater trochanter	Superior gluteal nerve (L4, L5, S1)	Abducts femur at hip joint; prevents pelvic drop during walking; medially rotates thigh
Gluteus medius	External surface of ilium	Greater trochanter		
Gluteus maximus	External surface of ilium, sacrum, coccyx, sacrotuberous ligament	Iliotibial tract and gluteal tuberosity of femur	Inferior gluteal nerve (L5, S1, S2)	Extensor and lateral rotator of femur at hip joint; stabilizer of hip and knee joint
Tensor fasciae latae	Crest of ilium	Iliotibial tract	Superior gluteal nerve (L4, L5, S1)	Stabilizes the knee in extension

Modified from Drake, RL, Gray's Anatomy for Students, 3rd ed, 2015, Churchill Livingstone, Elsevier (full table available in the e-book).

Table 7.2 Muscles of the anterior compartment of thigh

Muscle	Origin	Insertion	Innervation	Function
Psoas major	T12 to L5 vertebrae	Lesser trochanter of femur	Anterior rami of L1, L2, L3	Flexes the thigh at the hip joint
Iliacus	Iliac fossa	Lesser trochanter of femur		
Vastus medialis	Medial surface of femur	Quadriceps femoris tendon and patella		Extends the leg at the knee joint
Vastus intermedius	Anterior and lateral surfaces of femur	Quadriceps femoris tendon, patella, and lateral condyle of tibia		
Vastus lateralis	Lateral surface of femur	Quadriceps femoris tendon and patella	Femoral nerve (L2, L3)	
Rectus femoris	Anterior inferior iliac spine and superior to the acetabulum	Quadriceps femoris tendon		Flexes the thigh at the hip joint and extends the leg at the knee joint
Sartorius	Anterior superior iliac spine	Medial surface of tibia		Flexes the thigh at the hip joint and flexes the leg at the knee joint

Modified from Drake, RL, Gray's Anatomy for Students, 3rd ed, 2015, Churchill Livingstone, Elsevier (full table available in the e-book).

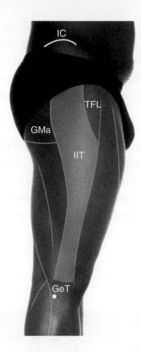

Fig. 7.5 Surface projections of the lateral aspect of the thigh. *GeT*, Gerdy's tubercle; *GMa*, gluteus maximus; *IC*, iliac crest; *IIT*, iliotibial tract; *TFL*, tensor fasciae latae.

To Do (Fig. 7.5)

Lateral aspect:

- While standing, locate the groove marked by the iliotibial tract. This can be more easily located in the upper thigh by stepping from one side to the other, which will tighten the tract
- Starting at the anterior superior iliac spine, draw a line inferiorly, curving the line toward the tibia at the knee, to represent the tract.

Femoral triangle

The femoral triangle is a region on the anterior surface at the junction of the thigh and abdominal wall. The area demarcated by the inguinal ligament forms the superior border. The sartorius muscle forms the lateral border, and the medial border is formed by the medial edge of the adductor longus muscle. The floor of the triangle, from medial to lateral, is comprised of the adductor longus, pectineus and iliopsoas muscles (Fig. 7.7). The roof is formed by the fascia lata, except at the saphenous opening, where the great saphenous vein enters the region. Lying within the femoral triangle are, from lateral to medial, the femoral nerve, femoral artery and femoral vein. Medial to the femoral vein is the femoral canal, which is a passageway for structures, such as lymph nodes, from the abdomen to the upper thigh. It also provides an expansion space for the femoral vein and is the location for femoral hernias. Access to the femoral artery is important for angioplasty.

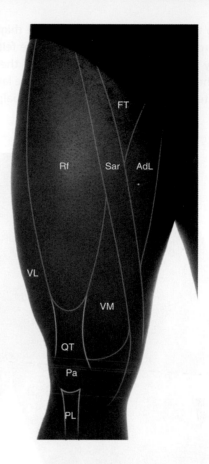

Fig. 7.6 Surface projections of anterior aspect of the thigh. *AdL*, adductor longus; *FT*, femoral triangle; *Pa*, patella; *PL*, patellar ligament; *QT*, quadriceps tendon; *Rf*, rectus femoris; *Sar*, sartorius; *VL*, vastus lateralis; *VM*, vastus medialis.

To Do (Fig. 7.6)

- Stand with one leg forward. Flex the knee joint of the forward leg to at least 30 degrees (such as during a lunge). Palpate the rectus femoris muscle in this limb.
- In the same posture, palpate the vastus lateralis and vastus medialis muscles.
- On the anterior surface of the thigh, trace the outlines of the quadriceps group: the rectus femoris, vastus medialis and vastus lateralis muscles.
- Trace the sartorius muscle form the anterior superior iliac spine to the medial side of the tibia.

Medial compartment

The muscles of the medial compartment of the thigh are the pectineus, adductor longus, adductor brevis, adductor magnus and gracilis muscles (Table 7.3). The adductor longus, adductor magnus and gracilis muscles are easily palpable. The tendon of adductor longus muscle can be palpated just   131 lateral to the pubis, particularly with the thigh flexed and laterally rotated. The muscle belly can be felt as it passes obliquely toward the posterior aspect of the shaft of the femur. The adductor magnus muscle is the largest in bulk, and the tendon of the hamstring part is palpable on the

medial side of the knee, deep to the vastus medialis muscle (Fig. 7.8). The adductor hiatus, which is formed by this tendon, lies about 10 cm superior to the adductor tubercle. This hiatus allows for the passage of the femoral artery and vein into the popliteal fossa where they continue as the popliteal artery and vein. The gracilis muscle, which is the most medial of the adductors, can be palpated on the medial side of the thigh. It inserts into the medial aspect of the proximal tibia as a conjoined tendon, together with the tendons of the sartorius and semitendinosus muscles, called the pes anserinus. The pes anserine bursa is situated between the pes anserinus, approximately 2.5 cm inferior to the tibial plateau.

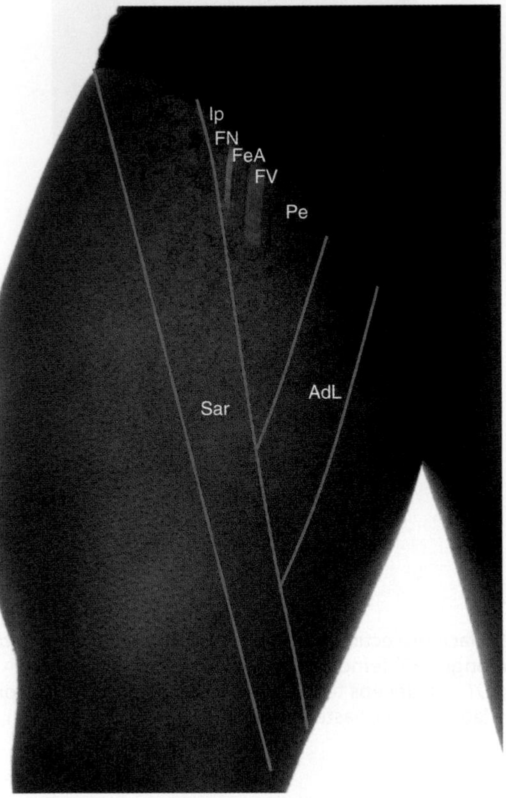

Fig. 7.7 Surface projections of the femoral triangle region. *AdL*, adductor longus; *FeA*, femoral artery; *FN*, femoral nerve; *FV*, femoral vein; *Ip*, iliopsoas; *Pe*, pectineus; *Sar*, sartorius.

To Do (Fig. 7.7)

Anterior aspect:
- Locate the position of the inguinal ligament lying between the pubic tubercle (see Chapter 4) and the anterior superior iliac spine.
- Using the medial border of the sartorius muscle and the medial border of the adductor longus muscle, draw the outline of the femoral triangle on a subject.
- Draw the positions of the femoral artery, femoral vein and femoral canal. The artery enters the triangle at the midinguinal point, passing inferiorly. To confirm the identity of the femoral artery, palpate its pulse.
- Draw a vertical line to represent the femoral nerve, which lies about 0.5–1 cm lateral to the femoral artery.

Table 7.3 Muscles of the medial compartment of thigh

Muscle	Origin	Insertion	Innervation	Function
Gracilis	Body of the pubis, the inferior pubic ramus, and ramus of the ischium	Medial surface of tibia	Obturator nerve (L2, L3)	Adducts thigh at hip joint and flexes leg at knee joint
Pectineus	Pectineal line and adjacent bone of pelvis	Posterior surface of femur	Femoral nerve (L2, L3)	Adducts and flexes thigh at hip joint
Adductor longus	Body of pubis	Linea aspera on femur		
Adductor brevis	Body of pubis and inferior pubic ramus	Linea aspera and posterior surface of femur	Obturator nerve (L2, L3, L4)	Adducts and medially rotates thigh at hip joint
Adductor magnus	Adductor part—ischiopubic ramus	Linea aspera and posterior surface of femur		
	Hamstring part—ischial tuberosity	Adductor tubercle	Sciatic nerve (L2, L3, L4)	

Modified from Drake, RL, Gray's Anatomy for Students, 3rd ed, 2015, Churchill Livingstone, Elsevier (full table available in the e-book).

Posterior compartment

The posterior compartment of the thigh contains the hamstring muscles (Table 7.4). These are the semitendinosus and semimembranosus muscles on the medial side, and the biceps femoris muscle on the lateral side. The biceps femoris and semitendinosus muscles can be easily palpated, whereas the semimembranosus muscle, which lies deep to semitendinosus muscle, cannot. With the leg partially flexed, the tendons of the semitendinosus and biceps femoris muscles can be identified on the medial and lateral aspect of the popliteal fossa, respectively (see popliteal fossa). The tendon of biceps femoris is a much larger, flatter tendon compared to that of the semitendinosus muscle (Fig. 7.9).

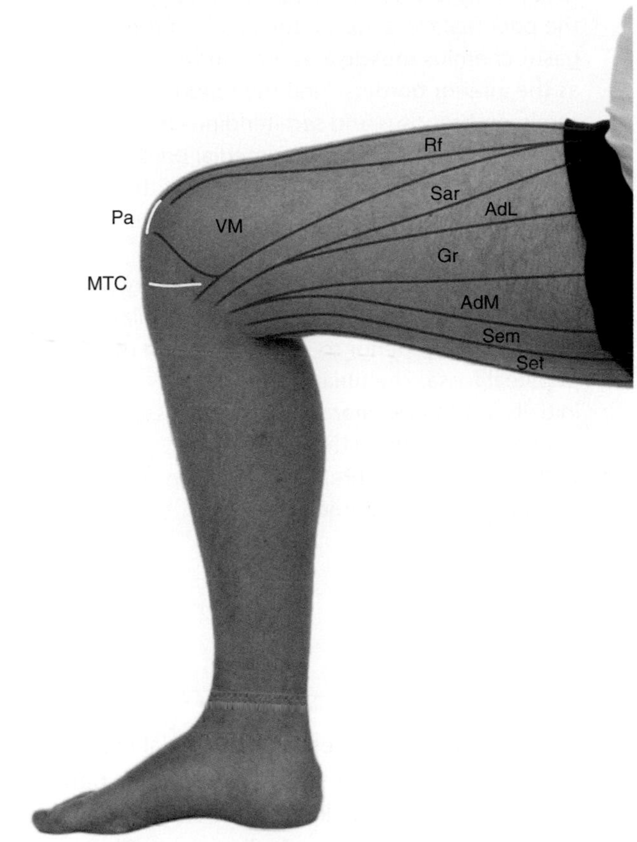

Popliteal fossa

The popliteal fossa is a diamond-shaped space on the posterior aspect of the knee joint. The superior borders are formed medially by the distal ends of the semitendinosus and semimembranosus muscles and laterally by the distal end of the biceps femoris muscle, which, except for the tendon of the semimembranosus muscle, can be easily palpated (Fig. 7.9). The inferior borders are formed by the lateral and medial heads of the gastrocnemius muscle. The typically fat filled fossa has a number of important

Fig. 7.8 Surface projections of the medial thigh. *AdL*, adductor longus; *AdM*, adductor magnus; *Gr*, gracilis; *MTC*, medial tibial condyle; *Pa*, patella; *Rf*, rectus femoris; *Sar*, sartorius; *Sem*, semimembranosus; *Set*, semitendinosus; *VM*, vastus medialis.

> **To Do** (Fig. 7.8)
>
> Medial aspect:
> - Determine the position of the boundary between the medial and posterior compartments of the thigh.
> - On a volunteer, locate the tendon of the adductor longus muscle during an isometric contraction of the muscle. This can be performed by asking the subject to adduct the thigh against resistance.
> - Locate the tendon of the adductor magnus muscle. This tendon can be palpated where it lies deep to vastus medialis muscle, close to its attachment to the adductor tubercle.
> - Draw outlines of the adductor muscles in the thigh.

Table 7.4 Muscles of the posterior compartment of thigh (spinal segments in bold are the major segments innervating the muscle)

Muscle	Origin	Insertion	Innervation	Function
Biceps femoris	Long head – ischial tuberosity; short head – linea aspera	Head of fibula	Sciatic nerve (L5, S1, S2)	Flexes leg at knee joint; extends and laterally rotates thigh at hip joint and laterally rotates leg at knee joint
Semitendinosus	Ischial tuberosity	Medial surface of tibia		Flexes leg at knee joint and extends thigh at hip joint; medially rotates thigh at hip joint and leg at knee joint
Semimembranosus	Ischial tuberosity	Medial tibial condyle		

Modified from Drake, RL, Gray's Anatomy for Students, 3rd ed, 2015, Churchill Livingstone, Elsevier (full table available in the e-book).

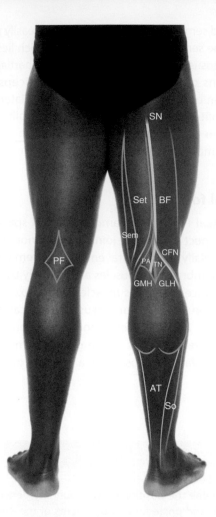

To Do (Fig. 7.9)

Posterior aspect:

- In a volunteer, palpate the hamstring muscles during an isometric contraction of the muscle group. This can be performed either standing or lying prone. Ask the subject to flex their leg at the knee joint to about 90 degrees against resistance.
- Draw in the diamond-shaped boundary of the popliteal fossa: locate the heads of the gastrocnemius muscle and draw in their arcs as the inferior borders. Find the tendons of the semimembranosus and semitendinosus muscles and mark these as the upper medial border. Palpate the tendon of the long head of the biceps femoris muscle and mark this as the upper lateral border.
- Draw lines to represent the popliteal artery, and vein, and the tibial and common fibular nerves passing from superior to inferior through the popliteal fossa. The tibial nerve initially lies on the lateral side of the vessels but crosses posteriorly to the medial side.
- With sufficient pressure, you should be able to feel the pulse of the popliteal artery.

Fig. 7.9 Surface projections of the posterior aspect thigh and popliteal fossa. *AT*, achilles tendon; *BF*, biceps femoris; *CFN*, common fibular nerve; *GLH*, gastrocnemius lateral head; *GMH*, gastrocnemius medial head; *PA*, popliteal artery; *PF*, popliteal fossa; *Sem*, semimembranosus; *Set*, semitendinosus; *SN*, sciatic nerve; *So*, soleus; *TN*, tibial nerve.

structures within or passing through it. These are the tibial nerve, popliteal vein, popliteal artery, small saphenous vein, common fibular nerve, sural nerve and the popliteal lymph nodes. The most medial structure within the fossa is the popliteal artery. The pulse of this artery is readily detectable. Sitting lateral to the popliteal artery is the popliteal vein. The popliteal artery and vein are a continuation of the femoral artery and vein passing through the adductor hiatus.

KNEE JOINT

The knee joint is a hinge joint formed between the condyles of the femur and tibia (Fig. 7.10). When the knee joint is

flexed, the margins of the femoral and tibial condyles can be palpated anteriorly on either side of the patella, or posteriorly. Stability of the knee is provided by a number of extracapsular and intracapsular ligaments. The principal extracapsular ligaments are the fibular (lateral) and tibial (medial) collateral ligaments (Fig. 7.11). The fibular collateral ligament is cordlike and attaches to the lateral femoral epicondyle and fibular head. It can be palpated on the lateral side of the knee. Passing deep to the fibular collateral ligament is the tendon of the popliteus muscle. The tibial collateral ligament is a broad flat structure attached to the medial femoral epicondyle and the medial aspect of the tibia. The main intracapsular ligaments are the anterior and posterior cruciate ligaments. These ligaments prevent anterior and posterior displacement of the femur on the tibia. The menisci are fibrocartilage plates lying between the femoral condyles and tibial plateau, which act as shock absorbers, reduce friction during movement and improve stability when standing. The medial meniscus is attached to the tibial collateral ligament. When the leg is flexed, the menisci are palpable superior to the anterior tibial plateau.

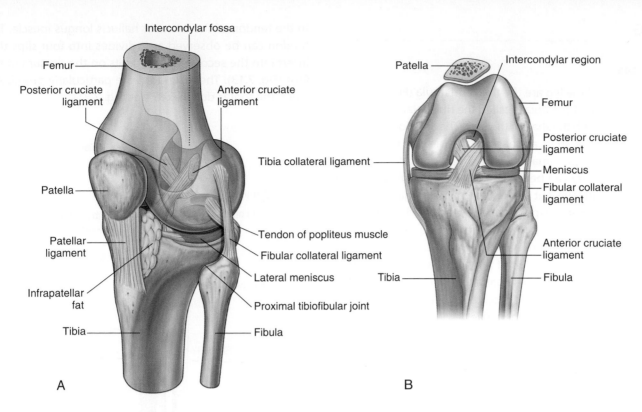

Fig. 7.10 Knee joint. A, Anterior view. B, Posterior view.
(Modified from Drake, RL, Gray's Anatomy for Students, 3rd ed, 2015, Churchill Livingstone, Elsevier.)

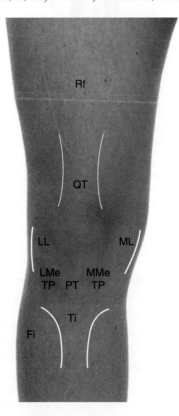

Fig. 7.11 Surface projections of the anterior aspect of right knee. *Fi*, fibula; *LL*, lateral ligament; *LMe*, lateral meniscus; *ML*, medial ligament; *MMe*, medial meniscus; *PT*, patellar tendon; *QT*, quadriceps tendon; *Rf*, rectus femoris; *Ti*, tibia; *TP*, tibial plateau.

To Do (Fig. 7.11)

- Examine flexion and extension of the leg at the knee joint.
- While sitting, raise one foot off the ground. In the limb that is raised, examine the extent of medial and lateral rotation at the knee joint.
- Palpate the femoral condyles when the knee is flexed. These can be located either side of the patella or posteriorly.
- Palpate the lateral and medial collateral ligaments at the sides of the knee. This can be more easily performed with the subject lying supine and knees flexed. Note the differences in shape. Palpate the ligaments during flexion and extension of the knee joint.
- While standing with weight on opposite limb, palpate the patella and observe how it moves from side to side when not weight bearing.
- Test the patellar reflex by tapping on the patellar tendon when the knee is at rest and observe the rapid extension of the knee joint.
- On a volunteer, position your fingers on the head of the fibula and the lateral epicondyle of the femur while they are sitting. Now ask your volunteer to stand. Note the medial rotation of the femur as the joint locks.
- Identify the patellar ligament in the midline.
- At the proximal end of the tibia, locate the tibial tuberosity.
- At the distal end of the tibia, palpate the medial malleolus.

LEG

Bones

The bones of the leg are the tibia and fibula (Fig. 7.12). The proximal end of the tibia is called the tibial plateau, which is continuous with the shaft of the tibia. The anterior and medial surfaces of the shaft are easily palpable. On the anterior surface of the proximal tibia, the bony prominence of the tibial tuberosity can be felt as a roughened protuberance. This is the attachment site for the patellar ligament. At its distal end, the tibia expands on the medial side of the ankle as the medial malleolus, which can be palpated. The fibula lies laterally to the tibia. Unlike the tibia, the fibula does not bear weight. The head of the fibula, along with part of the neck and shaft, is easily palpated. The distal end of the fibula is palpable where it projects as the lateral malleolus on the lateral surface of the ankle.

Muscles

Anterior compartment

The anterior compartment of the leg contains the tibialis anterior, extensor digitorum longus and extensor hallucis longus muscles (Table 7.5). The largest and most superficial of the muscles is the tibialis anterior muscle, which can be palpated in the anterior leg, adjacent to the shaft of the tibia. The distal tendons of the anterior compartment muscles pass under the 'Y' shaped extensor retinaculum as they cross the anterior ankle joint to the dorsum of the foot. Each tendon can be easily observed and palpated within the foot. The tendon of the tibialis anterior muscle is seen as it crosses toward the medial side of the foot. The relatively large tendon of the extensor hallucis longus muscle can be traced to the great toe. In the proximal foot, this tendon can be palpated immediately lateral to the tendon of the tibialis anterior muscle. The tendon of the extensor digitorum lies lateral to the tendon of the extensor hallucis longus muscle. The tendon can be observed as it divides into four slips that insert into the second to fifth digits on the dorsum of the foot (Fig. 7.13). These tendons are particularly prominent when the foot is dorsiflexed (see Fig. 7.21).

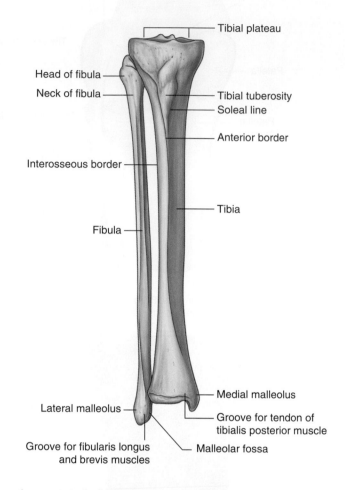

Fig. 7.12 Bones of the right leg, anterior aspect.
(Modified from Drake, RL, Gray's Anatomy for Students, 3rd ed, 2015, Churchill Livingstone, Elsevier.)

Table 7.5	Muscles of the anterior compartment of leg			
Muscle	**Origin**	**Insertion**	**Innervation**	**Function**
Tibialis anterior	Lateral surface of tibia and interosseous membrane	Medial cuneiform and metatarsal 1	Deep fibular nerve (L4, L5)	Dorsiflexion of foot; inversion of foot; support of medial arch of foot
Extensor hallucis longus	Medial surface of fibula and interosseous membrane	Distal phalanx of great toe		Extension of great toe and dorsiflexion of foot
Extensor digitorum longus	Medial surface of fibula and lateral tibial condyle	Distal and middle phalanges of lateral four toes		Extension of lateral four toes and dorsiflexion of foot
Fibularis tertius	Medial surface of fibula	Metatarsal 5		Dorsiflexion and eversion of foot

Modified from Drake, RL, Gray's Anatomy for Students, 3rd ed, 2015, Churchill Livingstone, Elsevier (full table available in the e-book).

the soleus and the plantaris muscles (Fig. 7.14 and Table 7.6). These superficial muscles plantarflex the foot at the ankle joint. The gastrocnemius muscle is the most superficial muscle of the posterior calf and has two heads, the medial and lateral. Standing on tip toes makes the two heads of gastrocnemius more prominent and palpable. Distally, they converge to form the calcaneal tendon, or Achilles tendon, which can be observed toward its attachment on the calcaneus. The soleus muscle lies deep to the gastrocnemius and also inserts into the calcaneal tendon. The soleus muscle can be palpated either side of the calcaneal tendon. The plantaris muscle is a small vestigial muscle with a long tendinous portion that passes between the soleus muscle and the gastrocnemius muscle. It cannot be palpated.

The deep group of posterior compartment consists of the popliteus, flexor hallucis longus, flexor digitorum longus and tibialis posterior muscles (Table 7.6). Although these muscles are not palpable, their tendons can be identified as they pass posterior and inferior the medial malleolus to enter the tarsal tunnel.

Tarsal tunnel

The tarsal tunnel is a depression on the posteromedial aspect of the foot. The tarsal tunnel runs between the calcaneus and the medial malleolus, the floor of which is formed by both of these bones and the talus. The roof of this tunnel is formed by the flexor retinaculum, which helps to prevent bowstringing of the tendons. The structures that pass through the tunnel are, from anterior to posterior, the tibialis posterior tendon, flexor digitorum longus tendon, posterior tibial artery and vein(s), tibial nerve and the flexor hallucis longus tendon (Fig. 7.15). The pulse of the tibial artery may be palpated as a point between the tendon of flexor digitorum and the tibial nerve, posterior to the medial malleolus.

Lateral compartment

The lateral compartment contains the fibularis (peroneus) longus and brevis muscles (Table 7.7). The more superficial fibularis longus muscle can be observed on the lateral side of the leg. The tendons of both muscles pass posterior and then inferior to the lateral malleolus under the fibular retinaculum before entering the foot (Fig. 7.16).

FOOT

Bones

There are 26 bones in the foot: seven tarsals (talus, calcaneus, cuboid, three cuneiforms and the navicular), five metatarsals and 14 phalanges (Fig. 7.17). All of the bones of the foot can be palpated, which includes the tarsal bones. The

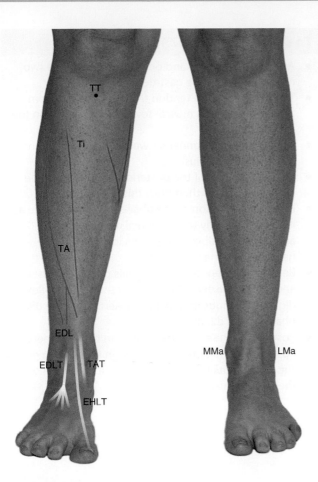

Fig. 7.13 Surface projections of the anterior aspect of the leg. *EDL*, extensor digitorum longus; *EDLT*, extensor digitorum longus tendon; *EHLT*: extensor hallucis longus tendon; *LMa*, lateral malleolus; *MMa*, medial malleolus; *TA*, tibialis anterior; *TAT*, tibialis anterior tendon; *Ti*, tibia; *TT*, tibial tuberosity.

To Do (Figs. 7.13 and 7.21)

- While dorsiflexing the foot, palpate the tibialis anterior muscle.
- Palpate the tendons of tibialis anterior, extensor hallucis longus and extensor digitorum longus muscles as they enter the dorsum of the foot.
- From the extensor retinaculum, draw lines that follow these tendons to their insertions. The tendon of the tibialis anterior muscle inserts into the first metatarsal and medial cuneiform; the tendon of the extensor hallucis longus muscle inserts into the distal phalanx of d1; the tendons of the extensor digitorum longus muscle insert into the distal phalanx of d2–d5. These tendons can be more easily identified by extending the toes.

Posterior compartment

In the posterior compartment of the leg there are superficial and deep muscles, which together form the bulk of the calf. The superficial group consists of the gastrocnemius,

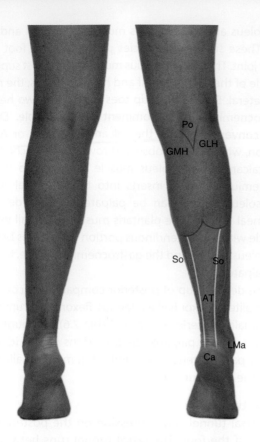

Fig. 7.14 Surface projections of the posterior aspect of the leg. *AT*, achilles tendon; *Ca*, calcaneus; *GLH*, gastrocnemius lateral head; *GMH*, gastrocnemius medial head; *LMa*, lateral malleolus; *Po*, popliteus; *So*, soleus.

To Do (Figs. 7.14 and 7.15)

- Ask a volunteer to stand on tiptoes. Locate the two muscle bellies of the gastrocnemius muscle.
- Trace the calcaneal tendon (Achille's tendon) from the gastrocnemius muscle toward its insertion on the calcaneus.
- Locate the tarsal tunnel between the calcaneus and the medial malleolus.
- Locate the pulse of the posterior tibial artery in the tarsal tunnel, and then draw this in.
- Draw in the tendon of the tibialis posterior muscle as it passes inferiorly to the medial malleolus and anterior to the tibial artery to its insertion on the navicular and medial cuneiform.
- Between the tendon of the tibialis posterior muscle and the tibial artery, draw in the tendon of the flexor digitorum longus muscle to its insertion on the distal phalanges of d2–d5.
- Posterior to the tibial artery, draw in the tibial nerve.
- Posterior to the tibial nerve, draw in the tendon of the flexor hallucis longus muscle to its insertion on the distal phalanx of the great toe.

Table 7.6 Superficial and deep group of muscles in the posterior compartment of leg

Muscle	Origin	Insertion	Innervation	Function
Superficial				
Gastrocnemius	Medial head—posterior surface of femur; lateral head—lateral femoral condyle	Via calcaneal tendon, to calcaneus		
Plantaris	Inferior surface of femur and oblique popliteal ligament of knee	Via calcaneal tendon, to calcaneus	Tibial nerve (S1, S2)	Plantarflexes foot and flexes knee
Soleus	Soleal line of tibia; fibula; tendinous arch between tibial and fibular attachments	Via calcaneal tendon, to calcaneus		
Deep				
Popliteus	Lateral femoral condyle	Posterior surface of tibia		Unlocks knee joint (laterally rotates femur on fixed tibia)
Flexor hallucis longus	Posterior surface of fibula and interosseous membrane	Distal phalanx of great toe		Flexes great toe
Flexor digitorum longus	Posterior surface of tibia	Distal phalanges of the lateral four toes	Tibial nerve (L4 to S1)	Flexes lateral four toes
Tibialis posterior	Interosseous membrane, tibia and fibula	Navicular and medial cuneiform		Inversion and plantarflexion of foot; support of medial arch of foot

Modified from Drake, RL, Gray's Anatomy for Students, 3rd ed, 2015, Churchill Livingstone, Elsevier (full table available in the e-book).

calcaneus can be easily identified at the posterior of the foot. A ridge of bone on the calcaneus, the sustentaculum tali, can be felt inferior to the medial malleolus. Anterior to the ankle joint, the head and neck of the talus are palpable. On the medial side of the foot, a bony prominence formed by the tuberosity on the navicular can be felt. Anterior to the navicular, the cuneiforms are palpable from the dorsal surface. On the lateral side of the foot, the cuboid can be identified. The metacarpals and phalanges are easily palpable from the dorsum. The bones of the foot are connected by ligaments that result in a strong, yet flexible, structure capable of supporting the body weight. The bones of the foot form arches that are important in shock absorbing, distributing weight and propelling the limb during walking and running (Fig. 7.18). The transverse arch is comprised of the cuboid, cuneiforms and metatarsals. The longitudinal arch is divided into medial and lateral components. The medial arch is higher

and is comprised of the calcaneus, talus, navicular, cuneiforms and the three medial metatarsals. The lateral arch is lower and is comprised of the calcaneus and the cuboid and the two lateral metatarsals. Body weight is spread between contact points on the foot. The forefoot (ball of the foot) contains six contact points: the two sesamoid bones of the first metatarsal and the heads of the lateral four

To Do (Fig. 7.16)

- Palpate the fibularis longus muscle during eversion of the foot.
- Palpate the tendons of the fibularis longus and brevis muscles as they pass posterior to the lateral malleolus.

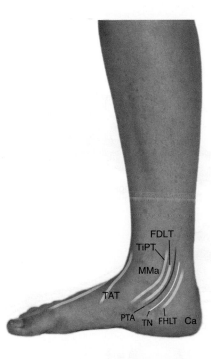

Fig. 7.15 Surface projections of the medial aspect of the leg. *Ca*, calcaneus; *FDLT*, flexor digitorum longus tendon; *FHLT*, flexor hallucis longus tendon; *MMa*, medial malleolus; *PTA*, posterior tibial artery; *TAT*, tibialis anterior tendon; *TiPT*, tibialis posterior tendon; *TN*, tibial nerve.

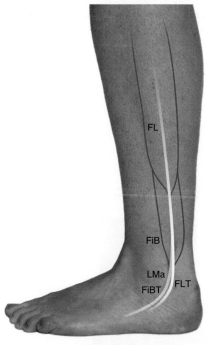

Fig. 7.16 Surface projections of the lateral aspect of the leg. *FiB*, fibularis brevis; *FiBT*, fibularis brevis tendon; *FL*, fibularis longus; *FLT*, fibularis longus tendon; *LMa*, lateral malleolus.

Table 7.7 Muscles of the lateral compartment of leg

Muscle	Origin	Insertion	Innervation	Function
Fibularis longus	Lateral surface of fibula	Medial cuneiform and metatarsal 1	Superficial Fibular nerve (L5, S1, S2)	Eversion and plantarflexion of foot; supports arches of foot
Fibularis brevis	Lateral surface of fibula	Metatarsal 5		Eversion of foot

Modified from Drake, RL, Gray's Anatomy for Students, 3rd ed, 2015, Churchill Livingstone, Elsevier (full table available in the e-book).

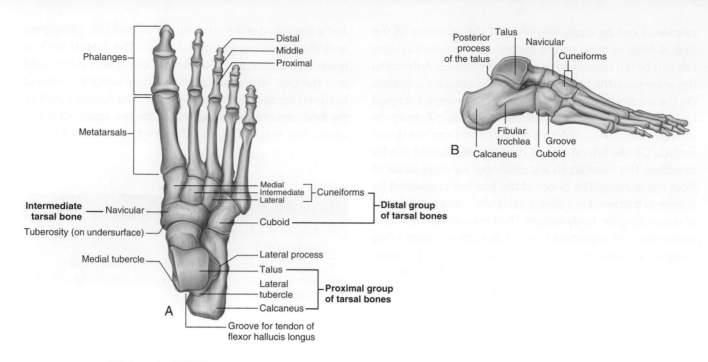

Fig. 7.17 Bones of the foot. A, Dorsum of foot. B, Lateral aspect of foot.
(From Drake, RL, Gray's Anatomy for Students, 3rd ed, 2015, Churchill Livingstone, Elsevier.)

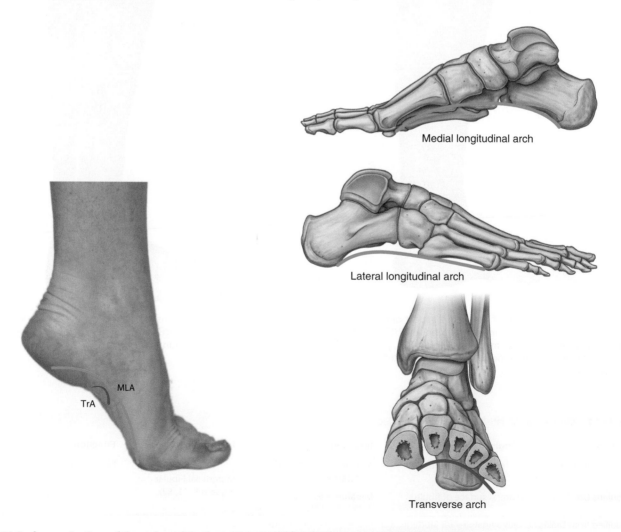

Fig. 7.18 Surface projections of the arches of the foot. MLA, medial longitudinal arch; TrA, transverse arch.
(Right images from Drake, RL, Gray's Anatomy for Students, 3rd ed, 2015, Churchill Livingstone, Elsevier.)

metatarsal bones. The hindfoot (heel) contains one contact point, the calcaneus (Fig. 7.19).

The joints of the foot are the ankle joint, intertarsal joints, tarsometatarsal joints, metatarsophalangeal joints and interphalangeal joints. The ankle joint (talocrural) is a mortice-like joint between the medial malleolus of the tibia, the lateral malleolus of the fibula and the talus (Fig. 7.20). It is supported medially by the fanlike deltoid ligament and laterally by three collateral ligaments, which are the anterior talofibular, posterior talofibular and calcaneofibular ligaments. These ligaments are not easily palpable. The ankle joint allows dorsiflexion and plantarflexion of the foot. Two important intertarsal joints are the subtalar and transverse tarsal joint. The subtalar joint is an articulation between the calcaneus and the talus. This joint allows inversion and eversion of the foot. The transverse tarsal joint is a compound joint between the calcaneus and cuboid, and the talus and navicular. This joint allows rotation along the long axis of the foot, which is important for pronation and supination of the foot, such as when walking over rough terrain.

Muscles

Dorsum of the foot

The dorsum of the foot is the area of the foot facing upwards while in the anatomical position (Fig. 7.21).

To Do (Fig. 7.21)

Dorsal aspect of the foot:
- With the toes extended, locate the extensor digitorum brevis muscle. This muscle can be identified on the dorsolateral side of the foot, directly over the cuboid.

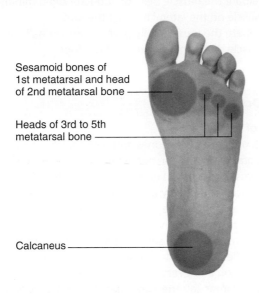

Sesamoid bones of 1st metatarsal and head of 2nd metatarsal bone

Heads of 3rd to 5th metatarsal bone

Calcaneus

Fig. 7.19 Weight-bearing areas of the foot.

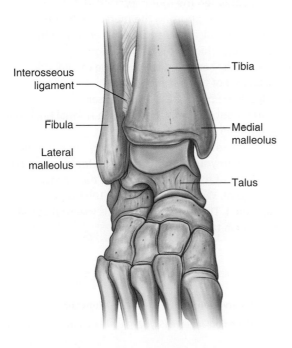

Interosseous ligament

Fibula

Lateral malleolus

Tibia

Medial malleolus

Talus

Fig. 7.20 Ankle joint.
(From Drake, RL, Gray's Anatomy for Students, 3rd ed, 2015, Churchill Livingstone, Elsevier.)

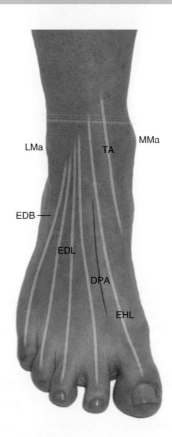

LMa TA MMa

EDB

EDL

DPA

EHL

Fig. 7.21 Surface projections of the dorsum of the foot. *DPA,* dorsalis pedis artery; *EDB,* extensor digitorum brevis; *EDL,* extensor digitorum longus; *EHL,* extensor hallucis longus; *LMa,* lateral malleolus; *MMa,* medial malleolus; *TA,* tibialis anterior.

Extrinsic muscles of the foot include all muscles of the anterior compartment of the leg that terminate in the foot (Table 7.5). The tendons of these muscles are easily observed in the dorsum foot as they pass to their insertions (see anterior compartment of leg and Fig. 7.21).

The intrinsic muscles of the foot lie within the foot. The two intrinsic muscles on the dorsal aspect of the foot are the extensor hallucis brevis muscle and extensor digitorum brevis muscle, which sit deep to the tendons of the extensor digitorum longus muscle on the dorsum of the foot (Fig. 7.21 and Table 7.8). The extensor digitorum brevis muscle can be palpated on the dorsolateral side of the foot.

Sole of the foot

The sole of the foot, or plantar aspect, is the area of the foot facing downwards while in the anatomical position (Fig. 7.22). Extrinsic muscles of the sole of the foot include all muscles of the posterior compartment of the leg that terminate in the foot (Table 7.6). It also includes the fibularis longus muscle, which has a tendon that runs obliquely across the sole of the foot to the medial side. The tendons of these muscles are not easily palpable within the foot.

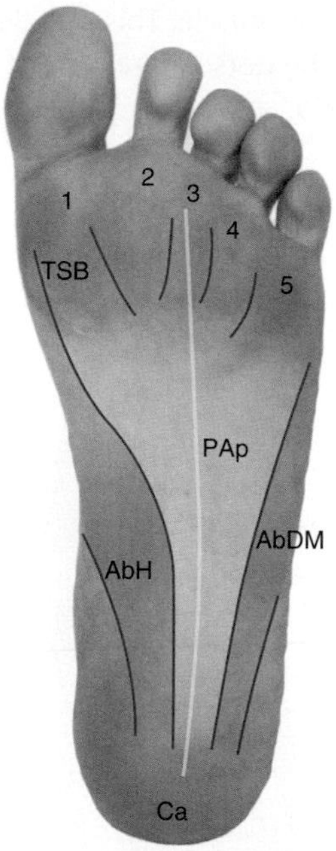

To Do (Fig. 7.22)

Sole of the foot:
- With the great toe extended, palpate the medial edge of the plantar aponeurosis distal to the calcaneus.
- Palpate the muscle belly of abductor digiti minimi muscle on the lateral edge of the foot.
- Palpate the muscle belly of the abductor hallucis muscle on the medial edge of the foot.

To Do (Fig. 7.22)

Sole of the foot:
- Identify the tarsal bones and metatarsals.
- Examine the foot arches, while checking for pes cavus (high arches) or pes planus (flat feet).
- Locate the ankle by palpating the distal ends of the tibia and fibula, the medial and lateral malleoli.
- Demonstrate the movements possible at the ankle joint as well as the subtalar joint. These include dorsiflexion and plantar flexion of the ankle, and inversion and eversion at the subtalar joint.
- The plantar calcaneonavicular ligament or spring ligament lies between the sustentaculum tali and the tuberosity of the navicular. Try to palpate this ligament when the foot is everted. It is an important ligament in supporting the medial arch of the foot.
- Locate the calcaneus and the tuberosity of the calcaneus, which projects posteriorly.
- Palpate the sesamoid bone on the medial side of the distal end of the first metatarsal.
- Palpate the heads of the metatarsals.
- Watch a subject walk, observing a normal heel strike and toe-off gait.
- While standing, move your feet together and then apart. With your feet together, the foot is pronated. The front of the foot is everted at the transverse tarsal joint. With your feet apart, the foot is supinated. The front of the foot is inverted at the transverse tarsal joint.

Fig. 7.22 Surface projections of the sole of the foot. *1*, first metatarsal head; *2*, second metatarsal head; *3*, third metatarsal head; *4*, fourth metatarsal head; *5*, fifth metatarsal head; *AbDM*, abductor digiti minimi; *AbH*, abductor hallucis; *Ca*, calcaneus; *PAp*, plantar aponeurosis; *TSB*, tibial sesamoid bone.

Table 7.8 Muscles of the dorsal aspect of the foot

Muscle	Origin	Insertion	Innervation	Function
Extensor digitorum brevis	Calcaneus	Tendons of extensor digitorum longus of toes 2 to 4	Deep fibular nerve (S1, S2)	Extension of toes 2 to 4
Extensor hallucis brevis	Calcaneus	Proximal phalanx of great toe	Deep fibular nerve (S1, S2)	Extension of great toe

 Modified from Drake, RL, Gray's Anatomy for Students, 3rd ed, 2015, Churchill Livingstone, Elsevier.

Table 7.9 Layer of muscles in the sole of the foot

Muscle	Origin	Insertion	Innervation	Function
First layer				
Abductor hallucis	Calcaneal tuberosity	Medial side of base of proximal phalanx of great toe	Medial plantar nerve (S1, S2, S3)	Abducts and flexes great toe
Flexor digitorum brevis	Calcaneal tuberosity and plantar aponeurosis	Middle phalanges of lateral four toes		Flexes lateral four toes
Abductor digiti minimi	Calcaneal tuberosity	Proximal phalanx of little toe	Lateral plantar nerve (S1, S2, S3)	Abducts little toe
Second layer				
Quadratus plantae	Calcaneus	Tendon of flexor digitorum longus	Lateral plantar nerve (S1, S2, S3)	Flexes toes 2 to 5
Lumbricals	Tendons of flexor digitorum longus	Extensor hoods of toes 2 to 5	Medial and lateral plantar nerves (S2, S3)	Flexion of metatarsophalangeal joint and extension of interphalangeal joints
Third layer				
Flexor hallucis brevis	Cuboid and lateral cuneiform; tendon of tibialis posterior	Proximal phalanx of the great toe	Medial plantar nerve (S1, S2)	Flexes great toe
Adductor hallucis	Transverse head—ligaments of metatarsophalangeal joints of lateral three toes; oblique head—metatarsals 2 to 4	Proximal phalanx of great toe	Lateral plantar nerve (S2, S3)	Adducts great toe
Flexor digiti minimi brevis	Metatarsal 5 and fibularis longus tendon	Proximal phalanx of little toe		Flexes little toe
Fourth layer				
Dorsal interossei	Sides of adjacent metatarsals	Extensor hoods and proximal phalanges of toes 2 to 4	Lateral plantar nerve; deep fibular nerve (S2, S3)	Abduction of toes 2 to 4
Plantar interossei	Metatarsals of toes 3 to 5	Extensor hoods and phalanges of toes 3 to 5	Lateral plantar nerve (S2, S3)	Adduction of toes 3 to 5

Modified from Drake, RL, Gray's Anatomy for Students, 3rd ed, 2015, Churchill Livingstone, Elsevier (full table available in the e-book).

The intrinsic muscles in the sole lie deep beneath the plantar aponeurosis, which is thick connective tissue that connects the tuberosity of the calcaneus to the heads of the metatarsals. The function of the plantar aponeurosis is to support the longitudinal arches of the foot. The plantar aponeurosis can be palpated on the medial side of the sole of the foot. The intrinsic muscles form four layers (Table 7.9). Muscles in the more superficial layers at the medial and lateral sides of the foot are palpable between the calcaneus and their insertions on the digits, such as the abductor hallucis and abductor digit minimi muscles (Fig 7.22).

NEUROVASCULAR STRUCTURES

Vasculature

The main arterial supply to the lower limb is the femoral artery, which arises from the external iliac artery, a branch of the common iliac artery in the pelvis (Fig. 7.23). The first branch of the femoral artery is the profunda femoris artery, which supplies the posterior thigh. The medial and lateral circumflex arteries branch off the deep artery of thigh shortly after its origin. These contribute to an anastomotic arrangement around the hip joint. The femoral artery passes medially down the thigh, through the adductor hiatus to the posterior aspect of the femur and into the popliteal fossa as the popliteal artery. In the leg, the popliteal artery divides into the anterior and posterior tibial arteries, which descend in the anterior and posterior compartments of the leg, respectively. At the ankle, the anterior tibial artery passes into the dorsum of the foot as the dorsalis pedis artery, which lies lateral to the extensor hallucis tendon. The posterior tibial artery passes through the tarsal tunnel into the plantar region of the foot, where it divides into medial and lateral plantar arteries (Fig. 7.24).

143

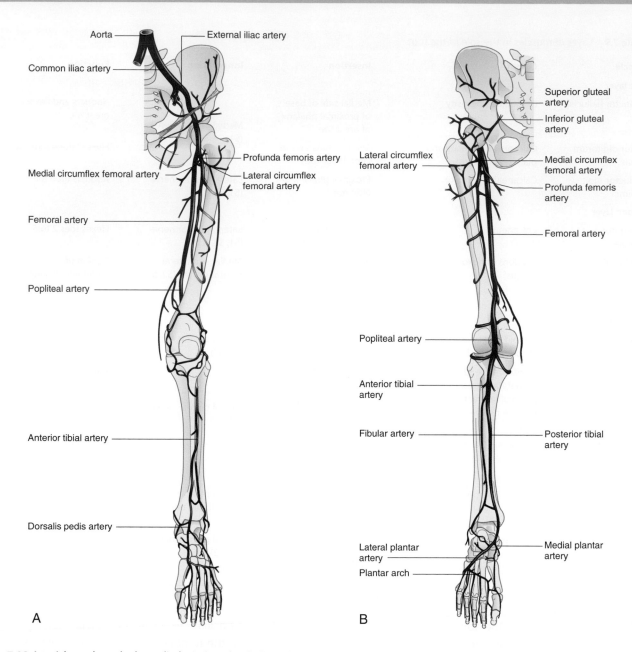

Fig. 7.23 Arterial supply to the lower limb. A, Anterior. B, Posterior.
(From Standring, S, ed. Gray's Anatomy, 41e, 2015, Elsevier.)

The pulse of the femoral artery can be palpated in the femoral triangle, allowing cannulation for angiography and angioplasty. Other sites where arterial pulses may be felt are the popliteal artery in the popliteal fossa, the posterior tibial artery in the tarsal tunnel, and the dorsalis pedis artery on the dorsum of the foot (Fig. 7.24). Because of the distance of the dorsalis pedis pulse point from the heart, it is often used to assess peripheral circulation (but is not always palpable in a normal subject).

Venous drainage

The venous drainage of the lower limb is provided by superficial and deep veins. The superficial veins lie in superficial fascia and are comprised of the great and small saphenous veins. These veins contain nonreturn valves, and when they become incompetent, varicosities develop that are referred to as varicose veins. The saphenous veins arise from the dorsal venous arch on the dorsum of the foot where they are easily visible. From there, passing anterior to the medial malleolus, the great saphenous vein then lies on the medial aspect of the lower limb in superficial fascia, until it drains into the femoral vein at the groin via the saphenous opening in the fascia lata (Fig. 7.25). The opening lies in the upper medial region of the femoral triangle about 3–4 cm inferolateral to the pubic tubercle. The small saphenous vein passes from

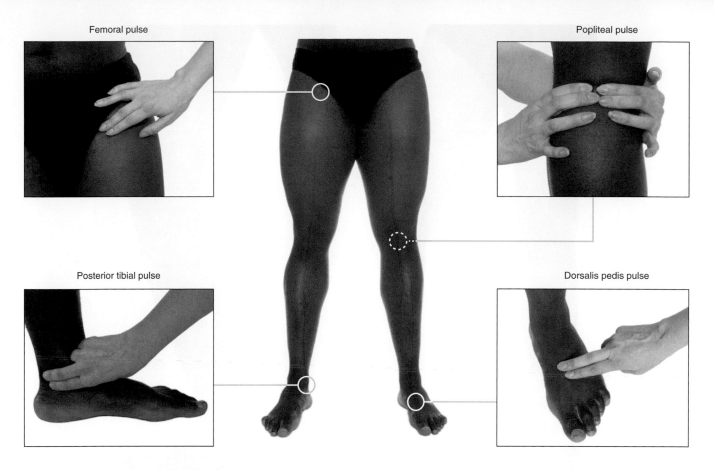

Femoral pulse

Popliteal pulse

Posterior tibial pulse

Dorsalis pedis pulse

Fig. 7.24 Surface projections of the arterial supply to the lower limb and pulse points.

To Do (Figs. 7.24 and 7.25)

- Trace out the position of the femoral artery, which lies two-thirds of the way along a line between the midinguinal point and the adductor tubercle. Note that the femoral vein lies on the medial side, and the femoral nerve on the lateral side of the femoral artery.
- Palpate the pulse of the dorsalis pedis artery on the dorsum of the foot. The vessel lies roughly midway between the two malleoli, just lateral to the extensor hallucis longus tendon.
- Palpate the pulse of the posterior tibial artery inferior to the medial malleolus.
- Locate the dorsal venous arch in the foot. Trace the great saphenous vein from the medial part of the dorsal venous arch toward the femoral triangle. Identify the position of the saphenous opening. Trace the small saphenous vein as it begins posterior to the lateral malleolus, then in the posterior midline part of the leg, to pierce the deep fascia at the posterior aspect of the popliteal fossa. Note that not all individuals display prominent superficial veins, though they are more easily observed if the subject is warm and if the limb is not elevated.

the dorsal venous arch, posterior to the lateral malleolus, toward the popliteal fossa, where it pierces the deep fascia in the roof of the fossa, between the two heads of the gastrocnemius, to drain into the popliteal vein.

Nerves

The nerves that innervate the lower limb originate in the lumbar and sacral plexus (L1 to S3). They include the femoral, obturator and sciatic nerves. In addition to innervating muscles, these nerves also supply the skin. Knowledge of the cutaneous nerves that supply the skin is important for testing for peripheral nerve lesions (Fig. 7.26).

Femoral nerve

The femoral nerve arises from the anterior rami of L2 to L4. It supplies muscles in the anterior compartment of the thigh, as well as overlying skin. It also supplies the iliacus and psoas major muscles, and the hip and knee joints (Fig. 7.27). Its cutaneous branch, the saphenous nerve, supplies the skin of the medial side of the leg. The femoral nerve lies immediately lateral to the femoral artery as it passes beneath the inguinal ligament to enter the femoral triangle (Fig. 7.28;

145

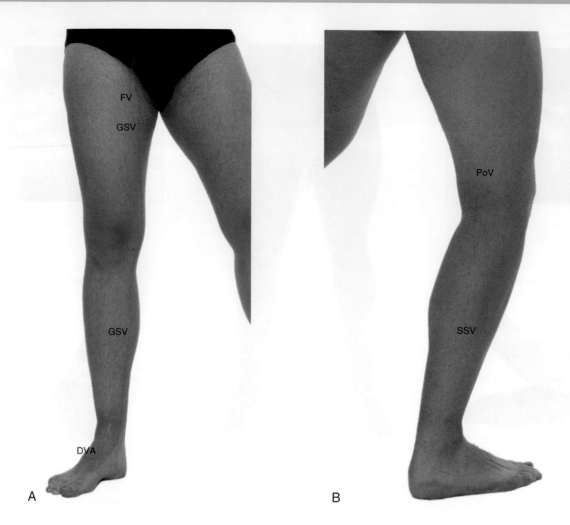

Fig. 7.25 Surface projections of the venous drainage of the lower limb. A, Anterior. B, Medial. *DVA*, dorsal venous arch; *FV*, femoral vein; *GSV*, great saphenous vein; *PoV*, popliteal vein; *SSV*, small saphenous vein.

also see Fig. 7.7). A femoral nerve block is performed at this location. The saphenous nerve passes with the femoral artery and vein under the sartorius muscle to reach the medial side of the knee.

Obturator nerve

The obturator nerve arises from the same spinal cord segments as the femoral nerve, namely the anterior rami of L2 to L4. The obturator nerve supplies the muscles of the medial compartment of the thigh (Fig. 7.27). It also supplies the hip and knee joints, and the skin overlying the medial compartment. The obturator nerve enters the medial compartment of the thigh through the obturator foramen (Fig. 7.28).

Sciatic nerve

The sciatic nerve arises from the anterior rami of L4 to S3. It supplies the muscles of the posterior compartment of the thigh, the whole of the leg and foot and the overlying skin, except for the skin on the medial side of the leg. The sciatic nerve also supplies the hip joint, and its lateral rotators. It divides into its tibial and common fibular branches at some point between where it emerges from under the piriformis

muscle and the level of the popliteal fossa (Fig. 7.27). The tibial nerve descends through the posterior compartment of the leg toward the tarsal tunnel. It supplies the posterior compartment muscles. The common fibular nerve curves inferiorly and anteriorly around the neck of the fibula to enter the lateral compartment of the leg where it divides into superficial and deep fibular nerves. The superficial fibular nerve supplies the muscles in the lateral compartment of the leg, whereas the deep fibular nerve supplies the muscles in the anterior compartment of the leg (Fig. 7.28). At the neck of the fibula, the common fibular nerve is superficial and can be easily palpated. It is frequently injured at this point, which can result in 'foot drop' with loss of cutaneous sensation on the dorsum of the foot and the anterior and lateral leg.

Lymph nodes

There are three main sets of nodes in the lower limb: the superficial and the deep inguinal nodes and the popliteal nodes. The superficial inguinal nodes lie in superficial fascia, parallel to the inguinal ligament, close to the great saphenous

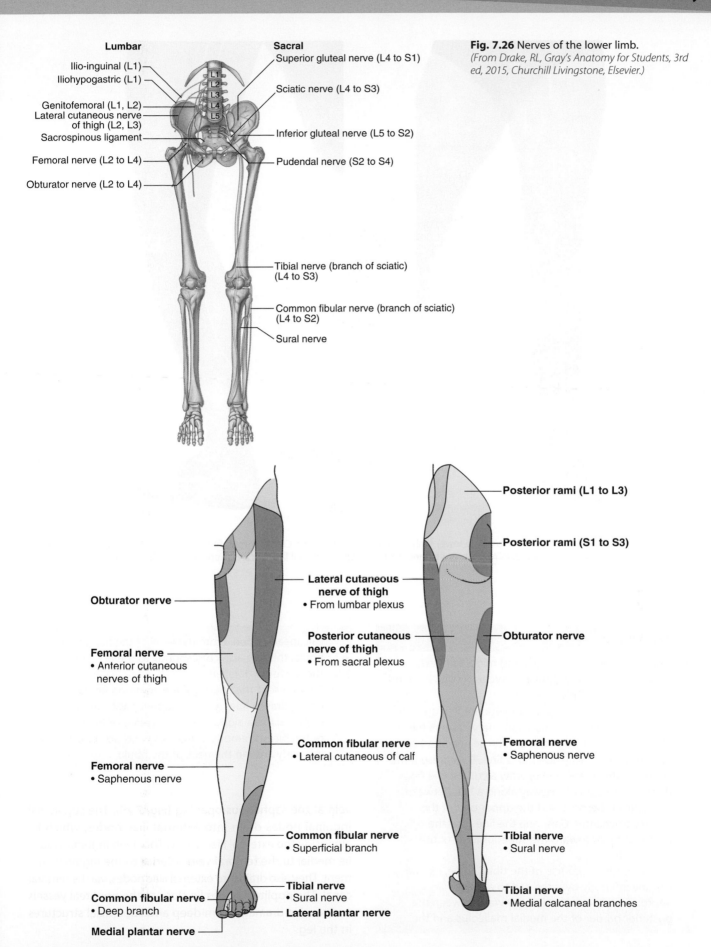

Lumbar
Ilio-inguinal (L1)
Iliohypogastric (L1)
Genitofemoral (L1, L2)
Lateral cutaneous nerve of thigh (L2, L3)
Sacrospinous ligament
Femoral nerve (L2 to L4)
Obturator nerve (L2 to L4)

Sacral
Superior gluteal nerve (L4 to S1)
Sciatic nerve (L4 to S3)
Inferior gluteal nerve (L5 to S2)
Pudendal nerve (S2 to S4)
Tibial nerve (branch of sciatic) (L4 to S3)
Common fibular nerve (branch of sciatic) (L4 to S2)
Sural nerve

Fig. 7.26 Nerves of the lower limb.
(From Drake, RL, Gray's Anatomy for Students, 3rd ed, 2015, Churchill Livingstone, Elsevier.)

Obturator nerve

Femoral nerve
• Anterior cutaneous nerves of thigh

Femoral nerve
• Saphenous nerve

Common fibular nerve
• Deep branch

Medial plantar nerve

Lateral cutaneous nerve of thigh
• From lumbar plexus

Posterior cutaneous nerve of thigh
• From sacral plexus

Common fibular nerve
• Lateral cutaneous of calf

Common fibular nerve
• Superficial branch

Tibial nerve
• Sural nerve

Lateral plantar nerve

Posterior rami (L1 to L3)

Posterior rami (S1 to S3)

Obturator nerve

Femoral nerve
• Saphenous nerve

Tibial nerve
• Sural nerve

Tibial nerve
• Medial calcaneal branches

Fig. 7.27 Regions of skin innervated by peripheral nerves (see Fig. 1.7).
(From Drake, RL, Gray's Anatomy for Students, 3rd ed, 2015, Churchill Livingstone, Elsevier.)

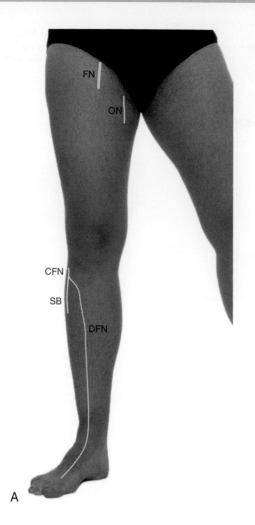
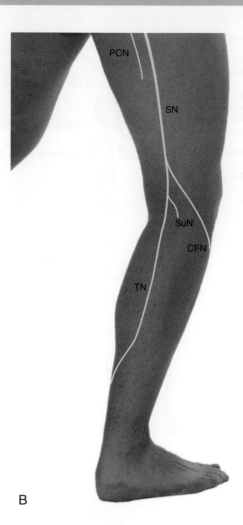

Fig. 7.28 Surface projections of the nerves of the lower limb. A, Anterior. B, Posterior. *CFN*, common fibular nerve; *DFN*, deep fibular nerve; *FN*, femoral nerve; *ON*, obturator nerve; *PCN*, posterior cutaneous nerve; *SB*, superficial branch; *SN*, sciatic nerve; *SuN*, sural nerve; *TN*, tibial nerve.

To Do (Fig 7.28)

- Using the tips of your index and middle fingers, palpate the common fibular nerve as it winds around the neck of the fibula.
- Draw a line from the posterior superior iliac spine to the ischial tuberosity. The sciatic nerve enters the gluteal region through the greater sciatic foramen one-third of the way down this line. To represent the course of the sciatic nerve, draw a curved line from this point to a point midway along a line between the ischial tuberosity and the upper part of the greater trochanter. Continue the line over the posterior thigh toward the superior apex of the popliteal fossa.
- To represent the course of the tibial nerve, extend the line inferiorly over the calf to a point approximately one-third of the way between the posterior border of the medial malleolus and the calcaneal tendon. From the level of the head of the fibula, this line also corresponds to the position of the posterior tibial artery.
- To represent the course of the common fibular nerve, draw a line from the superior apex of the popliteal fossa along the medial edge of the tendon of the biceps femoris muscle, to wind posteriorly and inferiorly around the neck of the fibula.

vein at the saphenous opening (Fig. 7.29). The superficial inguinal nodes drain into external iliac nodes, which lie alongside the external iliac artery. The deep inguinal nodes lie medial to the femoral vein, inferior to the inguinal ligament. They also drain into external iliac nodes, via the femoral canal. The popliteal nodes lie close to the popliteal vessels and receive drainage from deep and superficial structures in the leg.

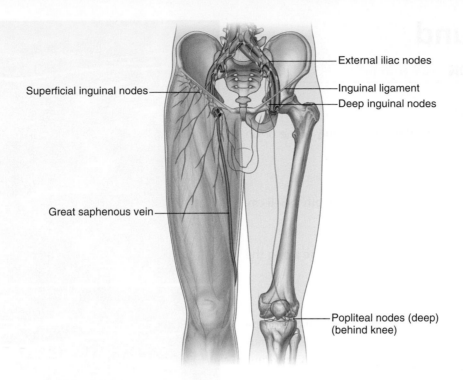

Fig. 7.29 Lymphatic drainage of the lower limb.
(From Drake, RL, Gray's Anatomy for Students, 3rd ed, 2015, Churchill Livingstone, Elsevier.)

To Do (Fig 7.29)

- Palpate the horizontal group of nodes inferior to the inguinal ligament. Extending further inferiorly you should be able to palpate the vertical group of nodes.

In the Clinic

Bursitis

Bursae are lubricating layers or 'sacs' found all over the body where there is the potential of friction from adjacent structures. These bags of synovium underlie structures like tendons or bony points, and are not normally palpable. If they become inflamed due to excess pressure or friction on the overlying structure they may be painful and palpable. In the gluteal region there are two bursae of note. The trochanteric bursa lies superficial to the greater trochanter, and the ischial bursa overlies the tuberosity of the same name. In the leg, there are many bursae related to the knee. There is a bursa around the attachments of the tendons of the sartorius, semitendinosus and gracilis muscles to the medial tibial condyle, known as the pes anserine bursa. There are also prepatellar, infrapatellar and suprapatellar bursae. The prepatellar bursa lies anterior to the patella and if inflamed, due to excessive kneeling, gives rise to

'housemaid's knee' or prepatellar bursitis. There are two infrapatellar bursae: a superficial and a deep bursa that lie anterior and posterior to the patellar ligament, respectively. Inflammation of one or both of these bursae is sometimes referred to as 'clergyman's knee' or infrapatellar bursitis, which is also brought on by excessive kneeling. The suprapatellar bursa lies above the knee as an extension of the synovial cavity, though if the knee is inflamed this bursa can also become swollen and palpable.

Popliteal aneurysm

A popliteal aneurysm is a palpable, pulsatile enlargement of the popliteal artery within the popliteal fossa. It is important to diagnose to avoid rupture. Nonpulsatile enlargements in the fossa that may be palpable include enlarged lymph nodes or Baker's cysts, which are synovial fluid-filled distensions from the bursae of the knee. Baker's cysts often occur in association with an arthritic knee joint.

Femoral herniae

The femoral canal is also notable because it has the potential to allow access of femoral herniae, which pass from the abdominal cavity into the upper anterior medial thigh. They are distinguishable from inguinal herniae because they are positioned lateral to the pubic tubercle. Femoral herniae are more common in elderly females, whereas inguinal herniae tend to occur in males.

Ultrasound

GLUTEAL REGION

Subject position

Imaging is performed with the subject lying prone or on their side.

Transducer

Use a linear array transducer. Set the image depth to 3–8 cm.

Transducer position

Position the transducer in the transverse plane along the gluteal crease.

Image features

A layer of subcutaneous fat will be seen at the top of the image. Below the subcutaneous fat, the gluteus maximus muscle can be inspected. Deep to the gluteus maximus muscle, the quadratus femoris muscle will be present. It can be seen originating from the ischial tuberosity on the medial side of the image and passing laterally toward the femur (Fig. 7.30). Located between the gluteus maximus and quadratus femoris muscles, the sciatic nerve will be in view in the short axis. The sciatic nerve can be tracked proximally, as it passes out from under the inferior border of the piriformis muscle, or distally toward the posterior thigh.

FEMORAL TRIANGLE

Subject position

Imaging is performed with the subject lying supine.

Transducer

Use a linear array transducer. Set the depth setting to 3–5 cm.

Transducer position

Position the transducer on the anterior thigh, just lateral of the pubic tubercle, where the femoral pulse can be palpated. This is just inferior to the inguinal ligament, which runs between the anterior superior iliac spine and the pubic tubercle. The neurovascular structures can be imaged in the short or long axis by positioning the transducer in the transverse plane (e.g. Fig. 7.31A) or sagittal plane (e.g. Fig. 7.31B), respectively. It is possible to track the vessels distally into the adductor canal.

Image features

In the transverse plane (Fig. 7.31A), the femoral artery and vein can be seen as two anechoic circles. The vein sits medial

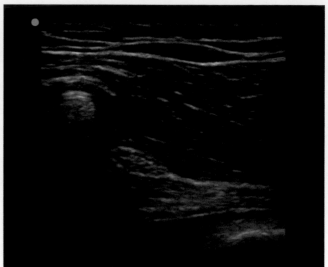

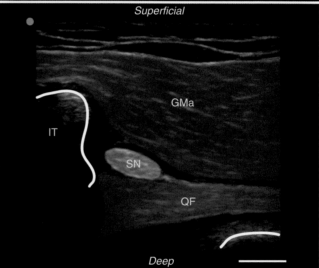

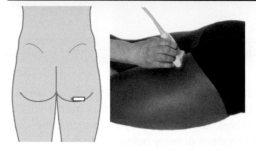

Fig. 7.30 Ultrasound of the right gluteal region. *GMa*, gluteus maximus; *IT*, ischial tuberosity; *QF*, quadratus femoris; *SN*, sciatic nerve. Scale bar = 1 cm.

to the artery and is usually larger. When scanning the patient during a Valsalva maneuver, the femoral vein will often dilate to three times the size of the artery. The femoral artery can be easily discerned from the vein by using gentle probe pressure to compress the vein. The femoral canal is subtle, but may also be in view and will appear as a small isoechoic feature, approximately one-quarter of the diameter of the

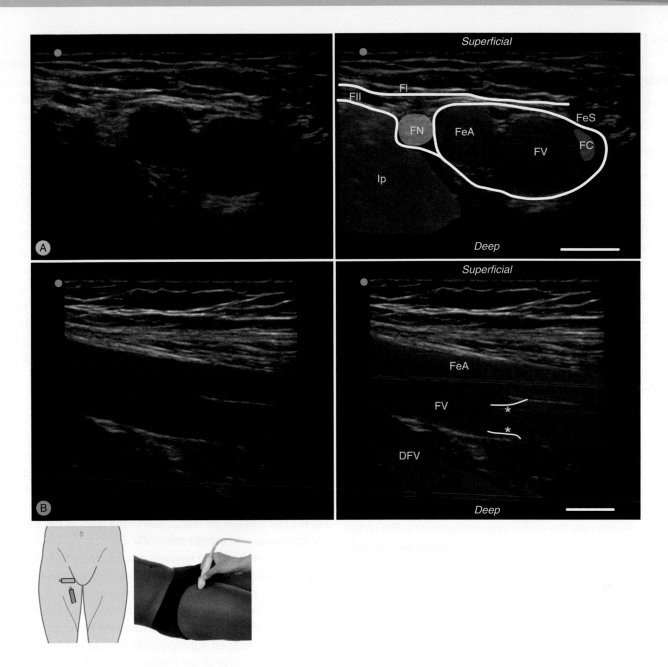

Fig. 7.31 Ultrasound of the right femoral triangle. A, Transverse view. B, Femoral vessels. *, valve; *DFV*, deep femoral vein; *FC*, femoral canal; *FeA*, femoral artery; *FeS*, femoral sheath; *FI*, fascia lata; *FII*, fascia iliaca; *FN*, femoral nerve; *FV*, femoral vein; *Ip*, iliopsoas. Scale bar = 1 cm.

femoral artery, toward the medial side of the femoral vein. The femoral sheath is visualized as a thickened hyperechoic fascial band surrounding the artery, vein and canal. Outside of the femoral sheath, immediately lateral to the femoral artery, the femoral nerve will be in view. Its medium-gray heterogeneous texture contrasts with the anechoic appearance of the vessels. Below these neurovascular structures, the muscular floor of the femoral triangle can be inspected. The iliopsoas muscle is seen on the lateral side of the image. The fascia iliaca extends over the surface of this muscle. Scanning medially, the pectineus and adductor longus

muscles will come into view. Sitting over the fascia iliaca and extending over the top of the femoral sheath, the fascia lata can be observed as a dense echogenic line. Above the fascia lata, there may be a layer of subcutaneous fat. In the sagittal plane (Fig. 7.31B), the femoral artery can be seen above the vein. It is possible to inspect the valves within the femoral vein, which appear as faint lines opening and closing. Doppler can be used to view blood flow within these vessels (Video 7.1). At the bottom of the image, the deep femoral vessels can be inspected as they descend toward the femur.

ANTERIOR THIGH

Subject position

Imaging is performed with the subject lying supine or sitting facing the operator.

Transducer

Use a linear array transducer. Set the depth setting to 4–8 cm.

Transducer position

Position the transducer over the distal third of the thigh in the transverse plane for short-axis views, where the muscle bulk becomes less (Fig. 7.32).

Image features

Scanning from the lateral to medial side of the thigh with the transducer positioned in the transverse plane, the organization of the anterior compartment can be examined. Each muscle belly is surrounded by myofascia, enabling delineation of the individual muscles. Towards the bottom of the image, the anterior surface of the femur will be in view. The vastus intermedius muscle can be seen wrapping over its surface. With the transducer toward the anterolateral side of the thigh (Fig. 7.32A), the vastus lateralis muscle can be inspected. The most medial part of this muscle lies partly over the vastus intermedius muscle. Moving the transducer more medially (Fig. 7.32B), the rectus femoris muscle is seen sitting directly over the vastus intermedius muscle. The rectus femoris muscle has a characteristic oval appearance. Towards the most medial side of the anterior compartment (Fig. 7.32C), the vastus medialis muscle will be in view, lying partly over the vastus intermedius muscle. Scanning in the direction of the knee, the quadriceps muscles can be seen converging on the patella as the quadriceps tendon. This is best observed with the transducer aligned longitudinally over the muscles (see Knee). The sartorius muscle can also be tracked through the anterior thigh from the anterior superior iliac spine to the medial aspect of the knee. It appears as a flat muscle, lying superficially over the quadriceps muscles and the femoral vessels. The distal part of this muscle forms the roof of the adductor canal (see Medial thigh).

KNEE

Subject position

Imaging is performed with the subject lying supine (leg extended) or sitting (leg flexed), facing the operator.

Transducer

Use a linear array transducer. Set the depth setting to 2–5 cm.

Transducer position

The quadriceps tendon and patellar ligament are best viewed along their long axis. Place the transducer in the sagittal plane immediately superior to the patella for the quadriceps tendon (Fig. 7.33A) or immediately inferior to the patella for the patellar ligament (Fig. 7.33C). With the knee flexed, the intracapsular structures can be viewed. By positioning the transducer in a transverse oblique plane on the medial side of the patella, with the orientation marker pointing to the left in a slight inferior direction, the oblique fibers of the vastus medialis muscle can be observed (Fig. 7.33B). The medial and lateral collateral ligaments are best imaged along their long axis by positioning the probe in the coronal plane between the medial epicondyle of the femur and the medial margin of the proximal end of the tibia (medial collateral ligament; Fig. 7.34A) or the lateral epicondyle of the femur and the head of the fibula (lateral collateral ligament; Fig. 7.34B). By positioning the transducer in a coronal plane immediately lateral to the patella, the lateral meniscus can also be viewed (Fig. 7.34C).

Image features

With the transducer superior to the patella in the sagittal plane (Fig. 7.33A), the quadriceps tendon can be observed. The tendon can be seen passing horizontally across the image. Compared to muscle, the tendon has a relatively hyperechoic texture. In this view, the linear arrangement of the fascicles can be seen. Deep to the tendon, the surfaces of the femur and patella are easily identifiable. The hyaline cartilage overlying the femur is also visible, which appears hypoechoic. The insertion of the quadriceps tendon into the patella can be inspected. The suprapatellar bursa can be seen between the quadriceps tendon and the hyaline cartilage of the femur. Sitting between the femur and patella, the triangle-shaped suprapatellar fat pad will be in view. Toward the surface of the image, subcutaneous fat may be present.

With the transducer positioned medial to the patella in a transverse oblique plane (Fig. 7.33B), the oblique fibers of the vastus medialis muscle can be inspected. The fascicles can be seen converging on the quadriceps tendon as it extends toward the patella. Both the surfaces of the femur and patella will be in view. It may also be possible to see the medial meniscus sitting below the tendon. It appears triangular in shape and has a homogenous medium-gray appearance.

With the transducer inferior to the patella in sagittal plane (Fig. 7.33C), the patellar ligament can be inspected. In the long-axis view, it has a striated appearance. The ligament can be seen extending from the patella to the tibia. Deep to the patellar ligament, the triangle-shaped infrapatellar

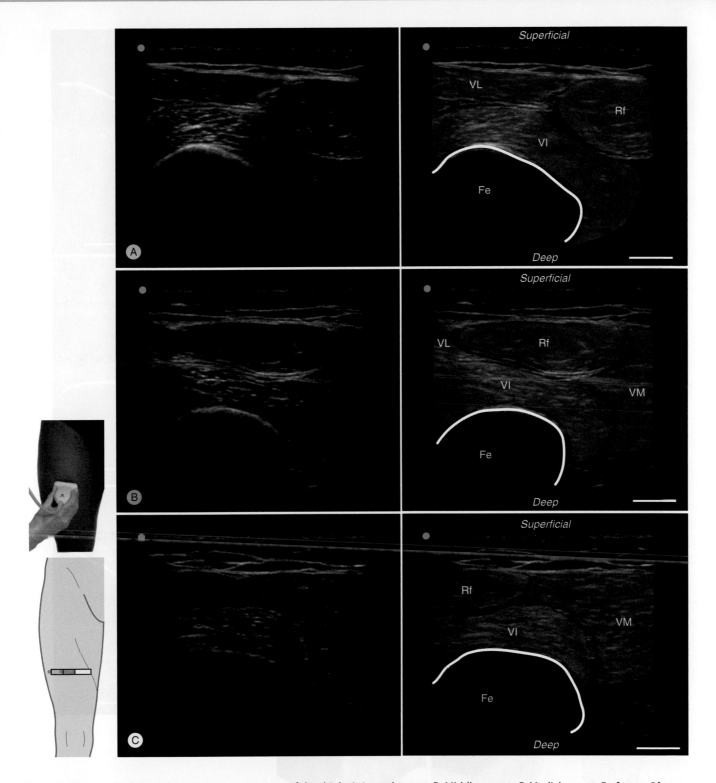

Fig. 7.32 Ultrasound of the right anterior compartment of the thigh. A, Lateral aspect. B, Middle aspect. C, Medial aspect. *Fe*, femur; *Rf*, rectus femoris; *VI*, vastus intermedius; *VL*, vastus lateralis; *VM*, vastus medialis. Scale bar = 1 cm.

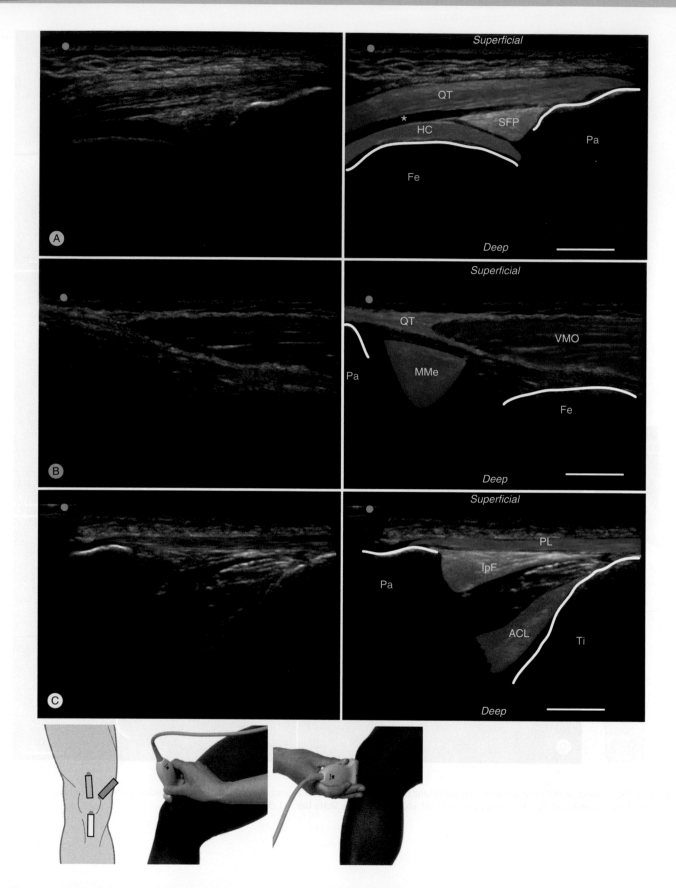

Fig. 7.33 Ultrasound of the right knee. A, Quadriceps tendon. B, Oblique fibers of the vastus medialis muscle. C, Patellar ligament. *, suprapatellar bursa; *ACL*, anterior cruciate ligament; *Fe*, femur; *HC*, hyaline cartilage; *IpF*, infrapatellar fat; *MMe*, medial meniscus; *Pa*, patella; *PL*, patellar ligament; *QT*, quadriceps tendon; *SFP*, suprapatellar fat pad; *Ti*, tibia; *VMO*, vasatus medialis oblique. Scale bar = 1 cm.

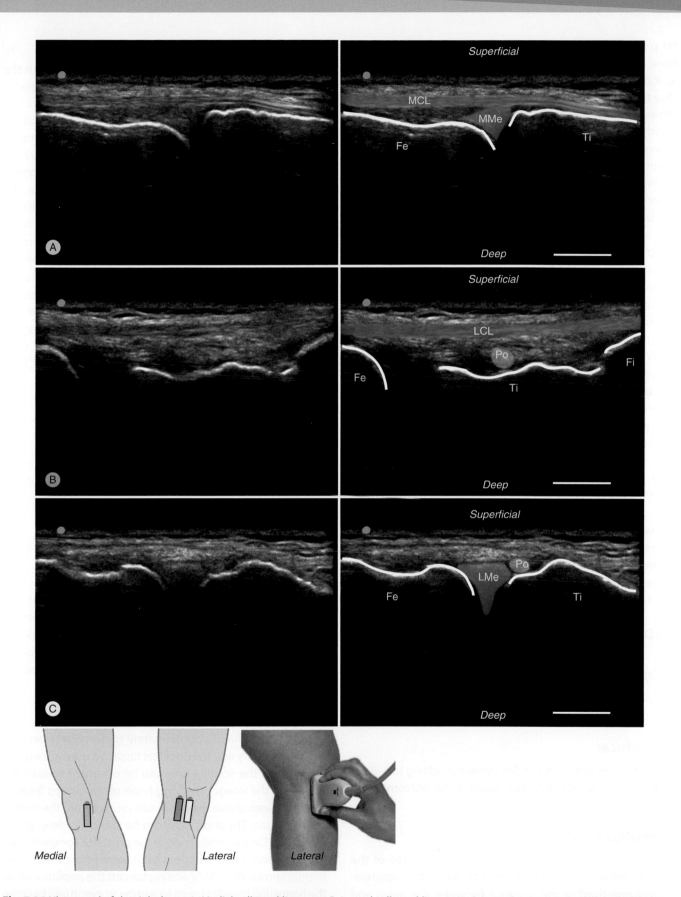

Fig. 7.34 Ultrasound of the right knee. A, Medial collateral ligament. B, Lateral collateral ligament. C, Lateral meniscus. *Fe*, femur; *Fi*, fibula; *LCL*, lateral collateral ligament; *LMe*, lateral meniscus; *MCL*, medial collateral ligament; *MMe*, medial meniscus; *Po*, popliteus; *Ti*, tibia. Scale bar = 1 cm.

fat pad will be in view. Deep to the fat pad, with a flexed knee, it is possible to observe the anterior cruciate ligament as it passes from the tibial plateau deep toward the femur. Due to the obliquity of the ligament to the direction of the ultrasound beam, it is relatively hypoechoic and not always clearly seen. The ligament will disappear out of view as it extends below the patella. The posterior cruciate ligament is not easily observed on ultrasound.

With the transducer on the medial side of the knee in a coronal plane (Fig. 7.34A), the medial collateral ligament can be inspected. In this long-axis view, it appears bandlike and can be seen extending superficially across the image. Deep to the medial collateral ligament, the surfaces of the femur and tibia will be visible. Note that in contrast to the lateral collateral ligament, the medial collateral ligament is in close proximity (adherent in places) to the bony surfaces. Sitting between the femur and tibia, within the joint capsule, the medial meniscus can be observed.

With the transducer on the lateral side of the knee in the coronal plane (Fig. 7.34B), the lateral collateral ligament will be in view. It appears cordlike, and can be observed extending between the femur and the head of the fibula. There is a noticeable space between the lateral collateral ligament and the underlying bony surfaces. Sitting within this space, between the ligament and the surface of the tibia, the tendon of the popliteus muscle can be seen.

With the transducer immediately lateral to the patella (Fig. 7.34C), the lateral meniscus will be in view sitting between the femur and tibia. Similar to the medial meniscus, it has a triangular shape. Directly inferior to the meniscus (right side on image), the tendon of the popliteus muscle is seen in passing between the lateral collateral ligament and the tibia.

MEDIAL THIGH AND ADDUCTOR CANAL

Subject position

Imaging is performed with the subject lying supine or sitting, facing the operator.

Transducer

Use a linear array transducer. Set the depth setting to 4–8 cm so that the shaft of the femur shows at the bottom of the image.

Transducer position

Position the transducer on the anteromedial side of the thigh in the transverse plane for short-axis views, approximately one-third of the distance between the pubis and the knee. Scan in the transverse plane in a medial direction (Fig. 7.35).

Image features

Starting on the anteromedial aspect of the thigh with the transducer in the transverse plane (Fig. 7.35A), the adductor canal can be observed. The artery and vein appear as two circles with the artery sitting above the vein. The walls of the adductor canal can be inspected. The narrow sartorius muscle can be seen forming the roof of the canal. The vastus medialis muscle will lie laterally and the adductor longus muscle, medially. Deep to the vastus medialis muscle, the femur may be visible. In a transverse plane, the adductor longus muscle, the most superficial of the adductors, has a characteristic oval shape that lies obliquely across the image, and can be traced back to its origin, the pubic tubercle. Scanning medially (Fig. 7.35B), the extent of the adductor magnus muscle can be examined. This muscle lies deep to adductor longus muscle, toward the bottom of the image. Located between the adductor longus and adductor magnus muscles, the adductor brevis muscle will be in view. With the transducer on the medial aspect of the thigh (Fig. 7.35C), the slender gracilis muscle can be inspected.

POSTERIOR THIGH AND POPLITEAL FOSSA

Subject position

Imaging is best performed with the subject lying prone or standing.

Transducer

Use a linear array transducer. Set the depth setting to 2–8 cm.

Transducer position

Place the transducer in the transverse plane for short-axis views, approximately midway between the ischial tuberosity and the popliteal fossa on the posterior thigh. The probe should be positioned close to the middle of the thigh so that the sciatic nerve can be tracked inferiorly toward the popliteal fossa (Fig. 7.36).

Image features

With the transducer approximately midway between the ischial tuberosity and the popliteal fossa in a transverse plane (Fig. 7.36A), the sciatic nerve can be observed toward the middle of the image. The long head of the biceps femoris muscle is seen above the nerve as it crosses from the medial to lateral side. The short head can be identified deep to the long head. On the medial side of the posterior compartment, the semitendinosus muscle is seen superficial to the semimembranosus muscle. Scanning toward the popliteal fossa, the hamstring muscles begin to narrow to eventually become tendinous. The tendon of the semitendinosus muscle can be identified on the surface of the semimembranosus muscle.

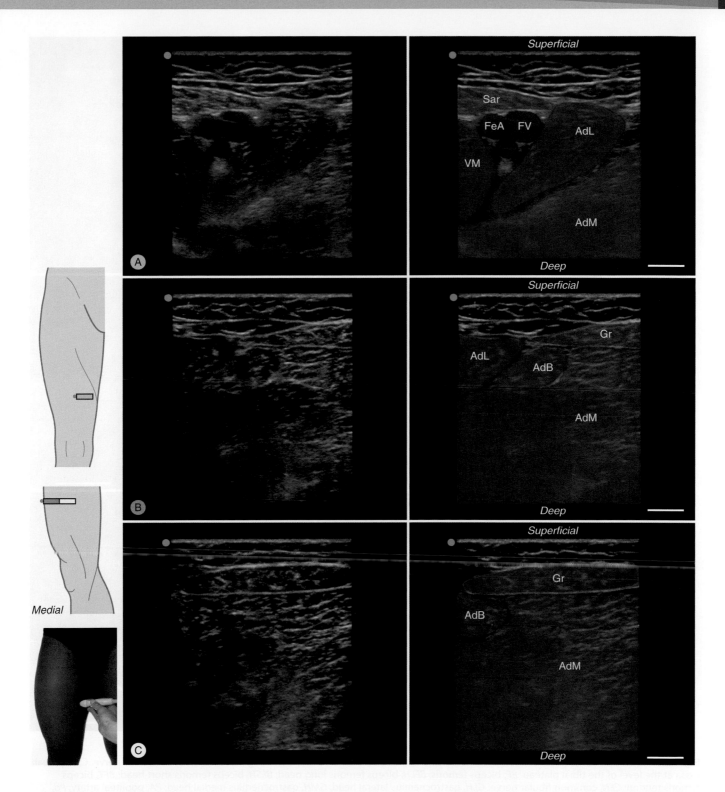

Fig. 7.35 Ultrasound of the right adductor canal and medial thigh. A, Adductor canal. B, Adductor magnus. C, Gracilis. *AdB*, adductor brevis; *AdL*, adductor longus; *AdM*, adductor magnus; *FeA*, femoral artery; *FV*, femoral vein; *Gr*, gracilis; *Sar*, sartorius; *VM*, vastus medialis. Scale bar = 1 cm.

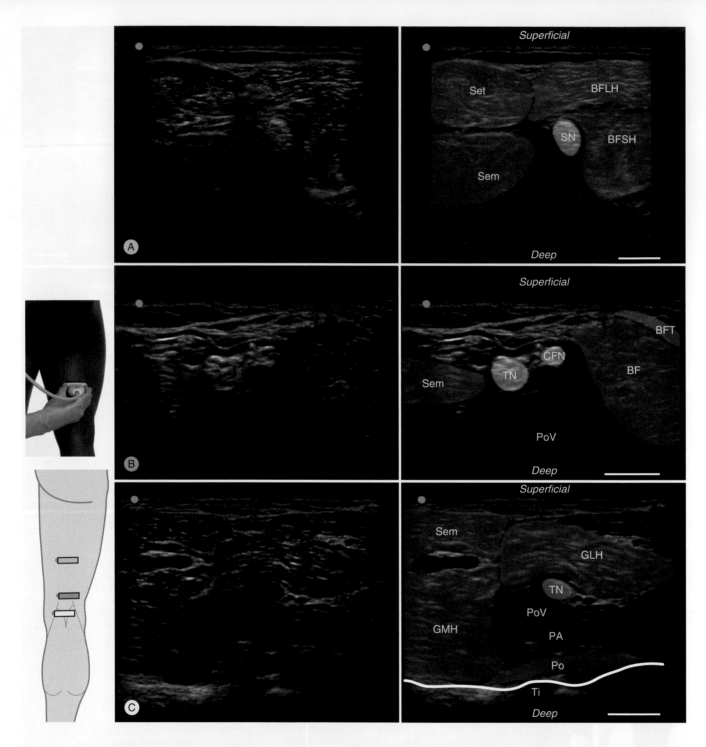

Fig. 7.36 Ultrasound of the posterior compartment of the thigh. A, Sciatic nerve in the midthigh. B, Division of the sciatic nerve. C, Popliteal fossa at the level of the tibial plateau. *BF*, biceps femoris; *BFLH*, biceps femoris long head; *BFSH*, biceps femoris short head; *BFT*, biceps femoris tendon; *CFN*, common fibular nerve; *GLH*, gastrocnemius lateral head; *GMH*, gastrocnemius medial head; *PA*, popliteal artery; *Po*, politeus; *PoV*, popliteal vein; *Sem*, semimembranosus; *Set*, semitendinosus; *SN*, sciatic nerve; *Ti*, tibia; *TN*, tibial nerve. Scale bar = 1 cm.

At a variable point above the popliteal fossa, the division of the sciatic nerve into the tibial and common fibular nerves can be observed (Fig. 7.36B). The tibial nerve is the larger of the two branches and lies to the medial side of the common fibular nerve, which descends laterally. It should be noted that there is substantial variation in the point of division, which can occur as proximal as the gluteal region. The popliteal vessels come into view from under the semimembranosus muscle on the medial side as they enter the fossa. The popliteal artery and vein are best viewed with the transducer aligned in a transverse plane across the middle of the popliteal fossa, at about the level of the tibial plateau (Fig. 7.36C). The vessels are seen as a series of circles with the popliteal artery lying deep to the vein. On either side of the image, the lateral and medial head of the gastrocnemius muscle will be in view. The semimembranosus muscle is lying over the medial head of gastrocnemius muscle. Towards the bottom of the image, the posterior proximal end of the tibia is observed as a horizontal line across the image. Sitting on the tibia, below the popliteal vessels, the flat popliteus muscle can be inspected.

ANTERIOR LEG

Subject position

Imaging is performed with the subject lying supine, sitting or standing facing the operator.

Transducer

Use a linear array transducer. Set the depth setting to 2–8 cm.

Transducer position

Position the transducer in the transverse plane for short-axis views approximately midway between the tibial tuberosity and the ankle. For the dorsum of the foot, position the transducer in the transverse plane (Fig. 7.37).

Image features

With the transducer positioned over the anterior compartment of the leg in a transverse plane (Fig. 7.37A), the surfaces of the tibia and fibula will be in view toward the bottom of the image. Sitting between these bones, the interosseous

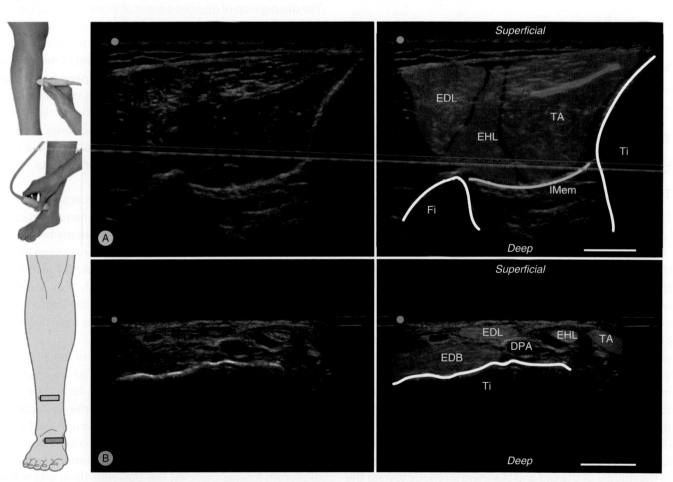

Fig. 7.37 Ultrasound of the anterior compartment of the right leg and dorsum of the foot. A, Anterior leg muscles. B, Dorsum of foot. *DPA*, dorsalis pedis artery; *EDB*, extensor digitorum brevis; *EDL*, extensor digitorum longus; *EHL*, extensor hallucis longus; *Fi*, fibula; *IMem*, interosseous membrane; *TA*, tibialis anterior; *Ti*, tibia. Scale bar = 1 cm.

membrane is seen as an arcing line. The three anterior compartment muscles will all be visible. The tibialis anterior muscle, the largest muscle, sits on the medial side, closest to the tibia. The extensor hallucis longs and extensor digitorum longus muscles sit lateral to this muscle. Although the muscle belly will be predominantly hypoechoic, tendinous parts will appear hyperechoic.

With the transducer positioned transversely over the dorsum of the foot (Fig. 7.37B), the hyperechoic dorsal surface of the tarsals (or more distally, the metatarsals) will be in view. Superficially, the tendons of tibialis anterior (medial), extensor hallucis longus (middle) and extensor digitorum longus (lateral) muscles will be visible. They may be surrounded by synovium, which will appear anechoic. Sitting between extensor hallucis longs and extensor digitorum longus muscles, the dorsalis pedis artery will be in view. With minimal probe pressure, it may be possible to see the superficial veins of the dorsal venous arch. Towards the lateral side of the foot, the extensor digitorum brevis muscle can be observed.

POSTERIOR LEG

Subject position

Imaging is performed with the subject lying prone or standing with their back to the operator.

Transducer

Use a linear array transducer. Set the depth setting to 2–6 cm.

Transducer position

The posterior compartment of the leg can be imaged in a transverse or sagittal plane.

To inspect the common fibular nerve as it passes toward the lateral compartment, position the transducer in the transverse plane for a short-axis view, on the lateral side of the posterior compartment at the level of the head of the fibula (Fig. 7.38A). To image the gastrocnemius muscle, place the transducer on the lateral head of gastrocnemius where the muscle bulk is thickest (Fig. 7.38B). Scan in the transverse plane in a medial direction (Fig. 7.38C). The deep muscles of the posterior compartment can be observed in the transverse plane toward the medial side of the compartment, approximately midway between the knee and ankle (Fig. 7.38D). The calcaneal tendon can be viewed along its long axis by positioning the transducer in the sagittal plane in the middle of the calf and scanning inferiorly toward the calcaneus (Fig. 7.39). By positioning the transducer in a coronal oblique plane between the medial malleolus and the calcaneus, the tarsal tunnel can be inspected (Fig. 7.40).

Image features

With the transducer positioned in the transverse plane on the lateral side of the posterior compartment of the leg at the level of the head of the fibula (Fig. 7.38A), the common fibular nerve can be inspected. It passes close to the prominent bony ridge on the fibula before crossing the bone to enter the lateral compartment. Note its proximity to the surface of the skin. With the transducer positioned over the lateral head of the gastrocnemius muscle in transverse plane (Fig. 7.38B), the relationship between this muscle and the soleus muscle, which lies deep, can be examined. On the lateral side of the image, the fibula can be observed. As the transducer is moved medially, the lateral head narrows to form an aponeurosis that connects the two heads (Fig. 7.38C). The medial head appears larger than the lateral head. Positioning the probe distal to the heads of the gastrocnemius muscle in transverse plane, the deep muscle can be visualized (Fig. 7.38D). At the bottom of the image, the tibia (medial) and fibula (lateral) will be in view. The soleus muscle can be seen extending over the deep muscle compartment. The deep group of muscles consist of (from medial to lateral) the flexor digitorum longus, tibialis posterior and flexor hallucis longus muscles. The tibialis posterior muscle is located between the tibia and fibula, adjacent to the interosseous membrane, which appears as a hyperechoic stripe between the bones. As the transducer is moved further distally toward the ankle, the tendon of flexor digitorum longus can be seen crossing over tibialis posterior. Directly above the deep muscles, below the soleus muscle, a neurovascular bundle is observed, consisting of the tibial nerve, posterior tibial artery and veins.

By rotating the probe longitudinally, the calcaneal tendon can be examined (Fig. 7.39). It is a relatively narrow structure that runs horizontally across the image directly below the subcutaneous tissue. The soleus muscle can be seen below the calcaneal tendon. The fibers of the soleus muscle run obliquely toward the tendon, into which they insert. A horizontal myofascial plane should be visible immediately below the soleus muscle, which separates the superficial and deep muscle groups.

With the transducer at the medial side of the ankle in a coronal oblique plane, the tarsal tunnel can be observed (Fig. 7.40). The flexor retinaculum, which forms the roof, runs superficially across the image as a continuous curved line. All of the main structures that pass through the tunnel can be inspected in their short axis. From anterior to posterior, these are the tendons of the tibialis posterior and flexor digitorum longus muscles, the posterior tibial artery and veins, the tibial nerve and the tendon of the flexor hallucis longus muscle. The medium-gray colored tendons contrast with the anechoic appearance of the synovium that can be

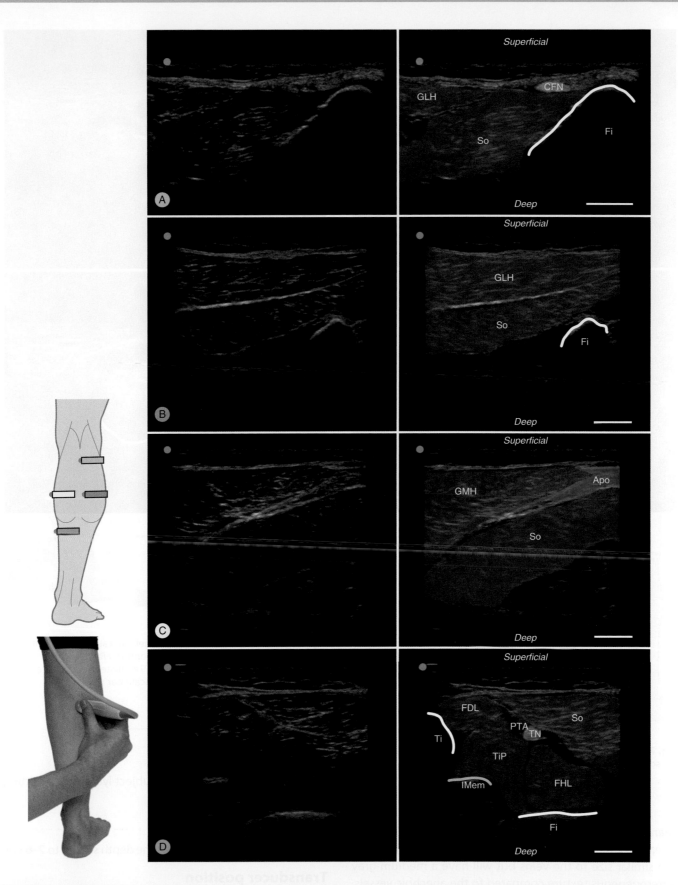

Fig. 7.38 Ultrasound of the posterior right leg. A, Common fibular nerve. B, Lateral head of gastrocnemius. C, Medial head of gastrocnemius. D, Deep muscles. *Apo*, aponeurosis; *CFN*, common fibular nerve; *FDL*, flexor digitorum longus; *FHL*, flexor hallucis longus; *Fi*, fibula; *GLH*, gastrocnemius lateral head; *GMH*, gastrocnemius medial head; *IMem*, interosseous membrane; *PTA*, posterior tibial artery; *So*, soleus; *Ti*, tibia; *TiP*, tibialis posterior; *TN*, tibial nerve. Scale bar = 1 cm.

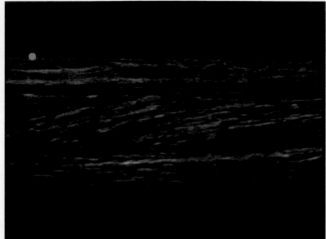

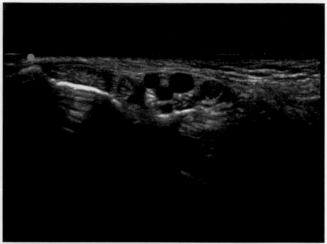

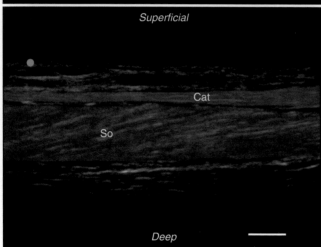

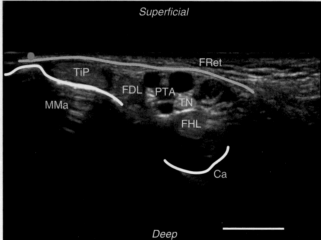

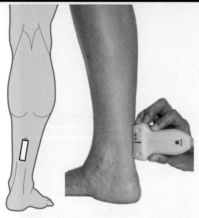

Fig. 7.39 Ultrasound of the calcaneal tendon. *Cat*, calcaneal tendon; *So*, soleus. Scale bar = 1 cm.

seen around many of these tendons. The posterior tibial artery is generally smaller than the veins. The tibial nerve is a similar size to the veins but will have a medium-gray heterogeneous texture compared to the anechoic vessels. Below these structures, the medial malleolus and calcaneus can be seen.

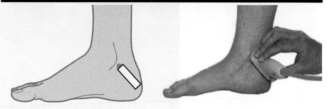

Fig. 7.40 Ultrasound of the tarsal tunnel. *Ca*, calcaneus; *FDL*, flexor digitorum longus; *FHL*, flexor hallucis longus; *FRet*, flexor retinaculum; *MMa*, medial malleolus; *PTA*, posterior tibial artery; *TiP*, tibialis posterior; *TN*, tibial nerve. Scale bar = 1 cm.

LATERAL LEG

Subject position

Imaging is performed with the subject lying supine, sitting or standing, facing to the side.

Transducer

Use a linear array transducer. Set the depth setting to 2–6 cm.

Transducer position

The lateral compartment of the leg and the dorsum of the foot can be imaged in the transverse (Fig. 7.41A) or coronal

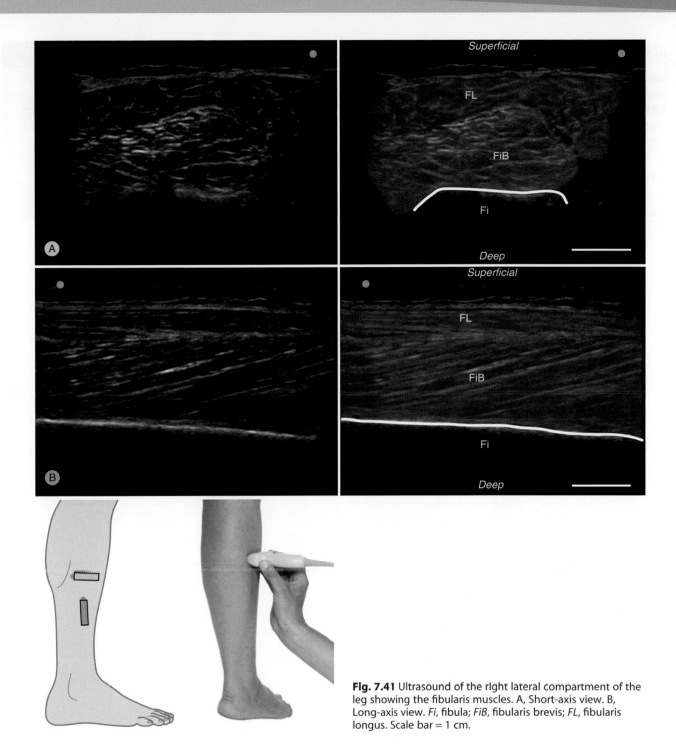

Fig. 7.41 Ultrasound of the right lateral compartment of the leg showing the fibularis muscles. A, Short-axis view. B, Long-axis view. *Fi*, fibula; *FiB*, fibularis brevis; *FL*, fibularis longus. Scale bar = 1 cm.

planes (Fig. 7.41B) for short-axis or long-axis views, respectively. Place the transducer on the lateral side of the leg, immediately below the head of the fibula. Scan in an inferior direction.

Image features

At the bottom of the image, in the transverse or coronal plane, the hyperechoic surface of the fibula will be prominent (Fig. 7.41A, B). Scanning in an inferior direction, the fibularis longus and brevis muscles will come into view. The fibularis longus muscle can be seen sitting over the fibularis brevis muscle. The two muscles should be relatively easy to identify; to confirm identity scan up or down the leg to the known origin or insertion. They are separated by a layer of echogenic myofascia. Towards the ankle, the muscles become thin and tendinous, the fibularis longus muscle has a much longer tendinous portion than the fibularis brevis muscle, appearing hyperechoic compared to the muscle fascicles. In the long-axis view, the organization of the muscle fascicles can be examined (Fig. 7.41B).

In the Clinic

Refer to upper limb chapter 'In the Clinic' for overview of ultrasound use in musculoskeletal clinics (page 127). Table 7.10 provides an overview of the some of the musculoskeletal conditions that can be diagnosed or monitored by ultrasound.

Table 7.10 Examples of musculoskeletal pathologies that are diagnosed by ultrasound

Region	Pathology
Hip and thigh	Greater trochanteric, ischial and iliopsoas bursitis; developmental dysplasia; iliotibial band syndrome; other tendinopathy; tears; contusions; soft tissue lesions
Knee	Knee effusion (water on the knee), quadriceps tendinopathy, patellar tendinopathy, prepatellar bursitis, infrapatellar bursitis, pes anserine bursitis, popliteal (Baker's) cyst, popliteal thrombus/ aneurysm
Leg and foot	Ankle effusion, ligament tears, sprains, Nerve pathology– (injury, lesions, extrinsic compression), stress fractures, tendon subluxation, ganglion cysts

Summary Checklist

- Surface projections of the bones related to the lower limb
- Surface projections of the muscles of the lower limb
- Surface projections of the inguinal canal
- Movement of the lower limb
- Ultrasound imaging of the gluteal region
- Ultrasound imaging of the thigh
- Ultrasound imaging of the popliteal fossa
- Ultrasound imaging of the leg and foot

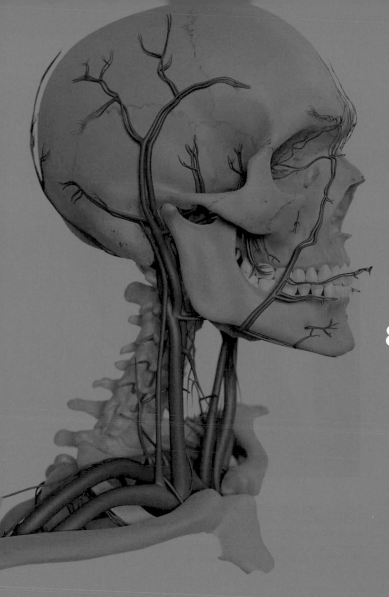

8 Head and neck

Conceptual overview

The head and neck region has important roles in protection, special senses and movement. It can be divided into the head, which consists of the neurocranium (brain case) and viscerocranium (facial skeleton), and the neck. The components of the head and neck include bones (cranium, maxilla, mandible and cervical vertebrae); viscera (brain, and cervical spinal cord, salivary and lacrimal glands, eyes and tongue); vasculature (carotid and vertebral arteries), nerves (cranial and spinal nerves) and lymphatics (cervical lymph nodes). Clinically, the head and neck are a key part of the physical examination for a range of conditions, including headache, stroke and common infections of the gastrointestinal and respiratory systems. The head and neck are easily accessible to palpate and to conduct further examinations, especially neurological.

Surface anatomy

HEAD

The head is divided into regions. Unpaired regions are the frontal, occipital, nasal, oral and mental regions. Paired regions are the parietal, temporal, mastoid, auricular, orbital, infraorbital, buccal, parotid and zygomatic regions (Fig. 8.1).

Bones

Neurocranium

The neurocranium provides the casing that encloses the brain. It consists of a series of flat bones (frontal, parietal, temporal, occipital) (Fig. 8.2). The dome of the neurocranium is known as the calvaria. Each of the cranial bones can be palpated as the scalp covering them is thin. Anteriorly is the frontal bone, posteriorly the occipital bone and laterally the paired temporal (inferior) and parietal (superior) bones. Associated with the posteriorly located occipital bone is the external occipital protuberance, which can be palpated in the midline. Extending laterally from this protuberance are the superior and inferior nuchal lines. The bones are joined by sutures that will all have fused by 30–40 years old. In some individuals the sutures can be palpated. The posterior boundary of the frontal bone articulates with the paired parietal bones at the coronal suture. The parietal bones articulate at the sagittal suture. The point where the sagittal suture intersects the coronal suture is known as the bregma. Posteriorly, the paired parietal bones and the occipital bone articulate at the lambdoid suture. The point where the sagittal suture

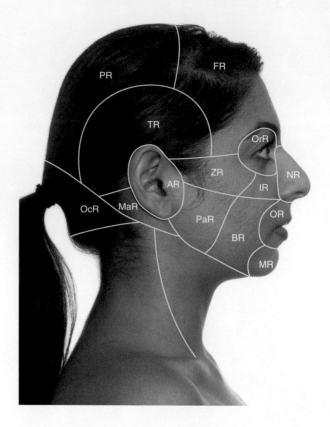

Fig. 8.1 Regions of the head. *AR*, auricular region; *BR*, buccal region; *FR*, frontal region; *IR*, infraorbital region; *MaR*, mastoid region; *MR*, mental region; *NR*, nasal region; *OcR*, occipital region; *OR*, oral region; *OrR*, orbital region; *PaR*, parotid region; *PR*, parietal region; *TR*, temporal region; *ZR*, zygomatic region.

intersects the lambdoid suture is known as the lambda. The lambda and bregma are the location of the fontanelles (soft spots). The anterior fontanelle (bregma) closes around 18 months and the posterior fontanelle (lambda) closes at 2–3 months. The fontanelles are important clinically during assessment of dehydration and raised intracranial pressure in an infant.

On the lateral aspect of the skull there is an H-shaped region, the pterion, where the frontal, parietal, sphenoid and temporal bones meet (Fig. 8.2). The pterion can be located 4 cm superior to the midpoint of the zygomatic arch. Part of the middle meningeal artery passes deep to the pterion (Fig. 8.3). It is not possible to palpate any of the brain and associated structures. The various regions of the cerebral cortex are named in relation to the overlying bones.

Facial skeleton

The bones forming the facial skeleton include paired nasal, maxillae, lacrimal, zygomatic, palatine and inferior conchae and the unpaired vomer and ethmoid bones (Fig. 8.4). The mandible is not part of the facial skeleton. Anteriorly, the

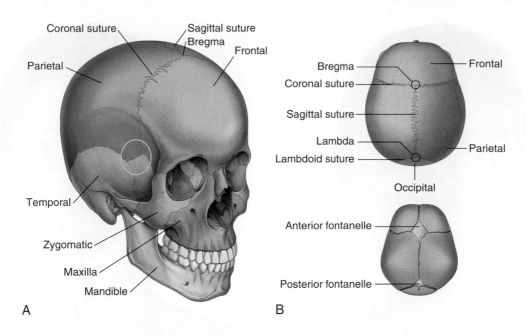

Fig. 8.2 Bones of the skull. A, Bones of the adult skull. B, Superior aspect of infant's skull.
(Modified from Drake, RL, Gray's Anatomy for Students, 3rd ed, 2015, Churchill Livingstone, Elsevier.)

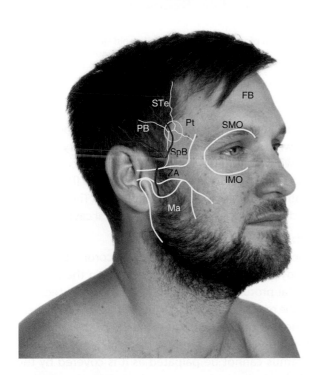

Fig. 8.3 Surface projections of the pterion. *FB*, frontal bone; *IMO*, inferior margin orbit; *Ma*, mandible; *PB*, parietal bone; *Pt*, pterion; *SMO*, superior margin orbit; *SpB*, sphenoid bone; *STe*, superficial temporal; *ZA*, zygomatic arch.

To Do (Fig. 8.3)

Anterior aspect:
- Palpate the frontal, parietal, temporal and occipital bones.
- Locate the bones of the midfacial skeleton; palpate the orbit (eye socket), zygomatic bone (cheek bone), and maxilla (upper jaw).
- Locate the region of the bregma by palpating the frontal bone in the midline and moving posteriorly. To locate the lambda palpate the occipital bone in the midline and move anteriorly until the sagittal suture is felt.
- Identify the region where the pterion is located. It can be difficult to locate the precise point. Work from the superior surface of the zygomatic arch at two finger breadths and one finger breath from the lateral edge of the orbit.
- Palpate the occipital bone, external occipital protuberance, and superior and inferior nuchal lines.

frontal bone forms most of the forehead and the superior boundary of the orbit. The frontal bone creates a slight protuberance, the glabella, in the midline. Below the glabella are the nasal bones. Inferiorly the nasal bones articulate with the nasal cartilages. The maxilla forms a substantial part of the anterior aspect of the mid-face. The maxilla forms the inferior margin of the orbit medially. Laterally, the zygomatic process of the maxilla articulates with the zygomatic bone to create the surface contours of the 'cheek bone'. Inferiorly, the upper teeth are embedded in the alveolar process of the maxilla. Laterally, the zygomatic bone articulates with the zygomatic process of the temporal bone. All of the landmarks described above can be palpated.

167

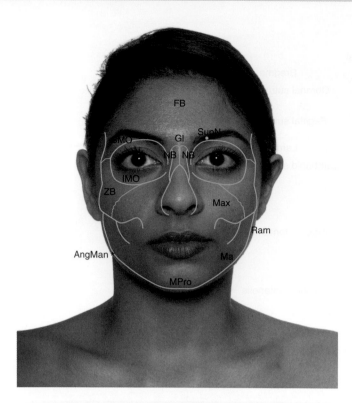

Fig. 8.4 Surface anatomy of the facial bones. **AngMan*, angle of mandible; *FB*, frontal bone; *Gl*, glabella; *IMO*, inferior margin orbit; *Ma*, mandible; *Max*, maxilla; *MPro*, mental protuberance; *NB*, nasal bone; *Ram*, ramus*SMO*, superior margin orbit; *SupN*, supraorbital notch; *ZB*, zygomatic bone.

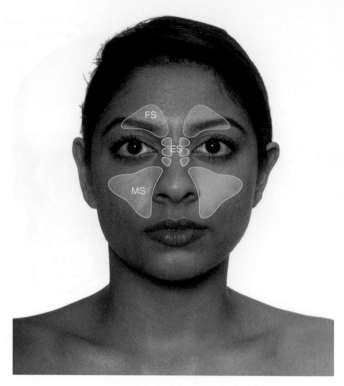

Fig. 8.5 Position of paranasal sinuses (sphenoid sinus not shown). *ES*, ethmoidal sinus (anterior group); *FS*, frontal sinus; *MS*, maxillary sinus.

To Do (Fig. 8.4)

- To examine the facial bones, start in the midline at the glabella, and move your fingers over the surface of the skin in a lateral direction, palpate the supraorbital notch of the frontal bone.
- Continuing laterally, palpate the zygomatic process and the zygomatic bone.
- In the midline palpate the paired nasal bones. The midline and slightly superiorly, palpate the paired nasal bones.

Sinuses

Sinuses are air-filled spaces lined by mucous membranes. The paranasal sinuses are located in the bones of their name: frontal, sphenoidal, ethmoidal and maxillary (Fig. 8.5). The right and left frontal sinuses are located in the anterior component of the frontal bone. The frontal sinus is approximately 1–2 cm high and 2–3 cm wide: male sinuses tend to be larger than female sinuses and there is considerable individual variation. The frontal sinuses are not of equal size and the midline septum can vary in its position. The sphenoidal sinus is deep within the body of the sphenoid bone and may extend into the wings of the sphenoid bones. The

ethmoidal sinus consists of anterior and posterior groups located within the ethmoid bone. The maxillary sinus is located within the maxilla lateral to the nasal cavity. The drainage point of the maxillary sinus is above its floor, which may contribute to the development of sinusitis. The paranasal sinuses drain into various meati of the nasal cavity.

Mandible

The mandible consists of a body, ramus, coronoid process and condylar process (Fig. 8.4). Anteriorly in the midline, the mental protuberance can be seen and palpated. The body of the mandible extends posteriorly to the angle, where it becomes continuous with the ramus. Both the angle and the inferior ramus can be easily palpated. The superior part of the ramus cannot be palpated as it is covered by the parotid gland.

Temporomandibular Joint

The temporomandibular joint is an articulation between the mandibular fossa of the temporal bone and the condylar process of the mandible (Fig. 8.6). Movements at this joint include protrusion and retraction, elevation and depression of the mandible. To open the mouth a forward movement first occurs followed by depression. To chew, movements on one temporomandibular joint are coordinated with the other side to create a grinding action. The muscles of

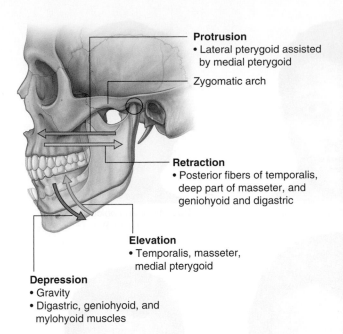

Protrusion
* Lateral pterygoid assisted by medial pterygoid

Zygomatic arch

Retraction
* Posterior fibers of temporalis, deep part of masseter, and geniohyoid and digastric

Elevation
* Temporalis, masseter, medial pterygoid

Depression
* Gravity
* Digastric, geniohyoid, and mylohyoid muscles

Fig. 8.6 Movements of the temporomandibular joint. *(Modified from Drake, RL, Gray's Anatomy for Students, 3rd ed, 2015, Churchill Livingstone, Elsevier.)*

mastication that act on the temporomandibular joint are the temporalis, masseter, and the medial and lateral pterygoid muscles. The temporalis muscle is a fan shaped muscle that originates from the temporal bone. Its is a powerful elevator of the mandible. Temporalis muscle can be palpated over the temporal bone when the teeth are clenched together. The masseter muscle is also responsible for closing the jaw and can be felt over the ramus of the mandible when the teeth are clenched. It is not possible to palpate the medial or lateral pterygoid muscles because they are more deeply located (Fig. 8.7).

To Do (Fig. 8.7)

* Palpate the temporalis muscle superior to the zygomatic arch by contracting and relaxing the jaw against closed teeth.
* Palpate the masseter muscle at the ramus of the mandible by contracting and relaxing the jaw against closed teeth.

Muscles

Muscles of the face form important sphincters for both the eyes and oral cavity, and enable emotions to be reflected through facial expression. The sphincter muscles include the orbicularis oculi muscle, which surrounds the orbit, and the orbicularis oris muscle, which surrounds the oral cavity. Muscles used in facial expression include the occipitofrontalis, corrugator supercilii, nasalis, levator labii superioris,

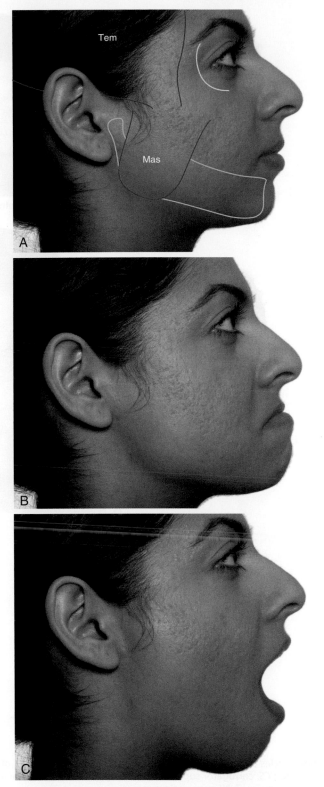

Fig. 8.7 Movements of the temporomandibular joint. A, Resting. B, Protraction. C, Depression. *Mas*, masseter; *Tem*, temporalis.

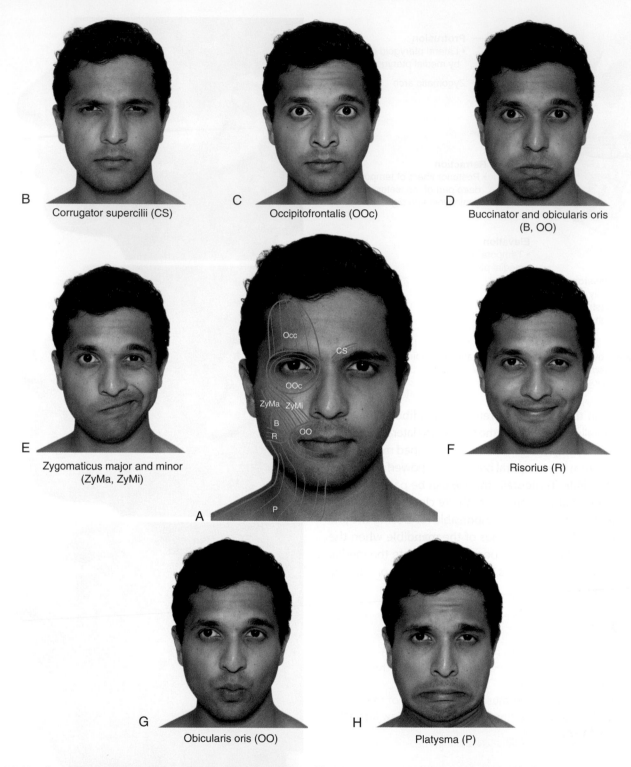

B Corrugator supercilii (CS)

C Occipitofrontalis (OOc)

D Buccinator and obicularis oris (B, OO)

E Zygomaticus major and minor (ZyMa, ZyMi)

A

F Risorius (R)

G Obicularis oris (OO)

H Platysma (P)

Fig. 8.8 Muscles of facial expression. A, Surface markings of muscles of facial expression. B–D, Facial expression highlighting muscles used. *B*, buccinator; *CS*, corrugator supercilli; *Occ*, occipitofrontalis; *OO*, obicularis oris; *OOc*, obicularis occuli; *P*, platysma; *R*, risorius; *ZyMa*, zygomaticus major; *ZyMi*, zygomaticus minor.

zygomaticus, risorius, depressor anguli oris, depressor labii inferioris and buccinator muscles (Table 8.1 and Fig. 8.8).

Eye

170 The eyeball is contained within the bony orbit and is bordered by the upper and lower eyelids that protect the

eye when closed. The eyelids are covered posteriorly by a thin membrane, the conjunctiva. On the margins of the eyelids are the eyelashes. The eyelashes protect the eye from debris. At the medial edge the eyelids merge to form the medial commissure (Fig. 8.9). This creates a space known as the lacrimal lake. On the medial side of the lacrimal lake

Table 8.1 Muscles of the face

Muscle	Origin	Insertion	Innervation	Function	Expression
Orbicularis oculi	Frontal bone and maxilla	Eyelid/eyebrow	Facial nerve	Closes eye	Sleeping
Orbicularis oris	Fascia of lips	Mucosa of lips	Facial nerve	Closes and purses lip	Kissing
Occipitofrontalis	Occipital bone	Eyebrow	Facial nerve	Elevates eyebrows, wrinkles forehead	Surprise or horror
Corrugator supercilii	Eyebrow	Root of nose	Facial nerve	Moves eyebrows toward midline	Frowning
Nasalis	Maxilla and nasal cartilage	Nose	Facial nerve	Widening external nares	Flaring nostrils
Levator labii superioris	Maxilla and zygomatic bone	Orbicularis oris	Facial nerve	Elevates upper lip	Seriousness
Zygomaticus (major and minor)	Zygomatic bone	Orbicularis oris	Facial nerve	Elevates corner of mouth and elevates upper lip	Laughing or smiling
Risorius	Fascia over maxilla	Orbicularis oris	Facial nerve	Moves angle of mouth laterally	Laughing or smiling
Depressor anguli oris	Mandible	Orbicularis oris	Facial nerve	Depresses corner of mouth	Sadness
Depressor labii inferioris	Mandible	Orbicularis oris	Facial nerve	Depresses lower lip	Doubt
Buccinator	Maxilla and mandible	Orbicularis oris	Facial nerve	Compresses cheek	Puffing out the cheeks i.e. in playing music

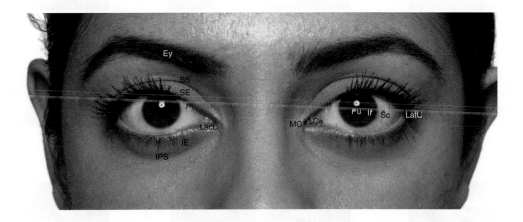

Fig. 8.9 Surface projections of the eye and the eyelids. *Ey*, eyebrow; *IE*, inferior (lower) eyelid; *IPS*, infrapalpebral sulcus; *Ir*, iris; *LacL*, lacrimal lake; *LatC*, lateral commissure; *LCa*, lacrimal caruncle; *MC*, medial commissure; *Pu*, pupil; *Sc*, sclera; *SE*, superior (upper) eyelid; *SS*, suprapalpebral sulcus.

is an elevated structure, the lacrimal caruncle. The lacrimal caruncle creates a fold at the edge of the sclera referred to as the lacrimal fold. Also on the medial side on the inner surface of the lower eyelid are the lacrimal papilla and lacrimal punctum. The papilla forms a raised mound. The punctum is the opening through which tears drain into the lacrimal sac. Tears are produced in the lacrimal gland on the lateral superior aspect of the bony orbit and are swept across the eye by blinking (Fig. 8.10). Laterally, the eyelids form the lateral commissure. Superior to the eyes are the eyebrows. These are regions of short hair that act to protect

To Do (Fig. 8.9)

- Examine the upper and lower eyelid and locate the medial and lateral commissures.
- Identify the lacrimal papilla and punctum.
- Locate the sclera, iris and pupil.
- Examine the nine positions of gaze.

the eyes from sweat and assist in communication through expression.

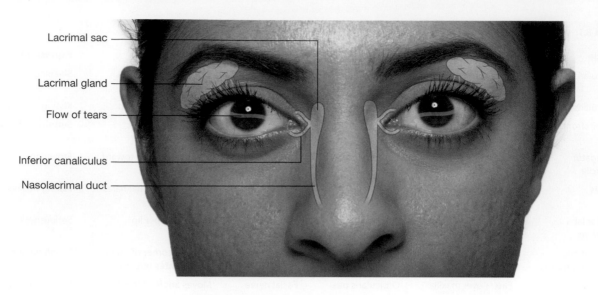

Lacrimal sac

Lacrimal gland

Flow of tears

Inferior canaliculus

Nasolacrimal duct

Fig. 8.10 Eye and lacrimal apparatus.
(From Drake, RL, Gray's Anatomy for Students, 3rd ed, 2015, Churchill Livingstone, Elsevier.)

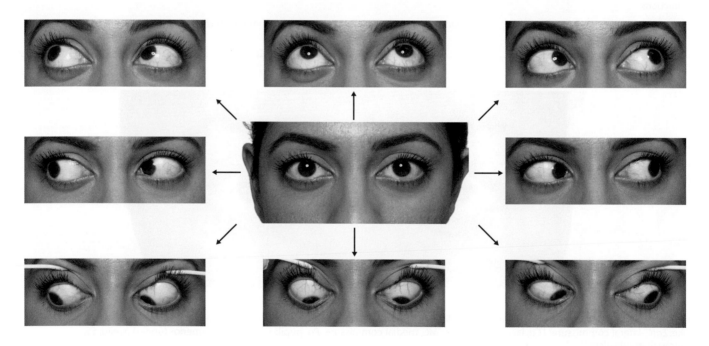

Fig. 8.11 A–H, Nine positions of gaze: elevation, depression, right abduction, left adduction and left abduction and right adduction.

The eyeball is located within the orbit, and is sphere-shaped with an anterior bulge. The eyeball is typically 2.5 cm in diameter. The eyeball contains a central opening known as the pupil. Surrounding the pupil is the iris. The iris is a circular structure that contains smooth muscle to control the size of the pupil. The iris varies in color between individuals. The sclera is the white connective tissue that is pierced by blood vessels and nerves and surrounds the iris (Fig. 8.9).

The eyeball is surrounded by orbital fat and six extrinsic (extraocular) muscles (superior rectus, inferior rectus, medial rectus, lateral rectus, inferior oblique and superior oblique), which are innervated by cranial nerves. The extrinsic muscles work to enable both eyes to follow an object. The opening of the orbit is angled slightly laterally. The extrinsic muscles work to correct this angle to enable us to look forward. The extrinsic muscles create the nine positions of gaze (Fig. 8.11).

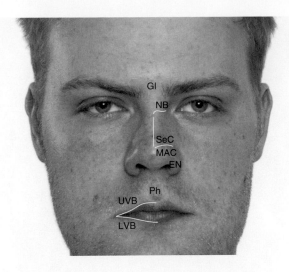

Fig. 8.12 Surface projections of the external nose and upper lip. *EN*, external nares; *Gl*, glabella; *LVB*, lower vermillion border; *MAC*, major alar cartilage; *NB*, nasal bone; *Ph*, philtrum; *SeC*, septal cartilage; *UVB*, upper vermillion border.

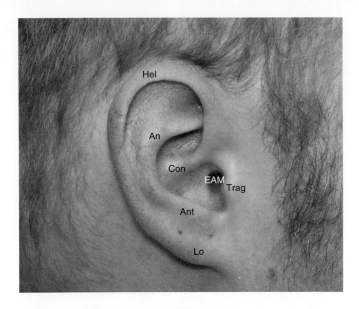

Fig. 8.13 Surface anatomy of the ear. *An*, antihelix; *Ant*, antitragus; *Con*, concha; *EAM*, external auditory meatus; *Hel*, helix; *Lo*, lobule; *Trag*, tragus.

To Do (Fig. 8.12)

- Begin in the midline at the glabella and palpate the nasal bones.
- Continue inferiorly and palpate the septal cartilage.
- Moving laterally, palpate the lateral part of the septal cartilage.
- Examine the external nares and philtrum.

To Do (Fig. 8.13)

- Examine the components of the auricle. Begin with the helix and work medially to the antihelix, concha and external auditory meatus.
- Palpate the tragus and antitragus.
- Palpate the lobule.

External Nose

The nose consists of two nasal bones and associated cartilages. In the midline, the septal (or quadrilateral) cartilage runs inferiorly, dividing the internal component of the nose. The septal cartilage has two lateral projections that are continuous superiorly with the nasal bones. Inferior to the lateral process of the septal cartilages are the major alar cartilages. Three or four minor alar cartilages complete the rest of the nose framework (Fig. 8.12). The external nares are the openings of the nasal cavity to the external environment. In the midline of the upper lip the vertical groove that can be seen and felt is the philtrum.

Ear

The ear consists of external, middle and internal components. Only a portion of the external ear can be examined without instrumentation. The external ear is attached to the lateral aspect of the head and consists of two parts: the auricle (or pinna) and the external acoustic meatus (Fig. 8.13). The auricle is important for directing sound waves and consists of cartilage covered with skin. The outer C-shape of the auricle is the helix, with the antihelix just medial. The central depression is the concha. Medial to the concha is the external acoustic meatus. On either side of the external acoustic meatus is an elevation. The anterior elevation is the tragus, and the posterior elevation is the antitragus. At the inferior pole of the auricle is the lobule.

The external acoustic meatus extends from the concha to the tympanic membrane. It is 2–4 cm in length and is slightly inclined, initially passing anteriorly and then turning posteriorly. This can make visualizing the tympanic membrane difficult. Visualization of the tympanic membrane can be improved by gently lifting the auricle posteriorly, superiorly and laterally. The external acoustic meatus wall consists of cartilage (lateral one third) and a bony tunnel with in the temporal bone (medial two thirds).

Oral Cavity

The oral cavity opens onto the face through the oral fissure. The oral cavity has great clinical relevance because it is involved in respiration, the first stage of digestion and in manipulating sounds produced by the larynx. It has a roof, which is formed by the hard and soft palates; walls, formed by the muscular cheeks; and a floor, formed by the tongue and various muscles (mylohyoid and geniohyoid muscles). Posteriorly, the cavity is continuous with a portion of the pharynx referred to as the oropharynx.

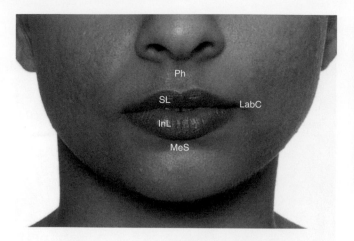

Fig. 8.14 Surface anatomy of the mouth. *InL*, inferior lip; *LabC*, labial commissure; *MeS*, mentolabial sulcus; *Ph*, philtrum; *SL*, superior lip.

To Do (Fig. 8.15)

In the oral cavity:
- Using your tongue, feel for the hard palate on the superior aspect of the oral cavity.
- Feel with the tongue for the opening of the parotid duct in the lateral cheek opposite the second upper molar tooth.
- Lift up the tongue and view the frenulum, sublingual caruncles and lingual vein.
- Examine the papillae of the tongue. A cotton tip containing blue food dye can be swept across the tongue to improve viewing of the papillae.

The lips are created from skin that becomes thinner as it merges with the oral mucosa. The red hue is due to blood vessels that lie close to the surface. The superior lip is indented in the midline by the philtrum (Fig. 8.14), a structure related to fusion of the medial nasal process in the embryo. The medial surfaces of both the upper and lower lips are connected to the gingivae by a median labial frenulum. At the lateral edge of the lips is the labial commissure. In the midline below the lower lip is the mentolabial sulcus.

Behind the oral fissure are the upper and lower dental arches that sit within a horseshoe-shaped region known as the oral vestibule. The parotid duct opens into the oral vestibule at the level of the second molar tooth. Superiorly, the hard and soft palates are covered with mucosa. Projecting from the soft palate in the midline is the uvula. The posterior of the cavity continues into the oropharynx. The junction (faucial isthmus) between the oral cavity and oropharynx is marked by the palatoglossal fold (anterior arch if the fauces). The palatine tonsil, a mass of lymphoid tissue, lies between the palatoglossal (anterior) and palatopharyngeal (posterior) arches (Fig. 8.15A).

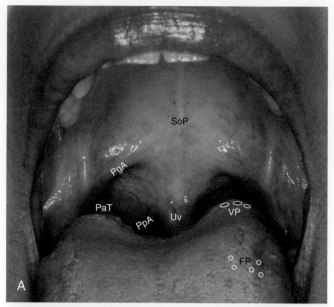

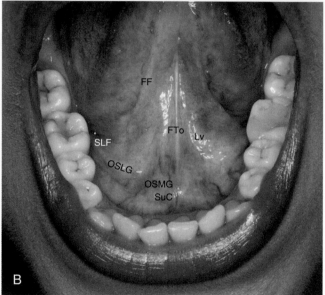

Fig. 8.15 A, Oral cavity. B, Inferior aspect of the tongue and floor of the mouth. *FF*, fimbriated fold; *FP*, fungiform papillae; *FTo*, frenulum tongue; *Lv*, lingual vein; *OSLG*, opening sublingual gland; *OSMG*, opening submandibular gland; *PaT*, palatine tonsil; *PgA*, palatoglossal arch; *PpA*, palatopharyngeal arch; *SLF*, sublingual fold; *SoP*, soft palate; *SuC*, sublingual caruncle; *Uv*, uvula; *VP*, vallate papillae.

The tongue is formed of highly vascularised muscle and is divided into an anterior two-thirds and a posterior one-third by a V-shaped sulcus terminalis. The anterior part is triangular in shape and located in the oral cavity, while the posterior third is located in the oropharynx. At the apex of the sulcus is the foramen cecum. The surface of the tongue is covered with papillae, of which there are three types: filiform, fungiform and vallate. The larger fungiform papillae can be identified on the superior surface and are more predominantly found scattered on the lateral edges and tip of the tongue. The vallate papillae lie immediately infront of the sulcus terminalis (Fig. 8.15A). The undersurface of the tongue is connected to the floor of the mouth by the lingual frenulum. Lateral to the frenulum are the sublingual caruncles, the openings for the submandibular glands. The lateral sublingual fold contains openings of the sublingual glands. The deep lingual veins may be observed on either side of the frenulum (Fig. 8.15B).

The teeth are attached to the mandible and maxilla through alveoli (sockets). At around 6 years of age the deciduous teeth begin to be replaced by 32 permanent teeth. This process occurs over time and may take until the late teens for all permanent teeth to be present. On each side are two incisors, one canine, two premolars and three molars (Fig. 8.16). Each type of tooth has characteristic features (Table 8.2).

NECK

The neck is the slender region between the clavicles inferiorly and the cranium and is a passageway for the respiratory and gastrointestinal systems as well as for essential neurovascular structures.

Bones

Hyoid

The hyoid bone is crescent shaped and is unique in that it is completely suspended by muscle (Fig. 8.17). It provides important attachments for a group of muscles collectively known as the strap muscles of the neck. The hyoid bone can be palpated on the anterior aspect of the neck at the point where the underside of the chin meets the neck. (palpating the hyoid can feel uncomfortable.)

Vertebrae

Posteriorly, there are seven cervical vertebrae. The most superior vertebra, the atlas (C1) forms a unique ring of

Table 8.2 Features of the adult teeth

Tooth	Features	Action
Incisor	Single root, chisel-shaped crown	Cutting
Canine	Single root, pointed cusp	Grasping
Premolar	Usually single root but may have two, bicuspid (buccal and lingual)	Grinding
Molar	Three roots, three to five cusps	Grinding

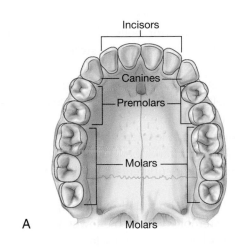

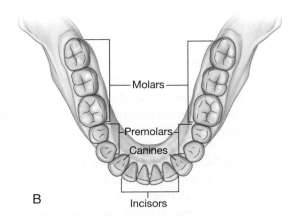

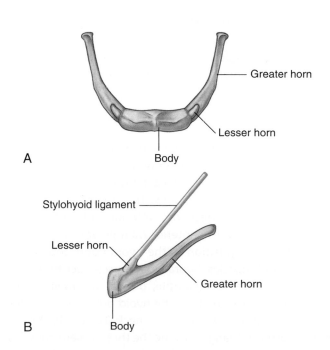

Fig. 8.16 Adult upper and lower permanent teeth. A, Upper. B, Lower. *(From Drake, RL, Gray's Anatomy for Students, 3rd ed, 2015, Churchill Livingstone, Elsevier.)*

Fig. 8.17 Hyoid bone. A, Anterior view. B, Lateral view. *(From Drake, RL, Gray's Anatomy for Students, 3rd ed, 2015, Churchill Livingstone, Elsevier.)*

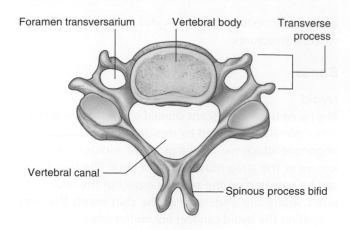

Fig. 8.18 Typical cervical vertebra.
(From Drake, RL, Gray's Anatomy for Students, 3rd ed, 2015, Churchill Livingstone, Elsevier.)

bone. The second cervical vertebra, the axis (C2), has a bony projection, the dens, that articulates with C1. The remaining cervical vertebrae have bodies, bifid spinous processes and a foramen transversarium, through which the vertebral arteries pass. Note that C7 may not have a foramen transversarium on one or both sides. If a C7 foramen is present, it rarely transmits the vertebral artery but may transmit the vertebral vein (Fig. 8.18). The spinous processes of C2 and C7 are especially prominent and can be palpated. The ligamentum nuchae can be palpated in the midline. This flat triangular ligament is attached to the external occipital protuberance and extends inferiorly to the spinous processes of C2–7. The apex of the triangle is located at C7 and can be palpated. Laterally, the splenius capitis muscle may be felt (see Chapter 5).

Muscles

The most superficial muscle of the neck is platysma, which runs as a sheet over the anterior aspect of the neck. The extent of platysma varies considerably between individuals and degenerates in the elderly. The sternocleidomastoid muscle divides the neck into anterior and posterior triangles. Muscles of the anterior triangle are described in relation to their position to the hyoid bone: suprahyoid or infrahyoid muscles. Suprahyoid muscles act to elevate the hyoid bone; for example, during swallowing. The infrahyoid muscles depress the hyoid bone and are often termed the 'strap' muscles of the neck (Table 8.3). Muscles of the posterior triangle include the three scalene muscles. The brachial plexus and subclavian artery pass between the anterior and middle scalene muscles, which are of clinical importance in procedures such as an interscalene nerve block.

Triangles

The anterior and posterior triangles are divided by the sternocleidomastoid muscle (Fig. 8.19). The anterior triangle is bordered by the sternocleidomastoid muscle posteriorly, the inferior border of the mandible inferiorly and the midline of the neck medially. The posterior triangle is bordered by sternocleidomastoid muscle anteriorly, the clavicle inferiorly and trapezius muscle posteriorly. The sternocleidomastoid muscle is broad and can be easily palpated as it extends from the mastoid process to the manubrium (sternal head) and the medial third of the clavicle (clavicular head). The sternocleidomastoid muscle is a significant muscle in movement of the neck. Acting unilaterally, it moves the head to the opposite side; acting bilaterally, it extends the neck at the atlanto-occipital joints and causes flexion at the cervical vertebrae bringing the chin to the chest.

The anterior triangle is further subdivided into four smaller triangles (Fig. 8.19):

- Carotid triangle: bounded by the posterior belly of digastric, the superior belly of omohyoid and the superior anterior border of the sternocleidomastoid muscles.
- Submandibular triangle: bounded by the anterior and posterior bellies of the digastric muscle and the inferior surface of the mandible.
- Submental triangle: located under the chin, which is bounded by the anterior belly of digastric muscle and continuous with the submental triangle on the opposite side.
- Muscular triangle: bounded by the superior belly of omohyoid, sternohyoid and the lower anterior border of the sternocleidomastoid muscles.

The posterior triangle is further subdivided into two triangles by the omohyoid muscle:

- Omoclavicular triangle: bounded by the clavicle and the inferior belly of omohyoid muscle.
- Occipital triangle: the largest triangle that is located superior to the inferior belly of omohyoid muscle. It is bounded by the sternocleidomastoid muscle and the trapezius muscle.

In a slender individual, the omohyoid muscle can be seen if the head is rotated to the side and flexed. It is important to note that the lung extends 3–4 cm above the medial third of the clavicle into the posterior triangle and that a pneumothorax may occur from trauma in this area.

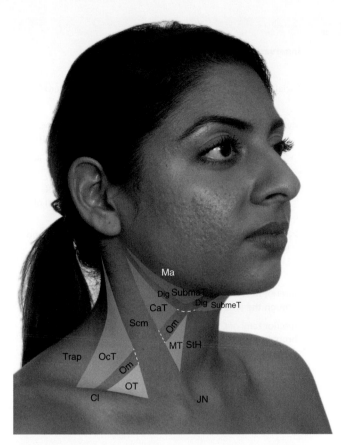

Fig. 8.19 Triangles of the neck. *CaT*, carotid triangle; *Cl*, clavicle; *Dig*, digastric (anterior belly); *JN*, jugular notch; *Ma*, mandible; *MT*, muscular triangle; *OcT*, occipital triangle; *Om*, omohyoid; *OT*, omoclavicular triangle; *Scm*, sternocleidomastoid; *StH*, sternohyoid; *SubmaT*, submandibular triangle; *SubmeT*, submental triangle; *Trap*, trapezius.

Viscera

The viscera of the neck consists of the thyroid, larynx, trachea, pharynx and esophagus. These structures are associated with the endocrine, respiratory and gastrointestinal systems, respectively. As part of the gastrointestinal system, the submandibular glands fill the submandibular triangle and are palpable as a soft mass.

Thyroid

The thyroid gland, is normally located between vertebral levels C5 and T1. It consists of two lobes joined across the midline by an isthmus (Fig. 8.20). It lies on the anterior surface of the larynx and trachea and extends posteriorly where it lies lateral to the pharynx and esophagus. The isthmus sits in front of the second to fourth tracheal rings. Anteriorly, the thyroid gland is covered by the infrahyoid 'strap' muscles. The gland is enclosed within two fascial capsules. The denser outer capsule is continuous with the pretracheal fascia, which covers the larynx and trachea. During a clinical examination, with the clinician's fingers placed over the thyroid gland,

To Do (Fig. 8.19)

Anterior and lateral aspect of the neck:
- Locate the sternocleidomastoid muscle. The anterior border may be traced from the manubrium to the mastoid process. Draw a line along its anterior border, which will form the posterior boundary of the anterior triangle, and a line along its posterior border, which will form the anterior boundary of the posterior triangle.

Draw the anterior triangle:
- Locate the midline of the neck and the inferior border of the mandible.
- Draw a line over the omohyoid muscle in the anterior triangle to create the carotid triangle and the muscular triangle.
- Palpate the digastric muscle and draw on the submandibular and submental triangles.
- Locate a point on the posterior border of the sternocleidomastoid muscle approximately one third from its origin. This point (sometimes called the 'nerve point') marks the general region where the cutaneous branches of the cervical plexus (lesser occipital, greater auricular, transverse cervical and supraclavicular nerves) emerge.

Draw the posterior triangle:
- Locate the trapezius muscle from its attachment at the mastoid process to the middle and lateral thirds of the clavicle. Draw a line along its anterior border creating the posterior boundary.
- Locate the clavicle. Draw a line along its superior border.
- Locate the omohyoid muscle to further subdivide the posterior triangle into the occipital and omoclavicular triangles.

the gland will be felt to move up when the patient is asked to swallow. An enlarged thyroid gland (goiter) may extend into the superior mediastinum, and in severe cases the goiter may compress the trachea, esophagus and veins, causing difficulty with breathing and swallowing. The thyroid gland is supplied on each side by a superior thyroid artery (a branch of the external carotid artery) and an inferior thyroid artery (from the subclavian artery or its branches). Thyroid veins drain superiorly and laterally into the internal jugular veins and some descend in front of the trachea and drain to the left brachiocephalic vein. The small, pea-sized parathyroid glands are usually embedded in the posterior surfaces of lobes of the thyroid gland.

Larynx

The larynx is a cartilaginous structure within the anterior of the neck that is continuous with the trachea inferiorly. The

Table 8.3   Anterior and posterior triangle of the neck

Muscle	Origin	Insertion	Innervation	Function
Anterior triangle of neck (suprahyoid and infrahyoid muscles)				
Stylohyoid	Styloid process	Hyoid bone	Facial nerve [7]	Pulls hyoid bone upwards.
Digastric				
—Anterior belly	Digastric fossa, inside of mandible	Tendon between two bellies to body of hyoid bone	Mylohyoid nerve [V3]	Opens mouth by lowering mandible; raises hyoid bone
—Posterior belly	Mastoid notch on mastoid process of temporal bone	Same as anterior belly	Facial nerve [7]	Pulls hyoid bone upward and back
Mylohyoid	Mylohyoid line on mandible	Body of hyoid bone	Mylohyoid nerve [V3]	Support and elevation of floor of mouth; elevation of hyoid
Geniohyoid	Inferior mental spine on mandible	Body of hyoid bone	Branch from anterior ramus of C1	Fixed mandible: elevates and pulls hyoid bone forward, fixed hyoid: pulls mandible downward and inward
Sternohyoid	Posterior sternoclavicular joint	Body of hyoid bone	Anterior rami of C1 to C3 through the ansa cervicalis	Depresses hyoid bone after swallowing
Omohyoid	Superior border of scapula	Body of hyoid bone	Anterior rami of C1 to C3 through the ansa cervicalis	Depresses and fixes hyoid bone
Thyrohyoid	Lamina of thyroid cartilage	Greater horn of hyoid bone	Anterior ramus of C1	Depresses hyoid bone, hyoid bone fixed: raises larynx
Sternothyroid	Posterior surface of manubrium of sternum	Thyroid cartilage	Anterior rami of C1 to C3 through the ansa cervicalis	Draws larynx downward
Posterior triangle of the neck; parentheses indicate possible involvement				
Sternocleidomastoid				
—Sternal head	Upper part of anterior surface of manubrium of sternum	Lateral one-half of superior nuchal line	Accessory nerve [11] and branches from anterior rami of C2 to C3 (C4)	Individually: tilt head toward shoulder on same side, acting together: draw head forward
—Clavicular head	Superior surface of medial one-third of clavicle	Lateral surface of mastoid process		
Trapezius	Superior nuchal line; external occipital protuberance; ligamentum nuchae; spinous processes of vertebrae C7 to T12	Lateral one-third of clavicle; acromion; spine of scapula	Motor—accessory nerve [11]; proprioception—C3 and C4	Elevate, adduct and depress scapula. Assists in rotating the scapula during abduction of humerus above horizontal.
Levator scapulae	Transverse processes of C1 to C4	Upper part of medial border of scapula	C3, C4; and dorsal scapular nerve (C4, C5)	Elevates scapula
Posterior scalene	Transverse processes of vertebrae C4 to C6	Upper surface of rib 2	Anterior rami of C5 to C7	Elevation of rib 2
Middle scalene	Transverse processes of vertebrae C2 to C7	Upper surface of rib 1	Anterior rami of C3 to C7	Elevation of rib 1
Anterior scalene	Transverse processes of vertebrae C3 to C6	Scalene tubercle and upper surface of rib 1	Anterior rami of C4 to C7	Elevation of rib 1
Omohyoid	Superior border of scapula	Body of hyoid bone	Ansa cervicalis; anterior rami of C1 to C3	Depress the hyoid bone

Modified from Drake, RL, Gray's Anatomy for Students, 3rd ed, 2015, Churchill Livingstone, Elsevier (full table available in the e-book).

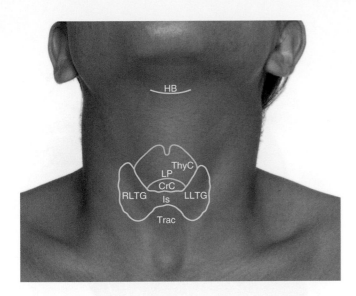

Fig. 8.20 Surface anatomy of the thyroid gland and larynx. *CrC*, cricoid cartilage; *HB*, hyoid bone; *Is*, isthmus; *LLTG*, left lobe thyroid gland; *LP*, laryngeal prominence; *RLTG*, right lobe thyroid gland; *ThyC*, thyroid cartilage; *Trac*, trachea.

To Do (Fig. 8.20)

Anterior aspect of the neck:
- Palpate the thyroid cartilage by gently placing the thumb and the forefinger finger on either side.
- Move your finger inferiorly to palpate the cricoid cartilage.
- Observe the movement of the larynx during swallowing.

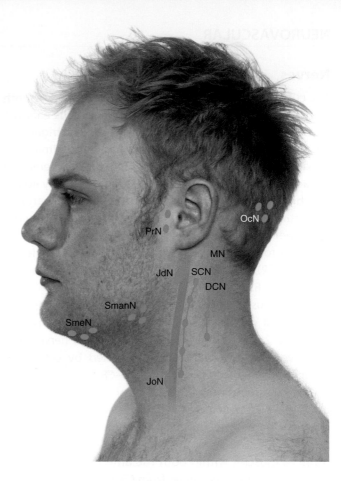

Fig. 8.21 Surface projections lymph nodes. *DCN*, deep cervical nodes; *JdN*, jugulodigastric node; *JoN*, jugulo-omohyoid node; *MN*, mastoid nodes; *OcN*, occipital nodes; *PrN*, preauricular/parotid nodes; *SCN*, superficial cervical nodes; *SmanN*, submandibular nodes; *SmeN*, submental nodes.

larynx is attached superiorly by a ligamentous membrane to the hyoid bone. The larynx is responsible for voice production and maintains patency of the airway. The larynx consists of three unpaired cartilages: thyroid, cricoid and epiglottis, and three smaller paired cartilages: arytenoid, corniculate and cuneiform. The thyroid cartilage can be palpated in the midline (Fig. 8.20), and in males the central laryngeal prominence (Adam's apple) can be seen. Inferior to the thyroid cartilage is the cricoid cartilage, which with gentle pressure may be palpated.

LYMPH

Lymph nodes within the head and neck are arranged into three groups: superficial, superficial cervical and deep cervical (Fig. 8.21). The superficial nodes include the occipital, mastoid, preauricular/parotid, submandibular and submental nodes. The superficial lymph nodes can be palpated in the corresponding region. For example, occipital nodes are palpated in the occipital region. Superficial cervical lymph nodes are a collection of nodes that run along the course of the external jugular vein and are palpated on the surface of the sternocleidomastoid muscle. Deep cervical lymph nodes are a collection of nodes that run along the course of the internal jugular vein. Two of the large deep cervical lymph nodes are of clinical importance. These are the jugulodigastric node and the jugulo-omohyoid node. The jugulodigastric node is located at the point where the internal jugular vein is crossed by the posterior belly of the digastric muscle. This node receives drainage from the palatine tonsils and may be enlarged in tonsillitis. The jugulo-omohyoid node is located at the point of the intermediate tendon of the omohyoid muscle (Fig. 8.21). This node receives drainage from the tongue and may be enlarged in carcinomas of the tongue. Clinically, lymph nodes in the neck are divided into 6 or 7 levels, which are used to describe the extent and spread of a tumor.

NEUROVASCULAR

Nerves

The cutaneous innervation to the head is formed by both cranial nerves and cervical nerves. Anterior to the ears, the face is supplied by the trigeminal nerve (V). The trigeminal nerve is divided into three branches: ophthalmic (V_1), maxillary (V_2) and mandibular (V_3) (Fig. 8.22). Innervation in each of these regions can be tested clinically by lightly touching the skin. The occipitofrontalis muscle and its aponeurosis is part of the scalp and is innervated by the facial nerve (C7). The nerves that innervate the scalp posterior to the ears are the great auricular (C2, C3), lesser occipital (C2), greater occipital (C2) and third occipital (C3) nerves (Fig. 8.22).

Cutaneous innervation to the anterolateral neck is from the cervical plexus (C1–C4), in particular the transverse cervical (C2, C3) and supraclavicular (C3, C4) nerves. The skin over the posterior neck is supplied by cutaneous branches of the posterior rami of C4–C8.

The cutaneous branches of the cervical plexus emerge from the posterior border of the sternocleidomastoid muscle, whereas the muscular branches are located more deeply. The ansa cervicalis, from C1–C3, is a loop that supplies muscles within both the anterior and posterior triangles. The phrenic nerve, from C3, C4 and C5, supplies the diaphragm and passes inferiorly through the posterior triangle on the anterior surface of the anterior scalene muscle.

The roots of the brachial plexus, formed from C5–T1, appear between the anterior and middle scalene muscles and pass as trunks through the posterior triangle, also giving off several branches.

The anterior triangle of the neck contains the glossopharyngeal, vagus and hypoglossal nerves. The vagus nerve enters the carotid sheath, which is a fibrous structure that also surrounds the common carotid artery, and internal jugular vein. The hypoglossal nerve passes medial to the internal jugular vein and hooks around the occipital artery to continue deep to the posterior belly of the digastric muscle. The accessory nerve runs predominantly in the posterior triangle, supplying sternocleidomastoid and trapezius muscles.

Vasculature

The arterial supply to the head and neck is derived from the common carotid and vertebral arteries. The right common carotid artery is a branch from the brachiocephalic trunk and the left common carotid artery from the arch of the aorta. Both ascend the neck in the carotid sheath. Around vertebral level C4, the arteries divide

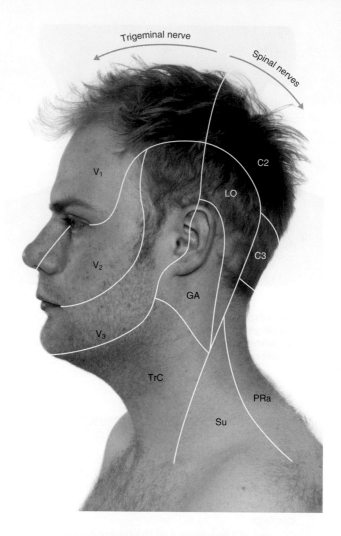

Fig. 8.22 Cutaneous innervation of the head and neck. *C2*, greater occipital; *C3*, third occipital; *GA*, greater auricular; *LO*, lesser occipital; *PRa*, posterior rami C4–C8; *Su*, supraclavicular; *TrC*, transverse cervical; *V₁*, ophthalmic nerve; *V₂*, maxillary nerve; *V₃*, mandibular nerve.

into internal and external. The internal carotid artery ascends into the skull without giving off any branches in the neck, and supplies the brain and spinal cord. The vertebral arteries arise from the subclavian arteries and ascends in the foramina transversarium of the cervical vertebrae to supply the cervical spinal cord and vertebrae and the brain. The head, neck and face is primarily supplied from the external carotid artery, which passes superiorly on the lateral aspect of the face. The external carotid artery extends along the angle of the mandible to continue as the superficial temporal artery anterior to the tragus of the ear giving an anterior branch, which continues to climb superiorly. The external carotid artery gives off several branches: superior thyroid, ascending pharyngeal, lingual, facial, occipital, posterior auricular, maxillary and superficial temporal (Fig. 8.23). A small region superior to the orbit is supplied by branches from the ophthalmic artery, which is a branch of the internal carotid artery. This provides communication between the branches of the external carotid artery and the internal carotid artery. There are five main pulse points in the head and neck: temporal, superficial temporal, anterior branch of superficial temporal, carotid and facial arteries (Fig. 8.24).

Veins of the head and neck drain into the internal and external jugular veins. The internal jugular vein begins at the jugular foramen and descends within the carotid sheath. The internal jugular vein joins the subclavian veins to form the right and left brachiocephalic veins. The external jugular vein is formed from the posterior auricular and retromandibular veins at the angle of the mandible. The external jugular vein passes inferiorly and superficial to the sternocleidomastoid muscle until it is posterior to the clavicle, where it joins the subclavian vein (Fig. 8.25). Clinically the path of venous drainage is important in relation to the spread of infection which may spread from the face to the

intracranial region through the vascular interconnections around the orbit and nose. The anterior jugular veins are paired channels, which descend anterior, to enter the subclavian vein. The anterior jugular veins may be connected by a jugular venous arch at the level of the suprasternal notch.

The subclavian vein is located anterior to the anterior scalene muscle and is frequently used for vascular access.

To Do (Fig. 8.23)

To draw out the arterial supply to the face and scalp.
- Draw a line passing from the sternoclavicular joint to the angle of the mandible. This line represents the common carotid artery. Terminate this line at the point where the common carotid artery usually bifurcates into the external carotid artery and the internal carotid artery, which normally occurs approximately 1.5 cm above the superior border of the lamina of the thyroid cartilage.
- Locate the facial pulse by compressing against the lower border of the mandible and add a red dot here.
- Continue a line superiorly from the carotid pulse to the level of the angle of the mandible. At this level create an anterior branch, the facial artery, that passes through the pulse point you have located to the lateral corner of the mouth.
- Take the main line superiorly as the superficial temporal artery.

In the Clinic

It is important to be familiar with the position of the subclavian and internal jugular veins as these are commonly used for central venous access. A potential complication when undertaking this procedure is a pneumothorax, since the pleura extends into the neck. To help avoid such complication, ultrasound is commonly used to guide the insertion of a central line.

Spread of infection and metastatic spread of head and neck cancers follows the lymphatic drainage to the relevant lymph nodes. The upper deep cervical or jugulo-digastric lymph nodes are often enlarged in tonsillitis.

Blunt trauma to the eye may result in a 'blow-out' fracture of the floor of the orbit resulting in entrapment of the inferior rectus muscle and orbital fascia causing restriction of upward gaze and diplopia (double vision). There may also be numbness of the cheek due to damage to the infraorbital nerve—a branch of the maxillary division of the trigeminal nerve (V_2).

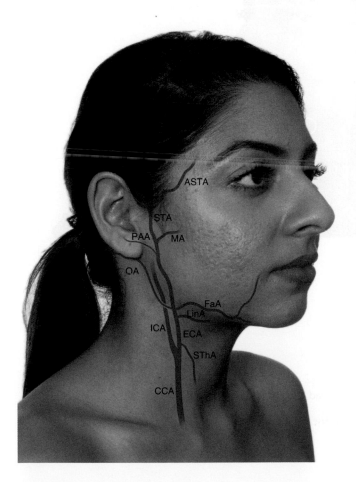

Fig. 8.23 External carotid artery. *ASTA*, anterior superficial temporal artery; *CCA*, common carotid artery; *ECA*, external carotid artery; *FaA*, facial artery; *ICA*, internal carotid artery; *LinA*, lingual artery; *MA*, maxillary artery; *OA*, occipital artery; *PAA*, posterior auricular artery; *STA*, superficial temporal artery; *SThA*, superior thyroid artery.

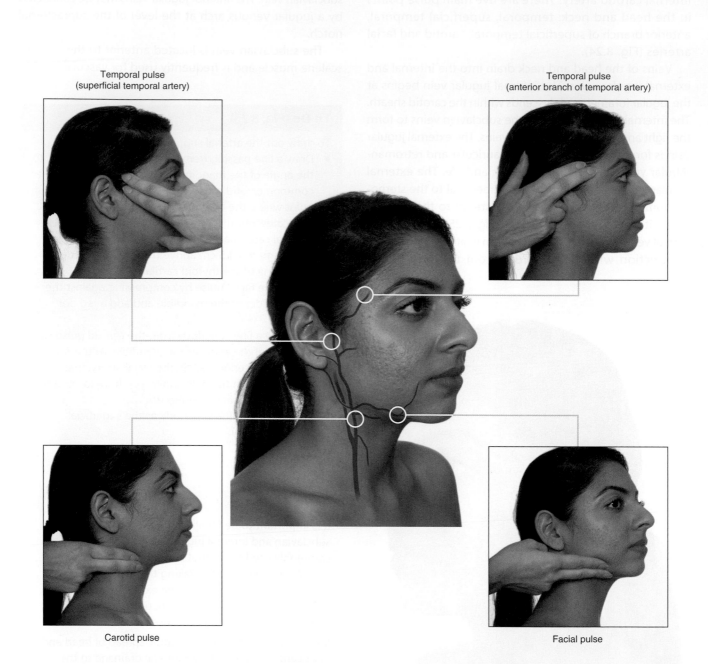

Temporal pulse
(superficial temporal artery)

Temporal pulse
(anterior branch of temporal artery)

Carotid pulse

Facial pulse

Fig. 8.24 Surface projections of the arterial supply and pulse points of the head and neck. A, Pulse points in the head and neck. B, Anterior superficial temporal. C, Superficial temporal. D, Carotid. E, Facial.
(A from Drake, RL, Gray's Anatomy for Students, 3rd ed, 2015, Churchill Livingstone, Elsevier.)

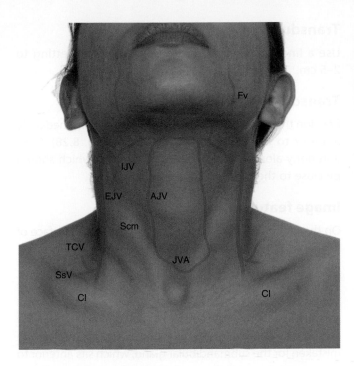

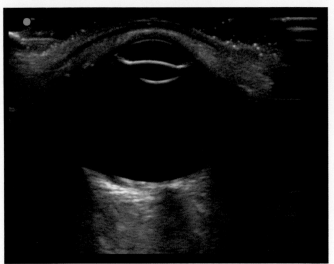

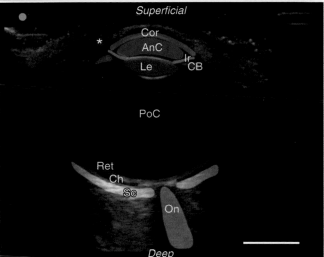

Fig. 8.25 Surface projections of the venous drainage of the head and neck. *AJV*, anterior jugular vein; *Cl*, clavicle; *EJV*, external jugular vein; *Fv*, facial vein; *IJV*, internal jugular vein; *JVA*, jugular venous arch; *Scm*, sternocleidomastoid; *SsV*, suprascapular vein; *TCV*, transverse cervical vein.

Ultrasound

EYE

Subject position

Imaging is performed with the subject sitting.

Transducer

Use a linear array transducer. Set the depth setting to 2–5 cm.

Transducer position

It is important that the eye remains closed and that sterile ultrasound gel is used. Apply adequate gel to the transducer and gently position the probe over the eyelid in transverse plane (Fig. 8.26). Tilt the probe slightly inferiorly. Avoid pressure onto the eye. After performing this examination, carefully wipe off any excess gel and rinse the eye with sterile saline.

Image features

The eyeball can be seen as a hypoechoic sphere-shaped ball (Fig. 8.26). The postremal (vitreous) chamber, which contains vitreous humor, fills much of the space. In front of the postremal chamber, the anterior chamber is in view. At

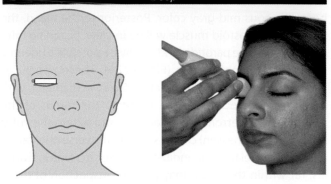

Fig. 8.26 Ultrasound of the right eye. ***, eyelid; *AnC*, anterior chamber; *CB*, ciliary bodies; *Ch*, choroid; *Cor*, cornea; *Ir*, iris; *Le*, lens; *On,* optic nerve; *PoC*, postremal chamber; *Ret*, retina; *Sc*, sclera. Scale bar = 1 cm.

the front of the eyeball, the cornea appears as a thin hyperechoic line following the curve of the anterior chamber. Sitting between the anterior and postremal chambers, the iris and lens can be seen. The iris appears as two short bright streaks behind which the conical-shaped lens sits. The surfaces of the lens produce bright reflections, which outline its shape. At the iris, the cornea becomes continuous with

183

the outer wall of the eyeball, called the sclera. The mid-gray colored ciliary bodies can be seen sitting lateral to the lens. The inner layer of the eyeball, the retina, has a mid-gray color compared to the underlying middle layer, the choroid, which is relatively hypoechoic. The outer dense layer of the eyeball, the sclera, appears as a mid- to light-gray thick layer. The three layers of the eyeball are best examined in the posterior wall of the eyeball. Behind the eye, the optic nerve will be in view as a hypoechoic shadow.

PAROTID GLAND

Subject position

Imaging is performed with the subject sitting.

Transducer

Use a linear array transducer. Set the depth setting to 2–5 cm.

Transducer position

Position the transducer in a transverse plane immediately inferior to the ear, posterior to the ramus of the mandible, with the orientation marker to the left. Scan inferiorly toward the angle of the mandible.

Image features

Towards the right side of the image, the hyperechoic surface of the ramus of the mandible will be in view (Fig. 8.27). Superficial to the mandible, the masseter muscle can be seen. Posterior to the mandible, the large parotid gland has a homogeneous mid-gray color. Posterior to the gland, the sternocleidomastoid muscle will be in view. Scanning inferiorly through the parotid gland, it may be possible to identify intraparotid lymph nodes (Fig. 8.27A). These appear as hypoechoic ovals, approximately 3–5 mm in diameter, with a central hyperechoic hilum. Close to the ramus of the mandible, the retromandibular vein and external carotid artery (deep to the vein) can be seen in transverse orientation running parallel to the mandible. However, in some individuals, fat within the gland may prevent inspection of these vessels. Note that the facial nerve can be inspected in the anterior portion of the gland as it passes through the gland, onto the surface of the masseter muscle. To observe the facial nerve, the transducer should be positioned anterior to the ear with the orientation marker pointing cephalic. In this view, the nerve appears in the short axis. It is 1–2 mm in diameter and has a notable hyperechoic border.

SUBMANDIBULAR GLAND

Subject position

Imaging is performed with the subject sitting. The head should be tilted posteriorly.

Transducer

Use a linear array transducer. Set the depth setting to 2–5 cm.

Transducer position

Position the transducer in the transverse plane immediately anterior to the angle of the mandible (Fig. 8.28). Scan anteriorly along the body of the mandible, which should be close to the lateral edge of the transducer.

Image features

On the lateral side of the image, the hyperechoic surface of the angle of the mandible will be in view (Fig. 8.28). Scanning from posterior to anterior, along the length of the body of the mandible, the submandibular gland will appear as a large triangular structure with a homogenous mid-gray color. It should be noted that the inferior portion of the parotid gland can be seen at the angle of the mandible and should not be mistaken for the submandibular gland, which sits anterior to the parotid. Towards the medial side of the submandibular gland, the facial artery can be observed. Deep to the facial artery, the submandibular duct will be in view. Both structures are observed in the transverse plane. Doppler can be used to distinguish the artery from the duct. In contrast to the artery, there will be no signal from the duct. Scanning toward the anterior of the gland, the mylohyoid muscle will be seen as a hypoechoic band passing obliquely across the image from the mandible toward the hyoid. Sitting either side of this muscle, the superficial and deep parts of the submandibular gland will be in view. Scanning anteriorly, the course of the facial artery can be inspected as it runs superficially over the gland toward the ramus of the mandible (Figs. 8.28B and C). The sublingual gland will come into view anterior to the submandibular gland.

FLOOR OF THE ORAL CAVITY

Subject position

Imaging is performed with the subject sitting. The head is best tilted posteriorly.

Transducer

Use a linear array transducer. Set the depth setting to 2–5 cm.

Transducer position

Position the transducer in the transverse plane immediately posterior to the chin (Fig. 8.29). Scan in a posterior direction toward the hyoid bone.

Image features

At either side of the image, shadows formed by the body of the mandible may be visible (Fig. 8.29). In this position,

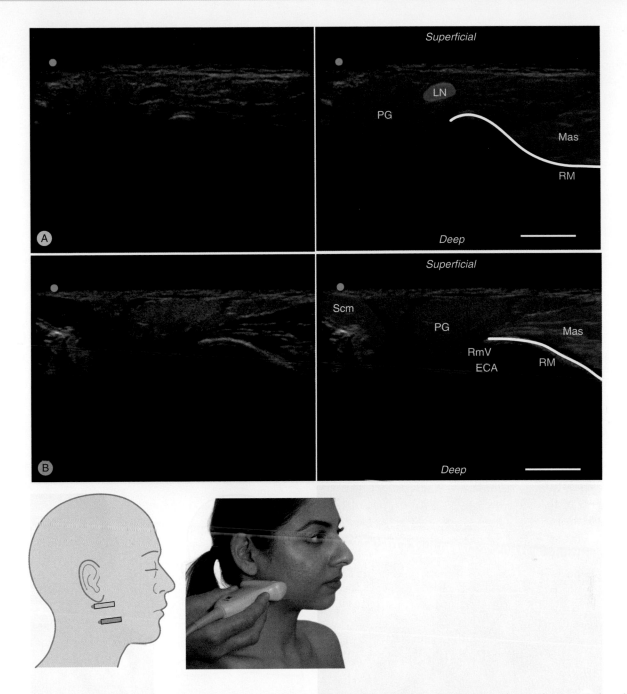

Fig. 8.27 Ultrasound of the right parotid gland. A, Immediately inferior to the ear. B, Inferior level. *ECA*, external carotid artery; *LN*, lymph node; *Mas*, masseter; *PG*, parotid gland; *RM*, ramus mandible; *RmV*, retromandibular vein; *Scm*, sternocleidomastoid. Scale bar = 1 cm.

the suprahyoid muscles in the floor of the oral cavity can be observed in short axis view. Superficially, the anterior bellies of the left and right digastric muscles can be seen. Deep to the digastric muscles, the two mylohyoid muscles form a narrow arc across the image. Sitting below the mylohyoid muscles, the geniohyoid muscles can be observed. Deep to the geniohyoid muscles, the genioglossus muscles will be in view. Swallowing will cause contraction of these muscles. Sitting lateral to the genioglossus muscles, the sublingual glands are visible, which have a homogenous mid-gray color, and are lighter compared to the adjacent

muscle. On the medial side of each gland, the sublingual vessels and submandibular duct may be visible.

CAROTID SYSTEM

Subject position

Imaging is performed with the subject sitting and the head rotated to the side.

Transducer

Use a linear array transducer. Set the depth setting to 2–5 cm.

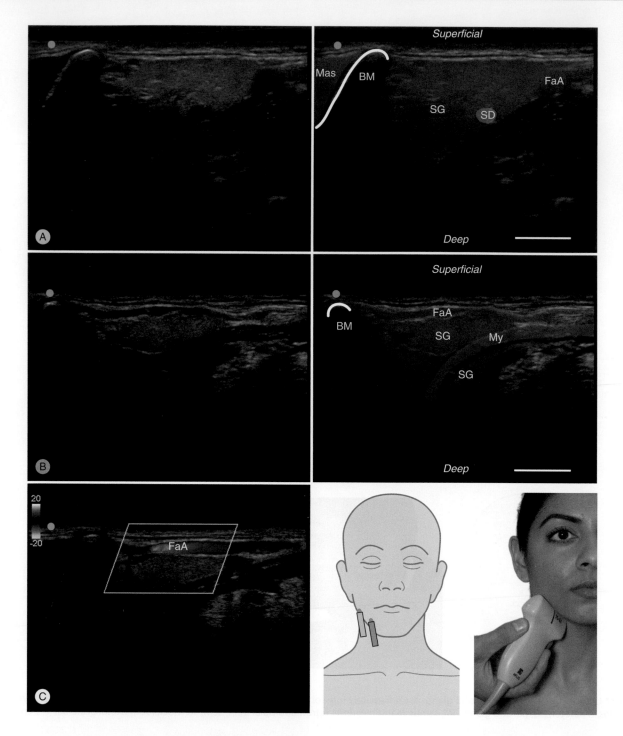

Fig. 8.28 A, B, Ultrasound of the right submandibular gland. A. Posterior mandible. B. Anterior mandible. C, Doppler of the facial artery. *BM*, body mandible; *FaA*, facial artery; *Mas*, masseter; *My*, mylohyoid muscle; *SD*, submandibular duct; *SG*, submandibular gland. Scale bar = 1 cm.

Transducer position

Position the transducer in transverse plane on the anterior surface of the neck, immediately superior to the clavicle, to the right or left side of the midline (Fig. 8.30). Scan in a superior direction following the sternocleidomastoid muscle.

Image features

Scanning in a superior direction from the lower part of the neck, the large sternocleidomastoid muscle can be observed in its short-axis (Fig. 8.30). It lies superficially across the image and has a flattened appearance. Immediately below the surface, above the sternocleidomastoid muscle, the thin layer formed by the platysma muscle will be visible. Deep to the sternocleidomastoid muscle, the common carotid artery and internal jugular vein can be inspected. The artery lies medial and deep to the vein, and is more rounded. The vein appears flattened. Doppler can be used to examine blood flow within these vessels (Video 8.1). Sitting between the artery and vein, the vagus nerve may be visible. These three structures are surrounded by the hyperechoic carotid sheath. Lateral to this neurovascular bundle (left on image), the anterior scalene muscle can be observed. Sitting on the anterior wall of this muscle, the small phrenic nerve can be seen as it descends over the surface of the muscle. In the inferior part of the neck (Fig. 8.30A), immediately postero-lateral to the anterior scalene muscle, the trunks of the brachial plexus can be seen in their short-axis. The trunks appear as three hypoechoic circles. Deep to the common carotid artery, the longus colli muscle will be visible. Towards the midline, the sternothyroid (inferiorly) and sternohyoid (superiorly) muscles can be seen medial to the sternoclei-domastoid muscle. Deep to the sternothyroid, the thyroid gland can be examined (see below).

Scanning superiorly, the course of the common carotid artery and internal jugular vein can be inspected. Immediately inferior to the level of the thyroid cartilage, the superior belly of the omohyoid muscle is observed extending immediately below the sternocleidomastoid muscle (Fig. 8.30B). Towards the midline of the neck, deep to the omo-hyoid, the sternohyoid and sternothyroid muscles can be inspected.

Scanning superior to the level of the thyroid cartilage (at the level of the C4 vertebra), the common carotid artery bifurcates into the internal and external carotid arteries. There is, however, considerable variability in the position of the bifurcation of this vessel. The thyroid cartilage appears anechoic and cannot easily be inspected on ultrasound. At the start of its course, the internal carotid artery sits lateral to the external carotid artery. At this location, the carotid sinus (a dilation in the wall of the internal carotid artery) can be inspected. Anterior to the carotid artery

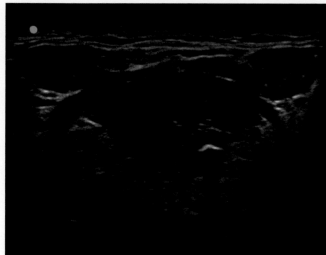

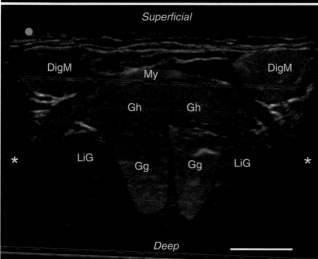

Superficial

DigM   My   DigM

Gh   Gh

*   LiG   Gg   Gg   LiG   *

Deep

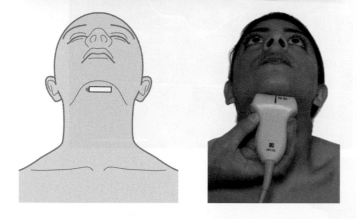

Fig. 8.29 Ultrasound of the floor of the oral cavity. *, shadows due to body of mandible; *DigM*, digastric muscle; *Gg*, genioglossus muscle; *Gh*, geniohyoid muscle; *LiG*, lingual gland; *My*, mylohyoid muscle. Scale bar = 1 cm.

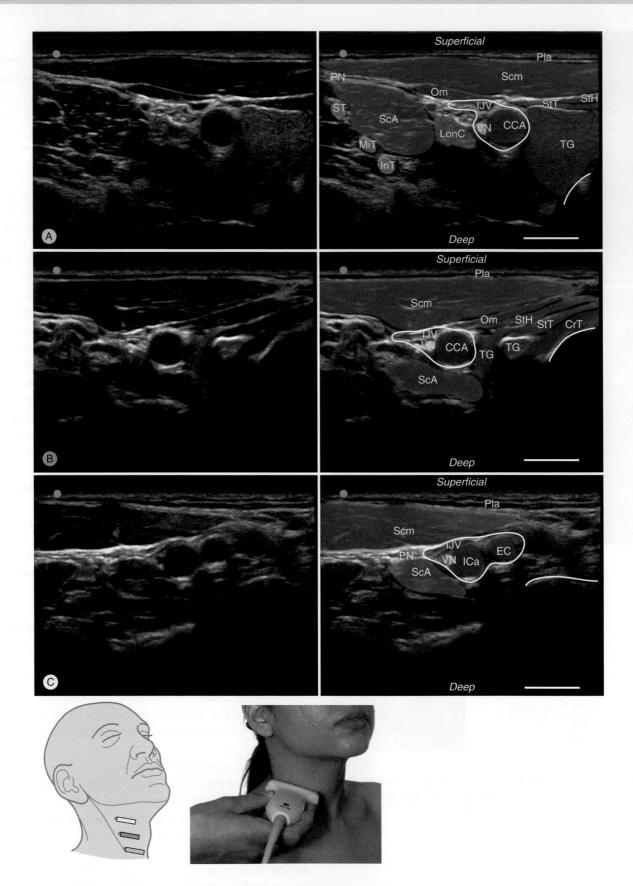

Fig. 8.30 Ultrasound of the right carotid system. A, Inferior neck. B, Mid neck. C, Superior neck. *CCA*, common carotid artery; *CrT*, cricothyroid; *EC*, external carotid; *ICa*: internal carotid; *IJV*, internal jugular vein; *InT*, inferior trunk; *LonC*, longus colli; *MiT*, middle trunk; *Om*, omohyoid; *Pla*, platysma; *PN*, phrenic nerve; *ScA*, scalenus anterior; *Scm*, sternocleidomastoid; *ST*, superior trunk; *StH*, sternohyoid; *StT*, sternothyroid; *TG*, thyroid gland; *VN*, vagus nerve. Scale bar = 1 cm.

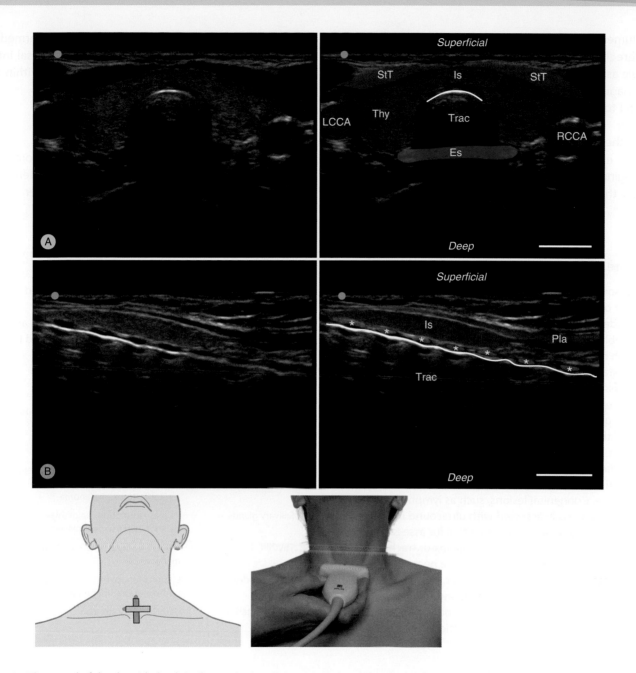

Fig. 8.31 Ultrasound of the thyroid gland. A. Short-axis view. B. Long-axis view. White line in B represents the air-mucosal interface. *, cartilaginous rings of the trachea; *Es*, esophagus; *Is*, isthmus; *LCCA*, left common carotid artery; *Pla*, platysma; *RCCA*, right common carotid artery; *StT*, sternothyroid; *Thy*, thyroid; *Trac*, trachea. Scale bar = 1 cm.

the flattened internal jugular vein is seen. Overlying the neurovascular bundle the sternocleidomastoid muscle will be in view.

THYROID GLAND

Subject position

Imaging is performed with the subject sitting.

Transducer

Use a linear array transducer. Set the depth setting to 2–5 cm.

Transducer position

Position the transducer across the midline immediately below the thyroid cartilage in the transverse plane for short-axis views or mid-sagittal plane for long-axis views (Fig. 8.31).

Image features

As with all glands, the thyroid gland has a homogenous mid-gray texture. In the transverse plane, the two lobes fill much of the image (Fig. 8.31A). The isthmus can be seen joining the lobes. Along the midline, the anterior surfaces of the tracheal rings appear as hyperechoic arcs, whereas

189

the lumen is anechoic. Posterior to the trachea, the lateral hyperechoic curved edges of the esophagus may be visible as it extends beyond the edges of the trachea. The esophagus cannot be observed directly behind the trachea. Lateral to the thyroid, the common carotid vessels will be in view.

In the sagittal plane, the isthmus of the thyroid gland can be inspected (Fig. 8.31B). Deep to the isthmus, the cartilaginous rings of the trachea will be in view. Immediately below the rings, a hyperechoic wavy line will be visible on the anterior wall of the trachea. This line is formed by the air-mucosal interface. Deep to the air-mucosal interface, a reverberation artifact can be observed within the trachea.

POSTERIOR TRIANGLE OF NECK

With the transducer positioned lateral to sternocleidomastoid muscle in line with the clavicle, the subclavian artery, vein and brachial plexus can be inspected (see Chapter 6).

In the Clinic

Ultrasound provides an effective tool for examining a range of structures within the head and neck. In particular, B-mode imaging is used to examine the glands and palpable masses in the neck. This includes the cervical lymph nodes, where ultrasound can be used to identify metastatic malignant nodes, as well as the presence of lymphadenopathy. The salivary glands are routinely assessed by ultrasound for signs of swelling, which may be associated with inflammation or obstructive calculi (sialolithiasis), as well as for the presence of cysts and neoplasms. In the thyroid gland, thyroid nodules are identified using ultrasound. Furthermore, fine needle aspiration of such nodules is performed under ultrasound guidance. Congenital lesions, such as lymphangiomas, can be relatively easily assessed with ultrasound in children. B-mode imaging also provides a tool for assessing trauma to the neck, such as injury to the larynx or trachea. Importantly, during assessment of the neck, Doppler imaging, in particular power Doppler, is used to assess the vascularity of localized masses and the glands to assist in diagnosis. Doppler ultrasound is also used to examine blood flow within the carotid arteries (carotid Doppler). In particular, it is used in the screening and evaluation of carotid artery stenosis or occlusion. Table 8.4 provides an overview of some of the head and neck conditions that can be diagnosed or monitored by ultrasound.

Table 8.4 Head and neck conditions that can be diagnosed or monitored by ultrasound

Structure	Pathology
Eye	Vitreous hemorrhage, cataracts, retinal detachment, lens implants, retinoblastoma, melanoma
Salivary glands	Abscess formation, sialolithiasis, sialadenitis, cysts, neoplasms
Thyroid	Thyroid nodules, adenomas, thyroid malignancy
Lymph nodes	Lymphadenopathy, malignant lymph nodes, core sampling for lymphoma
Carotid arteries	Carotid artery stenosis

Summary Checklist

- Surface projections of the bones of the skull
- Surface projections of eye, ear, nose and oral cavity
- Surface projections of the neuro-vasculature in the head and neck
- Ultrasound imaging of the vasculature in the neck
- Ultrasound imaging of the eye
- Ultrasound imaging of the glands of the neck

Index

Page numbers followed by "*f*" indicate figures, "*t*" indicate tables, "*b*" indicate boxes, and "*e*" indicate online content.

Index

Index

Index

Index